Handbook of Postanesthesia Nursing

Edited by

Mary Ellen Luczun, R.N., M.S.N.
Hunter College
Bellevue School of Nursing
New York, New York

AN ASPEN PUBLICATION
Aspen Publishers, Inc.

1987

Rockville, Maryland
Royal Tunbridge Wells

Library of Congress Cataloging-in-Publication Data
Handbook of postanesthesia nursing.

"An Aspen publication."
Includes bibliographies and index.
1. Postoperative care. 2. Anesthesia—Complications and sequelae. 3. Recovery room (Surgery) 4. Surgical nursing. I. Luczun, Mary Ellen. [DNLM: 1. Anesthesia—nursing. 2. Postoperative Care—nurses' instruction. 3. Recovery Room—nurses' instruction. WY 154 H236] RD51.H29 1987 617'.919 87-19272
ISBN 0-87189-864-0

Editorial Services: Carolyn Ormes

Copyright © 1987 by Aspen Publishers, Inc.
All rights reserved.

Aspen Publishers, Inc. grants permission for photocopying for personal or internal use, or for the personal or internal use of specific clients registered with the Copyright Clearance Center (CCC). This consent is given on the condition that the copier pay a $1.00 fee plus $.12 per page for each photocopy through the CCC for photocopying beyond that permitted by the U.S. Copyright Law. The fee should be paid directly to the CCC, 21 Congress St., Salem, Massachusetts 01970.
0-87189-864-0/87 $1.00 + 12.

This consent does not extend to other kinds of copying, such as copying for general distribution, for advertising or promotional purposes, for creating new collective works, or for resale. For information, address Aspen Publishers, Inc., 1600 Research Boulevard, Rockville, Maryland 20850

Library of Congress Catalog Card Number: 87-19272
ISBN: 0-87189-864-0

Printed in the United States of America

1 2 3 4 5

To Pamela Atwood, treasured friend and confidante

Contents

Contributors xi

Foreword xv
    Joseph F. Artusio, Jr., M.D.

Preface xvii

Acknowledgments xxi

Part I—INTRODUCTION 1

Chapter 1—The Operating Room Experience 3
    Sandra Del Pin Failla, R.N., B.S.N., M.P.A.

    Introduction 3
    The Perioperative Process 4
    Summary 10

Chapter 2—The Anesthesiologist and Surgeon as a Team 11
    Andrew F. Levitan, M.D., and
    Joseph F. Artusio, Jr., M.D.

    History and Background 11
    The Surgical Care Team 11

The Preoperative Period	12
The Intraoperative Period	15
The Postoperative Period	18

Part II—SURGICAL PROCEDURES AND RELATED PACU CARE 21

Chapter 3—Postanesthesia Care After Neurosurgery 23
Alan Van Poznak, M.D.

Introduction	23
Spine Surgery	23
Craniotomy	25
Carotid Endarterectomy	29

Chapter 4—Postanesthesia Care After Ophthalmalogic Surgery .. 31
Murk-Hein Heineman, M.D.

General Considerations	31
Pathophysiological Considerations	32
Surgical Procedures	35
Anesthetic Considerations	38
Postanesthesia Care	40

Chapter 5—Postanesthesia Care After Oral and Maxillofacial Surgery 43
David Behrman, D.M.D.

Introduction	43
Factors Influencing Postoperative Care	43
Airway Assessment	46
Other Aspects of Postanesthesia Care	47

Chapter 6—Postanesthesia Care After Head and Neck Surgery .. 51
Robert F. Ward, M.D.

Introduction	51
Anatomy and Physiology	51
Surgical Procedures	53
Intraoperative and Anesthetic Considerations	59
Postanesthesia Care	66
Conclusion	70

Chapter 7—Postanesthesia Care After Cardiac Surgery 73
Fun-Sun F. Yao, M.D.

    Introduction 73
    Cardiac Surgical Intervention and
      Anesthetic Management 73
    Postoperative Care 81

Chapter 8—Postanesthesia Care After Thoracic Surgery 99
John A. Lundberg, M.D.

    General Considerations 99
    Thoracic Procedures 106
    Postanesthesia Care 109

Chapter 9—Postanesthesia Care After Abdominal Surgery 111
Eugene Nowak, M.D., and
Douglas E. Paull, M.D.

    General Considerations 111
    Pathophysiology and Surgical Procedures 111
    Postanesthesia Care 123

Chapter 10—Postanesthesia Care After Vascular Surgery 125
Malcolm O. Perry, M.D.

    Introduction 125
    General Considerations 125
    Anesthetic Considerations 129
    Surgical Procedures 131
    Postanesthesia Care 132

Chapter 11—Postanesthesia Care After Burn Surgery 135
Michael Marano, M.D., and
Joseph M. Thomas, M.D.

    General Considerations 135
    Surgical Procedures 144
    Anesthetic Considerations 146
    Postanesthesia Care 149

Chapter 12—Postanesthesia Care After Orthopedic Surgery 155
    Ann Butler Maher, R.N., M.S.N.

    General Considerations 155
    Surgical Considerations 157
    Anesthetic Considerations 157
    Specific Problems and Techniques 158
    Complications 164

**Chapter 13—Postanesthesia Care After Urological
    and Renal Surgery** 169
    Karen D. Spadaccia, R.N., B.S.N.

    Introduction 169
    Anatomy of the Renal and Urological Systems 170
    Physiology of the Renal and Urological Systems 171
    History and Physical Findings 173
    Specific Disorders of the Urological System 176
    Anesthetic Management of the Patient
      with Renal Disease 184

**Part III—ADDRESSING THE SPECIAL NEEDS
    OF SELECT PATIENT GROUPS** 189

Chapter 14—Postanesthesia Care After Pediatric Surgery 191
    John R. Charney, M.D.

    Anatomic Considerations 191
    Physiological Consequences 192
    Monitoring 195
    Postanesthesia Assessment 196
    Ventilatory Management 198
    Fluid and Electrolyte Management 202
    Pain Control 205
    Unusual Problems 206
    Cardiopulmonary Life Support 210

Chapter 15—Postanesthesia Care After Obstetrical Surgery 217
    Farida Gadalla, M.D.

    General Considerations 217
    Surgical Procedures 217

Anesthetic Considerations	218
Postanesthesia Care	220

Chapter 16—Normal and Abnormal Hemostasis in the Surgical Patient **231**
Barry J. Zadeh, M.D.

Physiology of Hemostasis	231
Surgical Techniques	237
Abnormalities of Hemostasis	240
Abnormal Surgical Bleeding	247

Chapter 17—Surgical Patients with Respiratory Disease: Preventing Acute Respiratory Failure **255**
Virginia Schwend, R.N., M.S.N.

Introduction	255
The Settings of Acute Respiratory Failure	256
Pulmonary Diseases	266

Chapter 18—Surgical Patients with Infectious Diseases **291**
Lawrence C. Madoff, M.D.

General Considerations	291
Critical Aspects of Infectious Disease	291

Chapter 19—Surgical Patients with Coronary Artery Disease **311**
Mary Ellen Luczun, R.N., M.S.N.

General Considerations	311
Pathophysiology	311
Anatomy and Physiology	313
Preoperative Evaluation	313
Anesthetic Considerations	315
Postanesthesia Care	317

Chapter 20—Quality Nursing Care of Older Adults **321**
Marjorie A. Miller, R.N., M.S.N., A.N.P.

Introduction	321
General Concepts About the Aging Process	321

Areas of Concern	325
Subtle Influences on Nursing Care of Older Adults	332
A Real-Life Experience in Caring for the Aged	335

Part IV—TAKING CARE OF OURSELVES **339**

Chapter 21—Stress Management Techniques for PACU Nurse Practitioners **341**
Mary Ellen Luczun, R.N., M.S.N.

The Meaning of Stress	341
Stress is All Around Us	342
Stress and the Nursing Profession	343
Reactions to Stress	343
Stress in the PACU	344
Coping Measures	346

Index **353**

Contributors

Joseph F. Artusio, Jr., M.D.
Professor and Chairman of Anesthesiology
The New York Hospital-Cornell Medical Center
New York, New York

David Behrman, D.M.D.
Assistant Attending Surgeon
Oral and Maxillofacial Surgery
Assistant Professor of Surgery
The New York Hospital-Cornell Medical Center
New York, New York

John R. Charney, M.D.
Director of Cardiothoracic Anesthesia
Associate Director of Pediatric Intensive Care Unit
Adjunct Assistant Professor of Anesthesiology
Harbor/UCLA Medical Center
Torrance, California

Sandra Del Pin Failla, R.N., C.N.O.R., B.S.N., M.P.A.
Clinical Instructor, Operating Room
New York University Medical Center
New York, New York

Farida Gadalla, M.D.
Associate Attending Anesthesiologist
Assistant Professor of Anesthesiology
The New York Hospital-Cornell Medical Center
New York, New York

Murk-Hein Heineman, M.D.
Assistant Professor of Ophthalmology
The New York Hospital-Cornell Medical Center
New York, New York

Andrew F. Levitan, M.D.
Attending Anesthesiologist
Anesthesiologists of Central Florida
Orlando, Florida

Mary Ellen Luczun, R.N., M.S.N.
Clinical Instructor
Hunter College-Bellevue School of
    Nursing
New York, New York
Associate Editor-Research, *Journal
    of Post Anesthesia Nursing*

John A. Lundberg, M.D.
Assistant Professor of
    Anesthesiology
Harbor/UCLA Medical Center
Torrance, California

Lawrence C. Madoff, M.D.
Clinical Fellow in Medicine
Harvard Medical School
Clinical Fellow in Infectious
    Diseases
Brigham and Womens' Hospital
Beth Israel Hospital
Boston, Massachusetts

Ann Butler Maher, R.N., M.S.N.
Assistant Professor of Nursing
County College of Morris
Randolph, New Jersey
Editor, *Orthopaedic Nursing*

Michael Marano, M.D.
Clinical Burn Fellow
The New York Hospital-Cornell
    Medical Center Burn Center
New York, New York

Marjorie A. Miller, R.N., M.S.N., A.N.P.
Codirector
Geriatric Nurse Practitioner
    Program
The New York Hospital-Cornell
    Medical Center
New York, New York

Eugene Nowak, M.D.
Assistant Professor of Surgery
The New York Hospital-Cornell
    Medical Center
New York, New York

Douglas E. Paull, M.D.
Administrative Chief Resident in
    Surgery
The New York Hospital-Cornell
    Medical Center
New York, New York

Malcolm O. Perry, M.D.
Professor of Surgery
The New York Hospital-Cornell
    Medical Center
New York, New York

Virginia Schwend, R.N., M.S.N.
Assistant Clinical Instructor
Department of Operating Room/
    Postanesthesia Care Unit Nursing
The New York Hospital-Cornell
    Medical Center
New York, New York

Karen D. Spadaccia, R.N., B.S.N., C.C.R.N., C.E.N.
Critical Care Nurse Instructor
Northern Westchester Hospital
    Center
Mount Kisco, New York

Joseph M. Thomas, M.D.
Clinical Pain Fellow
Memorial Sloan Kettering Cancer
    Center
New York, New York
Clinical Fellow in Anesthesiology
The New York Hospital-Cornell
    Medical Center
New York, New York

Alan Van Poznak, M.D.
Professor of Anesthesiology and
Pharmacology
The New York Hospital-Cornell
Medical Center
New York, New York

Robert F. Ward, M.D.
Assistant Professor of
Otolaryngology
The New York Hospital-Cornell
Medical Center
New York, New York

Fun-Sun F. Yao, M.D.
Associate Professor of
Anesthesiology
Cornell University Medical College
Attending Anesthesiologist
The New York Hospital-Cornell
Medical Center
New York, New York

Barry J. Zadeh, M.D.
Instructor in Surgery and Cell
Biology
Cornell University Medical College
New York, New York

Foreword

Since its creation shortly after World War II, the postoperative recovery room has been one of the great advances in the care of the surgical patient. Prior to that time, most surgical patients were taken directly to their wards or private rooms, many floors away from the operating room and from personnel trained in resuscitation. Many patients died unnecessarily from respiratory arrest, aspiration of gastric or intestinal contents, or simply asphyxia from turning over and not being able to ventilate in that position or to right themselves. Calls for assistance were sent to the operating room, but trained personnel often could not arrive in time to resuscitate the patients.

The advent of the postanesthesia care unit (PACU) placed trained personnel in the immediate vicinity of the operating room, and the quality of postoperative care and postanesthesia care became directly related to the quality of the personnel trained for this particular area. Over the past 30 to 40 years, considerable experience has been gained in the care of patients recovering from anesthesia; and with the increased availability of trained personnel and the use of sophisticated monitors for these patients, postoperative morbidity and mortality have decreased significantly.

It is with great pleasure that I write this foreword to a book written by experts in each subspecialty of surgery, dealing with the particular needs of their individual patients in the postanesthesia recovery room. The PACU has paid tremendous dividends to modern surgery and anesthesia.

I would like to compliment Mary Ellen Luczun on her tireless efforts in putting this text together for the education of all who have the responsibility of postanesthesia care.

Joseph F. Artusio, Jr., M.D.,
Professor and Chairman of Anesthesiology,
The New York Hospital-Cornell Medical Center,
New York, New York

Preface

It is with great respect for postanesthesia nurses everywhere that I introduce yet another book devoted to this remarkable specialty, a book written by and for professionals.

This decade has demonstrated that PACU nurses are enterprising, resourceful, and knowledgeable. We have successfully applied the nursing process to our own practice. Assessment and planning began in the 1970s, as we identified problems that hampered our growth and proceeded to set goals. We have reached these goals; we have attained the autonomy that inevitably accompanies professional specialization. With the formation of the American Society of Post Anesthesia Nurses (ASPAN) in 1980, the implementation phase gained momentum. Since then, we have continued to evaluate our achievements and set new goals. By adhering to high standards of practice, we have gained prominent recognition by the health care community. We are to be commended!

Ten years ago it was a dream; today it is a reality. ASPAN has provided the major inspiration and vehicle for the progress we have made and exemplifies the power of unity and collaborative efforts. In this regard, the state of Florida merits special attention, since the nurses in that state were the pioneers during the assessment and planning phases, planting the seeds that led to national representation.

PACU nurses can now become certified, the evidence of excellence in practice. The *Journal of Post Anesthesia Nursing,* which came into being in February of 1986 and is the official publication of ASPAN, provides us with a suitable home for postanesthesia care manuscripts. Beyond this, many PACU nurses are currently writing for other specialty journals as well. Continuing education, academic advancement, and research proposals are further evidence of our dedication to professionalism and an unending search for knowledge.

In light of this scholarly climate, the need for additional publications related to postanesthesia care is great. The *Handbook of Postanesthesia Nursing* has been designed to meet this need, as it addresses the concerns of those who aspire to the elements of advanced practice. It ventures beyond basic considerations to a more comprehensive, in-depth presentation of the countless clinical problems we face on a daily basis.

The reader may notice that the majority of the handbook's chapter authors are physicians noted in their fields of specialty. The blend of their knowledge and expertise offer us comprehensive discussions on pathophysiology, surgical procedures, and anesthesia techniques and complications, both actual and potential. Edited by a nurse, each chapter concludes with a section specifically related to postanesthesia care. The perioperative approach is advocated to assist PACU nurses in acquiring an optimal comprehensive clinical picture of their patients in all care settings. I hope this will contribute to more effective communication and interaction among all health care professionals involved with the surgical patient.

Part I begins with a description of the operating room experience and acquaints us with the activities of a place from which we are generally absent. Chapter 2, concerning the anesthesiologist and surgeon as a team, lends vital insight into the importance of adequate cooperation and communication between these physicians—before, during, and after the surgical procedure. The remaining chapters in this part deal with each surgical specialty and related postanesthesia care. At first glance, Chapter 7, dealing with postanesthesia care after cardiac surgery, may seem unrelated to our specialty. It is included in this book because, as more and more PACUs expand and remain open on a 24-hour basis, caring for open-heart patients may very well become a future responsibility for us.

Part II addresses the needs of patients with specific preexisting illnesses. Depending on the disorder, these patients are at greater surgical or anesthetic risk than those without such preexisting problems. Thus, patients with coronary artery disease, respiratory and clotting defects, and infectious disease are presented; and strategies to prevent complications are explored. Another group of individuals, older adults, is also discussed in this context. Chapter 20 is a poignant account of the very special care geriatric patients require. This material may, therefore, be viewed as predictive of PACU nursing in the future. Due to today's advanced technology and modes of treatment, people with serious chronic diseases are surviving longer; and these are precisely the types of patients we are seeing more of. With these patients, it is crucial that we familiarize ourselves with the various postoperative complications that may ensue and be prepared to deal with them in the PACU.

PACU nurses wishing to augment their knowledge now have a powerful resource at their fingertips. The combined efforts of each of its contributing experts make this handbook a valuable reference for surgeons and anesthesiologists as well. Finally, any health professional who desires additional input into the care of the perioperative patient will most certainly benefit from its use and application.

Acknowledgments

First and foremost, I thank all of the authors who have contributed their time, effort, and expertise to this book; they are the ones responsible for its superior content.

A special thanks is extended to those who have patiently reviewed various chapters: Dr. Stanley Behrman, Dr. Peter Pruden, Dr. Jerry Halpern, and Dr. Martin Post.

I also thank the individuals I came into contact with throughout the many months of preparation. They were wonderful support: Cindy Colon, Manuela Colon, Evelyn Alberty, and Ruth Van Putten. Kenda Ward will always have my greatest respect for being the supreme liaison and organizer she was on behalf of her husband, Robert F. Ward, M.D.

I am truly indebted to Sue Pino, without whose help in retyping certain sections of this book I would have been in dire straits indeed.

For her valuable assistance in locating alien references, Betty J. Malino is someone I will never forget. Her knowledge of anesthesia publications is impeccable.

A special thank you to Douglas E. Paull, M.D., and David Behrman, D.M.D., for their conscientiousness, efficiency, and concern.

Barry J. Zadeh, M.D., deserves a very special acknowledgment in appreciation for the high standard (perfection) he subscribes to, and for giving me his chapter on a floppy disk! Thank you, Barry, for saving me a lot of time.

My close colleague and friend, John R. Charney, M.D., who wrote an outstanding chapter on pediatric surgery for the handbook, will always have my highest regard.

I also thank John Yanello for all his help in teaching me how to work a computer to my advantage and for helping me to keep my sanity during the final months of editing the book.

Two other computer experts are worthy of very affectionate mention: my brothers John and Peter. John, for giving me a superb printer as a gift; Peter, for assisting me in setting it all up!

Finally, I thank my parents: my mother, for her unwavering support and encouragement, and my father, for the same, and, more specifically, for his assistance in getting the chapters photocopied.

Thank you, one and all.

Mary Ellen Luczun, R.N., M.S.N.

Part I
Introduction

Chapter 1

The Operating Room Experience

Sandra Del Pin Failla, R.N., C.N.O.R., B.S.N., M.P.A.

INTRODUCTION

A successful operation depends on the smooth, efficient performance of the surgical team. A positive perioperative experience is determined by the multidisciplinary group of professionals called the perioperative team. This team is composed of nurses, surgeons, anesthesiologists, laboratory personnel, and support personnel.

This chapter is a basic introduction to a patient's perioperative experience. The perioperative experience described is limited to the time frame between the patient's preanesthetic medication and the patient's transfer to the PACU.

The purpose of this chapter is:

- to serve as a basic introduction to a patient's perioperative experience
- to identify and define the various roles and responsibilities of the perioperative team and to illustrate how the team works together to protect the patient's safety
- to describe the logical and systematic stages of the patient's perioperative experience
- to identify communication channels used by the team prior to, during, and after the patient's surgical intervention

The text is written from the perspective of a perioperative operating room nurse. Its content is drawn from professional experience at the New York University Medical Center's 17-room operating suite.

Recognizing that each patient will have an individualized perioperative care plan or series of care plans, the author's intent is to describe a generalized perioperative patient experience. However, adjustments can be made for patient variation, surgeons' preference, and architectural differences, thus rendering the described perioperative experience applicable to any hospital setting. As illustrated throughout the text, the patient's safety is the author's highest priority.

The following are members of the perioperative surgical team:

- Attending surgeon—primarily responsible for surgical intervention; performs surgery on the patient.
- Surgical resident—physician who assists the attending physician; performs surgery on the patient.
- Anesthesiologist—physician who specializes in the administration of anesthesia; administers anesthesia to the patient.
- Nurse anesthetist—nurse certified in the practice of assisting the anesthesiologist; administers anesthesia to the patient.
- Scrub nurse—technician or nurse who "scrubs," using a sterile gown and gloves, and sets up sterile supplies and instruments for the case; anticipates the surgeon's needs, passes instruments and supplies, and protects and maintains a sterile field.
- Circulating nurse—registered nonsterile nurse who coordinates the intraoperative phase of the perioperative experience; functions as the patient's advocate and coordinates the surgical team's actions to protect the patient from environmental hazards during the intraoperative stages of the perioperative experience.

THE PERIOPERATIVE PROCESS

The Preoperative Visit

The day before surgery, the patient is visited by several of the perioperative team members. The attending surgeon or surgical resident visits to review the operative procedure with the patient so that an informed consent can be obtained. The PACU nurse teaches the patient postoperative breathing exercises and reviews the operative day's routine. The anesthesiologist conducts a physical exam and reviews the patient's history and chart. The anesthesiologist pays particular attention to the patient's blood work (type and cross for transfusions, complete blood counts, bleeding and coagulation times, and electrolytes), chest x-ray, electrocardiogram, and urinalysis. The anesthesiologist also discusses with the patient the type of anesthesia planned (general, regional, local, or nerve block). The patient's attitude and anxiety level help to determine which preanesthetic medications will be ordered.

The preanesthetic medication should be administered 45 to 60 minutes prior to the patient's transport to the operating room or waiting room. This time allows the medication to reach its optimum effect. Some typical preanesthetic medications are:

- narcotics/analgesics—used as sedatives to relieve patient apprehension and resistance to the anesthetic
- tranquilizers—given to reduce anxiety and promote rapid induction
- anticholinergics—given to check secretions and prevent laryngospasm and for sedation; for example, atropine to decrease vagal stimulation and scopolomine to produce relaxation and amnesia

The Preoperative Transfer Routine

Approximately 30 to 45 minutes prior to patient pickup, the OR secretary calls the nursing unit and requests the nurse to "premedicate" the patient. At this time, the preoperative nurse properly identifies the patient, checks the chart for a signed consent, and administers the preanesthetic medication ordered by the anesthesiologist the previous day.

Within 30 minutes, the OR secretary calls the nursing unit to inform it that the OR orderly is on the way to pick up the patient. The OR orderly arrives at the nursing unit with an OR stretcher and a "patient pick-up slip." On occasion, the patient may go to the OR in the patient's own bed. The patient pick-up slip contains the correct spelling of the patient's name, the attending surgeon's name, and the patient's bed and room number. With the patient pick-up slip, the nurse accompanies the orderly to the patient's bedside and assists in the proper patient identification and transfer. Both the nurse and the orderly check the patient's identification band.

After proper identification, the nurse should assist the orderly with the safe transfer of the patient to the stretcher. Side rails should be lifted into the "up" position to protect the premedicated patient's safety. At this time, the nurse signs the preoperative checklist and gives the patient's identification plate and completed chart to the orderly. The orderly then pushes the patient from the head of the stretcher toward the elevator.

The OR Holding Area

Ideally, the anxious preoperative patient should not see preparations being made for the operation, nor should the patient be subjected to the noise and confusion of the OR corridor. Unfortunately, however, because of the layout of many OR suites, these two situations often cannot be avoided.

Patient holding or waiting areas are determined by OR space availability. Every OR has a waiting area of some sort; it may be an area in front of the entry elevator, or it may be a space in the corridor near the room itself. The more modern OR might have a quiet area, separate but proximal to the OR, that is monitored by nursing staff.

The circulating nurse uses the holding area to check in and admit the patient to the OR. In addition, the anesthesiologist might efficiently use the waiting time and space to place ECG leads and start intravenous lines on the patient.

Patient Admission to the OR Suite

The orderly alerts the circulator that the patient has arrived. The circulator greets the patient and asks for the patient's full name. The circulator simultaneously doublechecks with the chart the patient's identification band for name and identification number. The circulator then reviews the preop checklist and the chart. The preop checklist includes a synopsis of the patient's past medical/surgical history, against which the circulator reviews lab values and blood availability. While checking the chart, the circulator develops rapport with the patient by asking questions regarding patient allergies, personal belongings, and prostheses brought with the patient and enquiring whether the patient has eaten that day.

After this initial assessment is completed, the circulator explains briefly what the patient can expect to experience in the operating room. This explanation includes a brief description of the OR environment (for example, overhead lights) and temperature (cool), the method of transfer to and the feeling of the OR table, (narrow and firm), the use of a safety belt across the thighs for support, and the personnel present in the room (the number of nursing, surgical, and anesthesia personnel). This helps the patient overcome any fears, decreases the patient's anxiety level, and facilitates a smooth progression through the operative procedure.

The Case Begins

Patient Entry

Much of the preparation is done prior to patient entry. The anesthesiologist has assembled the anesthetics used on the anesthesia machine. The nursing team has assembled and set up the needed sterile supplies, such as instruments and sutures, in an organized fashion. And the nursing team has counted every sharp, needle, sponge, and instrument prior to patient entry.

The circulator pushes the patient into the room and assists with the safe transfer of the medicated patient onto the OR table. The anesthesiologist attaches ECG leads to the patient's chest and inserts intravenous lines. The anesthesiologist administers the anesthetics via intubation, epidural catheter, spinal injection, nerve block, or gas mask. After the patient has been induced, the surgeons leave the room to scrub their hands and arms. After the scrub, they return to the room to be gowned and gloved by the scrub nurse. The anesthesiologist gives permission for the surgeon to begin.

Patient Positioning and Surgical Preparation of the Site

At this point, the patient is positioned, and the operative site is prepared. The surgical team begins to paint the operative site with an antimicrobial solution. The surgeons drape the patient with a combination of sterile drapes. The final drape sheet is fenestrated to facilitate access to the operative site.

The anesthesiologist gathers and clips the edges of the drapes to two nearby intravenous poles, creating a tent-like barrier to the operative site. This barrier drape separates the nonsterile anesthesia team from the sterile field. It also facilitates easy access to the patient's airway. During surgery, the anesthesiologist will monitor the patient's progress and inform the surgeon of any changes in the patient's condition.

The Intraoperative Stage

The surgeon checks with the anesthesiologist prior to making the first incision. The scrub nurse's role, intraoperatively, is to assist by anticipating the surgeon's needs and by passing all instruments and supplies in a sterile, immediately usable position. This efficiency in action decreases the patient's anesthesia exposure and surgical time.

The surgeon may use electrical devices and power instruments. Electrosurgical units may be used to cut and coagulate tissue with minimal blood loss. Lasers may be used to destroy tissue. Drills and power instruments may be used on bone. The nursing team protects the patient by trouble-shooting and testing all electrical equipment prior to use. All defective equipment is removed from the room and reported to the electrical safety department.

Upon locating the disease-producing tissue, the surgeon removes it and passes it to the nursing team for proper disposal. The surgeon verbally identifies the tissue, and the circulator properly labels the specimen container. The circulator adds the appropriate solution and completes all paperwork, clearly communicating to the laboratory what the specimen is. The circulator transports the specimen to the lab refrigerator or specimen transport system and logs additional patient specimen labels in the OR specimen logbook.

Once the specimen has been removed, the surgeon checks for hemostasis. The surgical team begins to close the first layer. The nursing team simultaneously begins to count all sharps, needles, sponges, and instruments used. Such counts are done at least three times during each case—before the case begins, upon first closure, and at the beginning of the skin closure—to ensure patient safety.

The circulator is responsible for coordinating the efficient use of expensive OR time. During the first closure, the circulator informs the OR secretary at the nursing station that it is time to premedicate the next patient. The circulator pulls the patient's pickup slip and checks the patient's name against the OR schedule. Upon closure of the skin layer, the circulator directs the secretary to send an orderly to pick up the next patient. At this time, the circulator asks the secretary to call the postanesthesia care unit (PACU) and ask for "space" and permission to enter. If special equipment is required, such as ventilator or arterial Swan Ganz monitoring lines, the relevant requirement is also communicated to the PACU.

PACU management coordinates the patient's arrival and staggers nurse/patient assignments so that each case has one nurse to observe the patient closely during the first postoperative hour. The PACU can save the patient costly postoperative time by preparing for the incoming patient while the patient is still in the OR.

When the patient's skin is closed, a sterile gauze dressing is applied to the surgical site. Casts and plaster splints are applied after the surgical dressing has been secured.

The Case Ends

Patient Arousal

The anesthesiologist arouses the patient from the anesthetic state. The patient is often extubated in the OR and remains conscious but lethargic during transfer to the PACU.

During the arousal time, the nursing team evaluates the effectiveness of the intraoperative care plan and assesses the patient for injury (burns, skin alterations, decubiti). The patient groundplate is removed, and the patient is covered with warm blankets.

Once the patient is extubated and breathing normally and the patient's color and circulatory status appears satisfactory, it is usually safe to transport the patient to the PACU. The entire surgical team assists in the safe physical transfer of the patient from the OR table to a clean stretcher.

At the end of each case, the circulator must complete the OR worksheet. This worksheet is a legal document that contains important information describing what occurred in the OR and who was involved. Typically, information recorded on the OR worksheet includes the date; the room number; the service; the incision entrance-exit time; the full names of the participating surgical, anesthesia, and nursing personnel; the type of anesthetic given; preoperative and postoperative diagnoses; the operative procedure; implant information; electrosurgical devices used; the location of the patient groundplate; the name of the person who grounded the patient; a list of the catheters and drains inserted; the number and types of specimens sent to the lab; the patient's position and the person(s) responsible for the positioning; the names of the nurses responsible for sharp, needle, sponge, and instrument counts; and the number and accuracy of the counts performed. The OR record is a multipage carbon-copy document. One copy of the OR record is kept in the patient's chart. One copy is forwarded to the finance department for charging purposes and then to medical records for DRG coding. The remaining copy is placed in an OR worksheet log.

The circulator might complete additional intraoperative reports and notes that remain in the patient's chart. These reports and notes may provide additional information on the patient's arrival or departure or record vital signs and other intraoperative events not documented on the OR worksheet. These additional written communications assist other perioperative team members in understanding the patient's postoperative condition.

Patient Transfer to the PACU

After space has been granted by the PACU management, the anesthesiologist and surgical resident together transport the patient to the PACU. During the transfer, the anesthesiologist closely monitors the lethargic patient's airway for obstruction.

Upon arrival, PACU nurses assess the patient and check vital signs. The anesthesiologist gives a report to the PACU nurse. This report should include the patient's name, the anesthesia given, the surgical procedure used, an overall evaluation of vital signs, and the type and amount of solutions and drugs administered during the case. If the patient has any special conditions, either prior to surgery or because of surgery, the PACU nurse should be so informed. Also, all drains, tubes, and casts should be reviewed together at this time. Vital signs are checked every 15 to 20 minutes or more by the PACU nurse, depending on the patient's condition.

The anesthesiologist leaves promptly after giving the above report, informing the PACU nurse of where the anesthesiologist can be reached if needed. The PACU nurse is responsible for monitoring the patient's vital signs and condition and reporting any respiratory or medical alterations.

SUMMARY

A successful perioperative experience consists of the effective execution of a series of actions performed by the perioperative team. The process involves the following elements:

- close cooperation among the perioperative team members in implementing their roles and responsibilities
- successful progression through the various stages of the generalized and limited perioperative experience
- effective use of communication channels and routines by the perioperative team to facilitate and expedite the surgical patient's experience

A thorough understanding of each team member's role and responsibility will enable the perioperative team to deliver high quality care to the surgical patient.

Chapter 2

The Anesthesiologist and Surgeon as a Team

Andrew F. Levitan, M.D.
Joseph F. Artusio, Jr., M.D.

HISTORY AND BACKGROUND

Anesthesia has had a checkered history since the poet-physician Oliver Wendell Holmes first suggested the term to William Morton on 21 November 1846. However, the use of anesthesia in major surgery was actually initiated about a month earlier, on 16 October 1846, when the "anesthetist," William Morton, with great difficulty, convinced Dr. John C. Warren that the removal of a tumor from the mandible of Gilbert Abbott could be done without any pain through the use of ether. In fact, Abbott later reported that he had felt no pain during the operation.

Thus was anesthesiology born. And as quickly as steam and sail could carry the news around the world, the growing cooperation of anesthesiologist and surgeon began to free mankind forever from the fear of the knife. Within or outside the operating room, there is no area of cooperation that rivals in its benefits the symbiosis created between these two medical professionals.

As with all teams, the surgical team exists for the purpose of achieving a specific goal. Within this team, however, the surgeon and the anesthesiologist have a special interdependence, because extensive surgery cannot be performed without a means of providing relief from pain.

THE SURGICAL CARE TEAM

Modern surgery has become more complicated as it has been extended to all vital areas of the body. Thus, a combination of special skills must be used to accomplish the desired goal of correcting whatever may be impairing the function of one part with minimal damage to any other related part. The surgeon's efforts must be applied without interruption for the delicate operation being performed, without concern for vital functions or life-threatening signs. At the same time, the anesthesiologist must apply the skills of the clinical physiologist and pharmacologist to maintain respiration, circulation, and the metabolic homeostasis of the organism.

Smooth operation of the surgical team requires mutual confidence between the surgeon and the anesthesiologist. A surgeon who must be concerned constantly with the patient's respiration and circulation cannot be fully devoted to the task of operating. Similarly, the anesthesiologist cannot function properly if the anesthesiologist's warnings of danger go unheeded by the surgeon. In short, the morbidity and mortality of the surgical patient can be reduced only through close cooperation of the surgeon and anesthesiologist working as a team.

The postanesthesia care nurse receives the patient postoperatively from the surgeon and anesthesiologist. In a postoperative report, this nurse must be informed of the surgical procedure performed and of any potential complications. The relevant information must encompass the general condition of the patient, and include requirements for medications the patient may normally use or need in the immediate postoperative period. The postoperative report must also address the patient's hemodynamic status, including any intraoperative crystalloid and blood replacement. Finally, the PACU nurse must be informed of the type of anesthesia the patient received, particularly with regard to the administration of narcotics or muscle relaxants during the intraoperative period.

In addition to the PACU nurse and surgical nurses the surgical team may include specialists who are consulted outside the operating room when a patient requires specialized examinations, either preoperatively or postoperatively.

Within the surgical care team, the interaction between the surgeon and the anesthesiologist is a complex process, beginning with the preoperative evaluation of the patient and ending when the patient has fully recovered from the effects of surgery and anesthesia. This interaction is greatly facilitated when each member of the surgical team understands the individual responsibilities and problems faced by the other members of the team. The resulting cooperative effort increases overall efficiency in patient management and creates a climate of mutual confidence.

THE PREOPERATIVE PERIOD

Preoperative Evaluation

The preoperative evaluation begins with completion of a full history and physical examination of the patient. Particular emphasis is placed on the systems that will undergo the most stress in the presence of surgery and anesthesia. The history should include details relating to previous anesthetics experienced either by the patient or by the patient's relatives, as well as a careful review of organ system functions that may be altered by coexisting diseases. Specific points to elucidate include allergic reactions, sensitivity to muscle relaxants, bleeding tendencies, jaundice, and adverse responses to anesthetics among family members.

In evaluating the central nervous system, it is important to note the presence of cerebrovascular insufficiency and seizures. Specific information regarding cardiopulmonary disease is essential. Routine evaluation should consider coronary artery disease, hypertension, valvular heart disease, cardiac arrhythmias, dyspnea, orthopnea, asthma, cigarette smoking, chronic obstructive pulmonary disease, and recent upper respiratory tract infection. Other systems that require attention are the liver, genitourinary tract, skeletal muscle, and endocrine systems. Patients should also be questioned about their dentition.

Information regarding current drug therapy is of paramount importance during the preoperative evaluation. Because many types of interactions, some occasionally fatal, are known to occur among drugs administered during the perioperative period, the anesthesiologist must be fully aware of the possibility of adverse drug interactions in order to maintain the safety of current drug therapy in the perioperative period.

The physical examination performed by the anesthesiologist is primarily directed toward the cardiopulmonary system and the upper airway. The examination includes auscultation of the heart for rate, rhythm, and the presence of murmurs and auscultation of the lungs for the presence of abnormal breath sounds or wheezing. During the examination, the anesthesiologist focuses particularly on any characteristics that could make airway management difficult, such as abnormalities of the cervical spine, temporomandibular joint mobility, obesity, or a short neck. Also, at this time, patient mobility with regard to the proposed position of surgery should be evaluated. If regional anesthesia is planned, the site should be inspected for infection or anatomical anomalies.

In obtaining a complete history and physical examination, the collection of certain laboratory data is important. The relevant data should be ordered based on positive findings obtained from the history and physical examination. Certain laboratory tests are ordered routinely, since abnormalities may be associated with an increase in perioperative morbidity and mortality. In the authors' institution, the following data on adult patients are ordered routinely: a complete blood count, serum electrolytes, blood glucose and blood urea nitrogen concentrations, coagulation studies, urinalysis, electrocardiogram, and radiograph of the chest. Further testing depends on the individual needs of the patient.

After evaluating the history, physical examination, and laboratory data, the surgeon and anesthesiologist must turn their attention to the psychological and pharmacological preparation of the patient for surgery. Psychological preparation is accomplished during the preoperative visit and interview with the patient and family. At this time, the sequence of events in the perioperative period is described. This, combined with the proper choice of premedicant, results in a cooperative, drowsy, and relaxed patient who has a feeling of confidence in the surgical team.

Preoperative Medication Considerations

Ideally, the selection of premedication is individualized, depending on the patient's age and physical and psychological condition. By establishing patient confidence during the preoperative visit, premedication can be minimized, while maintaining an anxiety-free, cooperative, yet sedated, patient. Other goals of premedication may include amnesia, analgesia, an antisialagogic effect, or, in certain circumstances, an increase in gastric pH and allergy prophylaxis. In certain patients, such as those undergoing cardiac surgery, depressant pharmacological premedication is indicated. In other patients, such as the elderly or patients with severe chronic obstructive pulmonary disease, depressant pharmacological premedication should be minimized. Drugs administered as premedicants generally come from one or more of the following classes: the barbiturates, narcotics, benzodiazepines, butyrophenones, antihistamines, anticholinergics, histamine antagonists, and antacids.

Timing of administration of the premedicant is as important as its selection. For example, drugs that relieve anxiety and produce sedation are generally best given one to two hours prior to anesthetic induction, whereas an anticholinergic utilized for its antisialagogic effect is probably best administered just prior to transport to the operating room, in order to avoid the discomfort associated with a dry mouth.

During the preoperative period, the patient is physically optimized for surgery. The anesthesiologist must discuss with the surgeon the duration of the contemplated procedure and any postoperative problems or special care the patient may require. As the person responsible for intraoperative patient monitoring, the anesthesiologist must make a decision as to whether or not intraoperative invasive hemodynamic monitoring is necessary. The monitoring may be simple, or it may be complex, as in the case of intraarterial blood pressure measurement or Swan-Ganz catheterization. If it is felt that vigorous fluid resuscitation will be necessary intraoperatively, placement of a large bore intravenous cannula can be most helpful. Occasionally, the need for invasive monitoring first arises intraoperatively, for example, when there is an intraoperative surgical or anesthetic complication. Generally, in such cases, the need for further invasive monitoring is assessed by the anesthesiologist and is discussed with the surgeon prior to its intraoperative initiation.

Determination of Anesthetic Techniques

After discussing with the surgeon the type of surgery to be performed, its probable duration, and the likelihood of complications, the anesthesiologist decides on the anesthetic technique. Factors that guide selection of the appropriate anesthetic technique include the site of surgery, the position of the patient, airway availability, coexisting diseases, whether or not the surgery is emergent, and the preference of the patient. After evaluating the medical condition and unique needs of the patient, the anesthesiologist decides whether to perform general anesthesia, regional anesthesia, or a peripheral nerve block. In any event, prior to initiation of anesthesia, the chosen technique is discussed with the surgeon. If, during the preoperative evaluation of the patient, regional anesthesia or nerve block is contemplated, special attention must be focused on the site of injection to determine the feasibility of the contemplated procedure. Also, when planning a regional anesthetic technique, the emotional state of the patient is an important consideration, since not all patients are emotionally equipped to withstand the sights and sounds of the operating room.

Occasionally, regional anesthesia is the technique of choice because other types of anesthesia are contraindicated, for example, because of recent ingestion of food or the presence of severe metabolic or renal disease. Regional anesthesia may also be contraindicated in the presence of severe neurological disease or because the patient is being given anticoagulants.

From the above discussion, it should be clear that the interaction between surgeon and anesthesiologist begins long before the intraoperative period.

THE INTRAOPERATIVE PERIOD

Subspecialty Considerations

Intraoperatively, the interaction between the surgeon and the anesthesiologist is designed to maintain patient safety and avoid unnecessary delays. The interaction may differ in content in various subspecialties, but its maintenance is vital in maintaining optimal patient care. The following examples typify the importance of the surgeon-anesthesiologist relationship in various subspecialty contexts in maintaining optimal patient care.

In cardiac surgery, the complexity of the operative procedure and the function of the left ventricle often determine the intensity of the monitoring. Specifically, whether or not Swan-Ganz catheterization is necessary, or whether central venous pressure monitoring will suffice, is decided jointly by the surgeon and the anesthesiologist after reviewing pertinent clinical data. The selection of drugs given to the patient to induce and maintain anesthesia is solely a function of the anesthesiologist, but the anesthesiologist must notify the surgeon of abrupt changes in hemodynamic status that may demand the initiation of cardiopulmonary bypass. Likewise, the surgeon must inform the anesthesiologist when the heart is physically manipulated so that the anesthesiologist may be prepared for arrhythmias or large swings in blood pressure (the latter generally tend to be transient when due to physical manipulation of the heart and may or may not require treatment).

Prior to discontinuation of cardiopulmonary bypass, there are a number of essential parameters that must be analyzed by both surgeon and anesthesiologist. These include blood gases; hematocrit; body temperature; cardiac output, rate, and rhythm; blood pressure; ventilation of the lung; and venting of arterial air. With poor cardiac performance, an appropriate therapeutic regimen must be established; generally, this regimen is formulated jointly by the surgeon and anesthesiologist prior to its initiation.

In patients undergoing orthopedic surgery, the use of methyl methacrylate, a plastic resin-like material, is common. In such cases, it is crucially important that the orthopedist inform the anesthesiologist of such use, since it may be associated with profound hypotension. The anesthesiologist must be prepared to deal with this embolic phenomenon to prevent further complications.

In neurosurgical procedures, cooperation and communication between surgeon and anesthesiologist are essential for a smooth operation. An example of this is in the case of a patient who has increased intracranial pressure and who requires certain manipulations by the anesthesiologist to enable the surgeon to operate successfully. In such instances, therapeutic interventions involving cerebrospinal fluid drainage, the use of an osmotic agent such as mannitol, or hyperventilation are essential adjuncts to a successful operation.

Close communication between neurosurgeon and anesthesiologist is also essential in the prevention, diagnosis, and treatment of air emboli. This phenomenon is known to occur when the surgical field is above the right atrium, as in the patient undergoing posterior fossa surgery in the sitting position. The use of a precordial Doppler is essential in the diagnosis of air emboli.

In surgical procedures performed on pediatric patients, the establishment and maintenance of an adequate airway are crucial. In the presence of even transient hypoxia, pediatric patients rapidly become brachycardic, which, if untreated, may lead to cardiac arrest. In the pediatric patient, another possible complication is related to the short length of the trachea, in that intubation of the right mainstem bronchus can easily occur. Careful assessment by all members of the surgical team of blood loss is extremely important in these patients, especially in neonates. Intravenous fluid and blood administration should be performed using a soluset, giving small aliquots of fluid to prevent hypovolemia or fluid overload.

In obstetrical surgery, a good working relationship between anesthesiologist and surgeon contributes to the well-being of both the mother and the fetus. In nonobstetrical surgery for the pregnant patient, continuous monitoring of the fetal heart rate and maternal uterine activity is important in preventing premature labor.

During labor, the decision to perform epidural anesthesia is made following consultation by the obstetrician and anesthesiologist with the patient. For the patient who requires Cesarean section, a decision must be made about the type of anesthesia to be used—general, epidural, or spinal. The decision depends on the urgency and difficulty of the surgery, the medical status of the patient, and the patient's psychological state.

When a patient presents with an obstetrical complication, such as toxemia, joint obstetrical and anesthetic consultation is required. An example is in the case of a patient with placenta previa. Prior to the diagnostic examination, both surgeon and anesthesiologist must make preparations to replace acute blood loss and be ready to proceed with emergency Cesarean section.

In surgery of the genitourinary tract, such as transurethral resection of the prostate, the anesthetic regimen chosen for the patient, whether general or regional, must be individualized according to the needs of that patient. Regional anesthesia provides good analgesia intraoperatively, and is of great value in providing postoperative pain relief, particularly in cases where the transurethral catheter is on traction. During the operation, the irrigating solution enters the venous sinuses of the resected prostatic bed and may give rise to water intoxication and dilutional hyponatremia. Therefore, the surgeon should keep the actual resection under one hour. If the anesthetic method has been spinal or epidural, irritability, restlessness, and abdominal pain may herald perforation of the bladder.

In the trauma patient, the anesthesiologist must be prepared for a large amount of fluid resuscitation. Therefore, prior to the operative procedure, it is extremely important that the surgeon and anesthesiologist decide jointly on the need for invasive hemodynamic monitoring. The decision on arterial line placement, central venous pressure monitoring, or Swan-Ganz catheterization must be made with due regard for the medical status of the patient, the duration of anesthesia and surgery, and the site of the injury. Failure to maintain adequate fluid resuscitation in the face of continuing losses ultimately will lead to shock and/or death of the patient. Conversely, overzealous fluid resuscitation may lead to fluid overload and pulmonary edema. Thus, to ensure adequate resuscitation of the patient, the surgeon and anesthesiologist must remain in constant communication about blood and fluid loss.

In ophthalmic surgery, the anesthesiologist must be especially aware of systemic effects of certain eye medications and their interaction with anesthetic agents, particularly the anticholinesterases. The anesthesiologist must also carefully control intraocular pressure, particularly with an open globe, as a sudden increase in intraocular pressure may cause extrusion of the vitreous humor. Pressure on the globe of the eye, manipulation of the eye, or traction on the extraocular muscles may elicit the oculocardiac reflex, producing significant cardiac slowing.

In ear, nose, and throat surgery, the close proximity of the surgeon to the patient's airway makes communication between the surgeon and anesthesiologist essential. This is particularly important in preventing inadvertent extubation.

THE POSTOPERATIVE PERIOD

Postoperatively, the anesthesiologist must report to the PACU nurse if any drug reversals were used, since the original drug given will occasionally outlast the duration of action of the antagonist drug. An example of this situation is when naloxone (Narcan) is given to reverse a narcotic and the effects of the narcotic may outlast the reversal. In such cases, the PACU nurse must be aware of the possible effects of the initial drug given that may manifest themselves during the postoperative period. If there was significant blood loss during the procedure, the amount lost must be reported. It is routine practice to check a hematocrit either after transfusing a patient postoperatively or on arrival in the PACU.

Immediate postoperative airway problems—including hypoxemia, hypoventilation, airway obstruction, bronchospasm, and aspiration—are usually managed by the anesthesiologist in conjunction with the PACU nurse.

The management of circulatory complications, such as hypotension, requires prompt diagnosis and treatment and is often performed jointly by the surgeon and anesthesiologist. The surgical wound must be examined to make sure there is no further bleeding at the surgical site. Occasionally, invasive hemodynamic monitoring must be instituted, enabling the surgical team to identify decreased ventricular preload or reduced myocardial contractility as the etiology of the hypotension.

Treatment of acute hypertension postoperatively is usually managed by the anesthesiologist in conjunction with the surgeon. The management generally consists of alleviating pain, correcting hypoventilation or hypoxemia, and treating fluid overload, or of treatment by appropriate vasodilation.

Cardiac arrhythmias occur occasionally postoperatively and require prompt investigation of their etiology. Patients who complain of chest pain that is felt to be of cardiac origin and patients with life-threatening cardiac arrhythmias are usually seen by a cardiologist in the PACU. In patients with cardiac arrhythmias, factors that must be investigated include electrolyte abnormality, insufficient pulmonary gas exchange, metabolic abnormalities, and preexisting heart disease. Life-threatening cardiac arrhythmias must be treated immediately, often before the physician has time to determine their etiology.

Postoperative pain is a common occurrence in the PACU, and its treatment is generally performed by the anesthesiologist in conjunction with the PACU nurse. Narcotic analgesics are the mainstay of treatment. In such cases, the PACU nurse must carefully observe the patient following administration of the narcotic analgesic, watching for possible circulatory and respiratory depression.

Postoperative agitation is also common in the PACU. Prior to its pharmacologic treatment its etiology must be sought. Occasionally, such agitation is drug-induced, as in the patient who received ketamine intraoperatively; other etiologies include urinary or gastric distention. More commonly, however, postoperative agitation is due to inadequate pulmonary gas exchange. Thus, it is the responsibility of the surgeon and anesthesiologist in the PACU to assess the patient's airway and, if necessary, to obtain an arterial blood gas prior to sedating the patient. This procedure is extremely important, since further sedation of an hypoxic or hypercarbic patient could result in respiratory and cardiac arrest.

In high-risk patients in the PACU, an indwelling urinary catheter is necessary for early identification of oliguria. Its diagnosis is important, since most patients who develop renal failure often present initially with oliguria. Most cases of oliguria in the PACU are prerenal, usually secondary to hypovolemia or cardiac failure. Invasive hemodynamic monitoring often becomes necessary to distinguish between the two; its institution usually derives from a joint decision by the surgeon and the anesthesiologist who is caring for the patient during the postoperative period. Postoperatively, oliguria may also be of renal or postrenal origin.

Prior to discharge from the PACU, the patient is again evaluated by the anesthesiologist to ensure that most of the effects of the anesthetic have worn off and that the patient is stable enough to go to the floor.

In the evening of the day of surgery, or on the day following surgery, the patient is again visited by the anesthesiologist to confirm that the patient has fully recovered from anesthesia and that no anesthetic complications have occurred. Following discharge from the PACU, the surgeon is responsible for the day-to-day care of the patient. Thus, the interaction between the surgeon and anesthesiologist begins preoperatively, continues during the intraoperative process, and is maintained in the postanesthetic care period.

BIBLIOGRAPHY

Dripps, R.D., Eckenhoff, J.E., and Vandam, L.D. *Introduction to Anesthesia, The Principles of Safe Practice,* 6th ed. Philadelphia: W.B. Saunders, 1982, 1–7, 15–44.

Miller, R.D. *Anesthesia,* 2nd ed. New York: Churchill Livingstone, 1986, 3–48, 1463–1598.

Stoelting, R.K., and Dierdorf, S.F. *Anesthesia and Co-Existing Disease.* New York: Churchill Livingstone, 1983, 683–810.

Stoelting, R.K., and Miller, R.D. *Basics of Anesthesia.* New York: Churchill Livingstone, 1983, 103–125, 419–432.

Yao, F.S., and Artusio, J.F. *Anesthesiology: Problem-Oriented Patient Management.* Philadelphia: J.B. Lippincott, 1983, 189–200, 263–272.

Part II
Surgical Procedures and Related PACU Care

Chapter 3
Postanesthesia Care After Neurosurgery

Alan Van Poznak, M.D.

INTRODUCTION

Cooperation between competent practitioners is essential for successful treatment of the neurosurgical patient. In particular, close cooperation between surgeon, anesthesiologist, and operating room nurse is essential in the operating room; and this must be followed by equally close cooperation between surgeon, anesthesiologist, and postanesthetic recovery personnel if optimum results are to be achieved. It is also important that PACU staff be aware of what was done in the operating room, since that will affect the diagnostic and therapeutic activities conducted in the postanesthetic recovery setting.

In this chapter, we outline some commonly performed neurosurgical procedures, with special emphasis on the effects that operating room activities may produce on the patient who arrives in the PACU.

SPINE SURGERY

Operation for herniated disc is the most commonly performed neurosurgical procedure. Although disc herniation can occur at any level, the most commonly herniated discs are in the lumbar or cervical region. Patients are troubled with pain in the distribution of the nerve roots affected by the herniated disc and may have muscle spasm and motor impairment in the affected areas as well.

Surgery for herniated lumbar or lumbosacral disc may be performed with the patient in a number of different positions. Our preference at the New York Hospital/Cornell Medical Center is to use the knee-chest position. This position affords the advantages of excellent anatomical exposure and minimal venous bleeding, since the operative site is at the highest point of the patient's body and therefore has the lowest venous pressure. The patient's abdomen and chest are free to move easily, ensuring adequate spontaneous respiration in all but the most obese patients. Whenever possible, we prefer to use spontaneous respiration in the presence of a light level of inhalation anesthetic, such as isoflurane (Forane). In this way, the pattern of the patient's respiration can be observed. If the patient appears to be in pain, small amounts of intravenous narcotic can be titrated until there is an adequate expiratory pause.

While it is difficult to speak of the perception of pain in an unconscious patient, there nevertheless is respiratory response to the reception of noxious stimuli. This is expressed in the lightly anesthetized, spontaneously breathing patient by shortening or disappearance of the expiratory pause. If patients are properly titrated with narcotic while lightly anesthetized, they will awaken from anesthesia with a reasonable degree of comfort. They will certainly not be in agony after they have breathed out the small residual amount of isoflurane and nitrous oxide. They may require a small additional amount of narcotic to be made comfortable again.

Operations on the cervical spine may be done with the patients either in prone or in supine position. Operations done in the prone position involve the removal of muscles from their attachments to the spine and possibly the posterior portion of the skull. These procedures can be quite painful, leaving the patient with a literal "pain in the neck" that should be treated with adequate titration of intravenous narcotic. In addition, the cervical region of the spinal cord contains nerves that are essential to proper respiratory function. The thoracic nerves to the intercostal muscles pass through the cervical cord, and the innervation of the diaphragm comes from cervical Segments 3, 4, and 5. Patients who have had intraspinal manipulation in the high cervical level should be closely watched for adequate respiratory function.

Patients operated on in the supine position for the anterior approach to the cervical disc are usually much more comfortable, since the large muscles that hold the head and neck together do not have to be divided. The incision is placed between the sternocleidomastoid muscle laterally and the trachea and esophagus medially, then down to the subcutaneous tissue and platysma, and on to the transverse processes of the cervical vertebrae. The vertebrae are often pulled apart either by weights attached to the Gardner-Wells tongs embedded in the skull during the operative procedure, or the vertebrae may be separated with a special distracting tool. Postoperatively, these patients are usually more comfortable than those who have had a posterior approach to a cervical disc.

CRANIOTOMY

Intracranial surgery places special demands on the anesthesiologist and eventually on the staff in the PACU. In addition to keeping the patient physiologically safe and free from pain and anxiety, the anesthesiologist must provide satisfactory operating conditions for the neurosurgeon. One of these conditions is adequate room for the surgeon to work. Another is the control of excessive bleeding.

Making room for the surgeon to work inside the head involves four specific procedures:

1. hyperventilation
2. administration of hypertonic solutions
3. spinal fluid drainage
4. induction of deliberate hypotension

By deliberately hyperventilating the patient, the carbon dioxide content of the blood is lowered. The decrease of carbon dioxide content causes cerebral vasoconstriction. Although the cerebral vessels make up only a small percent of the intracranial volume, their vasoconstriction throughout the brain causes a reduction in brain bulk and may allow the surgeon the few extra millimeters needed to work in safety without having to retract the brain with excessive force. Vigorous retraction of the brain is one of the leading causes of postoperative complications, since petechial hemorrhages and edema may follow the application of excessively vigorous retraction. The carbon dioxide level is reduced from its normal of about 40 millimeters of mercury down to a level of 25–30 millimeters. This decrease will produce significant brain shrinkage, and yet it is not so low as to be dangerous.

The second means of shrinking the brain to provide the neurosurgeon more room to work is by the administration of hypertonic solutions, such as 20-percent mannitol. About one gram of mannitol per kilogram of the body weight of the patient is administered. The hypertonic solution circulates in the blood stream and draws water from all cells with which it comes in contact. Since about 16 percent of the cardiac output goes to the brain, the brain cells see the mannitol first and so are exposed to its action. The water drawn from the brain cells is eventually excreted by the kidney. This makes it necessary to install an in-dwelling catheter during the procedure and during the early postoperative period to monitor the amount of urine produced and to permit satisfactory replacement by intravenous fluid. While mannitol is largely an innocuous substance, an extreme overdose may draw so much water from the cardiac cells that they cease to function. This can produce a cardiac arrest from which resuscitation is extremely difficult, if not impossible.

The third method of giving the surgeon additional room to work consists of spinal fluid drainage. Lumbar puncture needles are placed after the induction of anesthesia, and spinal fluid is drained at the time the surgeon begins to open the dura. This allows the normally fluid-filled ventricles of the brain to collapse, enabling retraction of a lobe of the brain to be done more easily and without the danger of the trauma previously mentioned.

The fourth method to provide adequate room for the surgeon to work is the induction of deliberate hypotension. This produces a less tense brain that is easier to retract.

Hemostasis

Venous Bleeding

Venous bleeding is controlled by proper tilt of the table. Venous pressure is lessened as the patient approaches the upright position. By judiciously elevating the head of the table, the venous pressure in the head is decreased and the circulating blood volume tends to pool in the dependent lower extremities. However, one must be careful not to position the head so high that the venous pressure becomes negative. This will introduce the danger of venous air embolism. Since the venous pressure within the dural venous sinus would be subatmospheric, an opening made in a dural venous sinus could invite the entrance of atmospheric air, producing bubbles and foam in the right side of the heart and the pulmonary circulation. This could be a serious or even fatal complication.

Arterial Bleeding

There are four factors to be sequentially considered in controlling arterial pressure:

1. the depth of the anesthetic agent
2. the tilt of the table
3. the relative blood volume of the patient
4. the use of deliberate hypotension-inducing drugs

If the first three of these factors are carefully considered, there will rarely be any need for the fourth.

By deepening the anesthesia with an inhalation agent, such as isoflurane, enflurance (Ethrane), or halothane (Fluothane), there will be peripheral vasodilation and decreased myocardial contractility. Sufficient tilt of the table will cause the patient's blood volume to move toward the dependent lower extremities. If there is blood pooled in the feet, there will be less venous return to the right atrium of the heart. Whatever blood the heart does receive will be pumped out less forcefully, due to myocardial depression from the anesthetic. The blood that is pumped out will go into the periphery that has been vasodilated by the action of the anesthetic. In this way, the amount of blood going to the head will be lessened, and the amount of arterial bleeding and capillary oozing will be significantly diminished.

The third factor, the relative blood volume of the patient, is influenced by the fact that patients who have brain tumors frequently neglect their food and fluid intake, especially if they live alone. It may be hazardous to anesthetize deeply these hypovolemic patients with depleted circulating volume; when tipping the head up sharply, their small blood volume may go into their lower extremities, and there may be insufficient venous return to maintain an adequate cardiac output. Thus, it may be necessary to administer intravenous fluids a bit more liberally to these patients, even though in general it is our preference to fluid-restrict craniotomy patients.

There are several reasons for this fluid restriction. First, it is easier to induce hypotension in a patient who does not have a large circulating volume. Second, because postoperative cerebral edema is one of the principal problems seen in the early postoperative period, by restricting the amount of fluid to a reasonable amount, it is possible to lessen the incidence of this problem postoperatively. Remember, one can't have edema without water.

If careful attention is paid to the anesthetic depth, the tilt of the table, and the relative blood volume of the patient, it is rarely necessary to resort to hypotension-inducing drugs. If such drugs are needed, it will be only in small amounts. The danger of toxicity from these drugs will then be small to nonexistent.

The principal drugs used in the recent past for induction of hypotension in neurosurgery include trimethaphan (Arfonad) and sodium nitroprusside (Nipride). Both of these drugs have the capacity to lower the arterial pressure. Neither of them is perfect, however. Trimethaphan may cause decreased renal blood flow; and sodium nitroprusside, if given in large amounts, may produce cyanide toxicity. For these reasons, we avoid these drugs whenever possible. Instead, we prefer to use the first three simple methods in the above list to keep the blood pressure sufficiently low to enable the neurosurgeon to do the operation safely and with a minimum of blood loss. In an operation involving the clipping of an aneurysm under the microscope, even a few cubic centimeters of blood loss may be too much, since it can obscure the surgeon's vision and make his task difficult, if not impossible.

All of the above factors are important considerations for the staff of the PACU. If deep anesthesia with inhalation agents has been used, it may be expected that the patient will take longer than usual to emerge. However, if the patient continuously becomes lighter and more responsive, it can be considered to be a satisfactory recovery. The patient who emerges and then goes back to sleep even though no drugs have been administered should be the object of immediate and serious concern, since the deterioration in neurological function may be the result of bleeding within the cranium. Vigorously hyperventilated patients also take longer to emerge. This should not be of concern as long as the patient is continuously becoming more responsive.

Following an operation in which hypotension has been deliberately induced, there may be a period of rebound hypertension. The hypertension can have several possible causes. Pain can produce hypertension and should be treated with an appropriately titrated dose of intravenous narcotic. If adequate medication for pain does not control the hypertension, it is reasonable to proceed to the use of antihypertensive drugs such as hydralazine (Apresoline), nifedipine (Procardia), nitroglycerin paste (Nitrol), propranolol (Inderal), or, in extreme cases, trimethaphan or sodium nitroprusside. The urine output should be closely monitored and appropriate replacement administered. Some patients, especially those who have had operations around the pituitary or hypothalamic region, may exhibit diabetes insipidus. A sudden outpouring of large-volume, low-specific-gravity urine may require treatment with oxytocin (Pitocin), as well as replacement of fluid that has been lost.

Posterior Fossa Surgery

The cerebellum is the coordination center for many simple learned acts. Tremors or disturbance in motor function may be observed following operations upon the cerebellum. Beneath the cerebellum are the brain stem and medulla. This is of special interest in that the respiratory surgery and vasomotor centers are located there. Patients who have had posterior fossa surgery should be observed very closely for proper respiratory and cardiovascular function, as well as the ability to maintain their airway. This is because the ninth and tenth cranial nerves, which control swallowing, coughing, and other laryngeal and pharyngeal functions, are located in the posterior fossa.

Transphenoidal Surgery

Transphenoidal operations are done through the nose. Strictly speaking, these operations are not intracranial procedures in the same sense as the previously discussed operations. They do however frequently involve the pituitary gland and thus deserve the same considerations with regard to hormonal balance, salt and water balance, temperature, and other functions that are centered in that area of the brain. Spiral-wire, armored endotracheal tubes are usually used to minimize the danger of kinking of the tube during the procedure. Secretions from the operative area may run down the back of the pharynx and accumulate around the endotracheal tube; thus, these should be carefully suctioned out before the cuff on the endotracheal tube is deflated. Sometimes blood and cerebrospinal fluid may be swallowed by the patient. If this happens, the fluid may be vomited up from the stomach.

CAROTID ENDARTERECTOMY

Carotid endarterectomies are done to increase the blood flow to the brain. Most patients referred to neurosurgeons for this procedure have already had transient ischemic attacks, and some may have had strokes. For these patients, it is important to optimize blood flow throughout the anesthesia and surgery. Anesthetic induction that will not cause hypotension or hypertension is chosen, and the level of blood pressure is closely monitored throughout the procedure. During the operative procedure, electroencephalograph-monitoring of brain function may also be employed by some neurosurgeons. In the PACU, it is important to watch the patient for level of neurological function, as well as for any evidence of arterial or venous bleeding in the neck. If bleeding should occur, it may be necessary to return the patient to the operating room.

Many patients are heparinized during the procedure, and some of them will be only incompletely reversed before they come to the PACU. Rarely, in extreme cases, compression of the airway may result from rapid accumulation of a hematoma in the neck, necessitating immediate opening of the wound and, if endotracheal intubation cannot be promptly accomplished, possibly performing a tracheotomy. Patients who present for carotid endarterectomy often have many other problems present in their circulatory systems; they may also have had myocardial infarction, renal insufficiency, and/or peripheral vascular problems. The nursing staff in the PACU should be alert to any of these other cardiovascular problems that may be present.

Chapter 4

Postanesthesia Care After Ophthalmalogic Surgery

Murk-Hein Heineman, M.D.

GENERAL CONSIDERATIONS

Ophthalmic surgical procedures, although confined to small anatomical areas, involve tissues of considerable delicacy and complexity. The eye and its adnexal structures, including the orbit, lids, and lacrimal apparatus, are subject to a wide variety of pathological conditions and injuries that often require surgical intervention or diagnostic evaluation of the need for anesthesia. Most ophthalmic surgical and diagnostic procedures can be carried out under topical or infiltrative anesthesia. General anesthesia is usually reserved for cases in which prolonged or extensive surgery is contemplated, procedures are to be performed upon children, or patients refuse local anesthesia.

Topical anesthetics, such as proparacaine (Ophthaine), tetracaine (Pontocaine), and cocaine, are used for minor diagnostic or surgical procedures, such as measuring intraocular pressure or removing superficial corneal foreign bodies. These surface active agents are also commonly used with local, infiltrative anesthesia in the majority of ophthalmic surgical cases. Of historical interest is the fact that the anesthetic properties of cocaine, the first effective local anesthetic, were initially reported by Carl Koller, a medical student working with Freud in Vienna.

In most cases, ophthalmic surgery is of sufficiently short duration to allow for the use of local, infiltrative anesthesia. Not only are the intra- and postoperative risks of general anesthesia avoided, the administration of local anesthesia is also simpler and less expensive to the patient. However, the use of infiltrative anesthetics is not without risk. Systemic reaction to the drugs used may occur; and the administration of the anesthetic may be complicated by hemorrhage, perforation of the globe, or localized tissue damage.

The use of general anesthetic drugs carries with it the attendant risk of circulatory and respiratory collapse, profound changes in metabolic function, and postoperative complications, such as uncontrolled vomiting. In addition, certain drugs, such as nitrous oxide and succinylcholine (Anectine), may not be appropriate in certain ocular surgical situations.

PATHOPHYSIOLOGICAL CONSIDERATIONS

Anterior Segment

Cataract

Cataract is one of the most common ocular conditions requiring surgery. A cataract may be defined as a clouding or opacification of the lens in the eye. Not all cataracts require surgery; the decision whether or not surgery is necessary is made largely on the basis of the degree of functional disability for the particular patient. The vast majority of cataracts are found among older patients; however, cataracts may occur at any age and may even be congenital. Certain systemic diseases, such as diabetes mellitus, predispose patients to earlier onset and more rapid progression of cataracts. Cataracts may also complicate medical therapy, as in cases of prolonged systemic corticosteroid use and radiation therapy.

The development of a cataract is usually a gradual process. Mild cataracts may cause only minor symptoms, such as glare, and do not require surgery. Cataract surgery is usually elective; but, in some rare instances, advanced cataracts may produce glaucoma or inflammation requiring prompt surgical intervention.

There are many different types of cataract surgery, but all such operations involve the removal of the lens, either in toto or in pieces. Subsequent visual rehabilitation depends upon such factors as whether an intraocular lens has been implanted or if glasses or contact lenses are to be used.

Corneal Disease and Injury

Diseases and injuries to the cornea may require primary repair or more extensive surgery, such as corneal transplantation (penetrating keratoplasty). The cornea, along with the lens, refracts or bends the incoming light to form a focused image on the retina. If the cornea is irregularly shaped, scarred, clouded, or otherwise damaged, good vision is impossible. The cornea is avascular; as a result, successful transplantation with donor tissue can usually be achieved with a low risk of tissue rejection.

Common conditions that may require corneal transplantation include hereditary diseases, such as keratoconus (abnormally steeped cornea), and a wide variety of corneal dystrophies. The cornea may also be scarred following trauma or infection, or it may become cloudy and edematous following previous cataract surgery if the endothelial cell layer is damaged.

The shape of the cornea may be changed surgically to correct refractive errors. One procedure, radial keratotomy, is becoming increasingly popular for the correction of near-sightedness (myopia). This involves the careful placement of radial incisions around the central visual axis, thereby changing the shape (flattening) of the cornea.

Glaucoma

Glaucoma is a group of diseases caused by elevations of the intraocular pressure. Most cases of glaucoma are the result of impaired outflow of intraocular fluids (aqueous humor), which are being produced continuously. Subsequent elevation of the intraocular pressure can result in the gradual, insidious damaging of the optic nerve, eventually leading to visual loss and even blindness. These cases of so-called open-angle glaucoma come to surgery only if medical therapy or photocoagulation (laser) treatment fail. Much more rarely, the intraocular pressure can rise suddenly, resulting in an attack of angle-closure glaucoma. In this condition, the eyeball may become hard and painful, and vision may deteriorate rapidly. This is an ophthalmic emergency; and, after the attack has been stabilized, using topical and systemic medication, surgery (peripheral iridectomy) is usually required to correct the underlying anatomic deficit.

Posterior Segment

Disease of and injuries to the retina and vitreous body often require surgical intervention. The central cavity of the eye is filled with a gel-like substance, the vitreous humor. This tissue plays an important role in the development of many types of retinal detachment and can complicate intraocular surgery, ocular trauma, or vascular diseases, such as diabetes mellitus. Vitrectomy, or removal of the vitreous, may be performed as part of a trauma or retinal detachment repair or by itself, if intraocular hemorrhage or infection is present.

Retina

The retina is the extremely delicate, light receptive layer lining the posterior part of the eye. It is a highly complex neural tissue that is actually part of the central nervous system. The retina sometimes detaches from its underlying pigment layer (retinal detachment) and may require surgical repair. Retinal detachments may occur spontaneously, especially among patients with high myopia or a strong family history of peripheral retinal disease. Retinal detachments may also occur following ocular trauma or as a complication of proliferative diabetic retinopathy.

Lids and Orbit

The orbit or eye socket is the cavity, made up of seven bones of the skull, which contains the eye, extraocular muscles, lacrimal (tear) gland, fat, nerves, and blood vessels. Surgical procedures involving the orbit are most commonly performed in order to repair traumatic injuries, to remove orbital mass lesions, or to decompress the orbit to prevent damage to the optic nerve or other vital structures. Although the orbital rim is very durable, trauma to this region may result in damage to the weak floor or medial wall of the orbit, necessitating surgical repair. A wide variety of tumors and inflammatory conditions may involve the orbit; and, because the volume of the orbit is finite, such mass lesions may impair normal ocular and optic nerve function, necessitating decompression. In addition, resection or biopsy of orbital masses is performed when orbital tumors are suspected.

Abnormalities of the eyelids often require surgical treatment. In both adults and children, ptosis or drooping of the eyelid may often be repaired surgically. Ptosis may be congenital, it may be acquired, or it may be the result of mechanical or neurogenic abnormalities. Cosmetic procedures, such as blepharoplasty, in which redundant skin and prolapsed orbital fat are excised, are commonly performed. Tumors of the eyelids may require excision and the subsequent reconstruction of remaining tissue.

Tears normally drain through the puncta (small orifices in each lid) and the nasolacrimal duct into the lacrimal sac and out through the nose. Obstructions of the system, the result either of an anatomic defect or of infection, may require surgical correction. Congenital abnormalities of the nasolacrimal system are common among children, whereas chronic infection and secondary scarring are usually seen among the elderly.

Strabismus

Good binocular vision depends upon the accurate coordination of extraocular movements. Incoordinate action of the muscles that control these movements is known as strabismus. In many cases, the attachments of the extraocular muscles can be adjusted surgically in order to straighten the eyes. Such procedures are usually performed on infants and children, although, in some cases, ocular deviations among adults are also repaired.

Trauma

Trauma may involve any combination of the orbital, intraocular, or extraocular structures discussed thus far. Surgical procedures may involve repair of bone and soft tissue injuries as well as microsurgical repair of the eye and intraocular structures. In such cases, the repair of penetrating ocular injuries and the removal of intraocular foreign bodies are usually given the highest priority, and repair of all the injuries may have to be staged accordingly.

SURGICAL PROCEDURES

Cataract Surgery

The goal of cataract surgery is to remove the opacified lens and clear the visual axis. Cataracts may be removed in toto, through so-called intracapsular surgery, or in such a way that the lens capsule is left in place, using an extracapsular technique. The latter technique has the advantage of allowing for the placement of a posterior chamber lens implant (placed behind the iris). It also has the theoretical advantage of reducing some of the risks of cataract surgery, such as retinal detachment or edema of the fine vision area.

All types of cataract surgery require that an incision be made in the eye at the junction between the clear cornea and the white sclera. This area is known as the limbus. Cataracts may be aspirated with a phacoemulsifier (using high frequency sound waves) through a small incision, or they may be aspirated through a larger incision to allow for the insertion of a lens implant. Many modifications of these techniques exist. In any case, following removal of the clouded lens and implantation of the artificial lens, the eye is closed with fine suture material. During this procedure, especially when the eye is opened, it is critical that the patient not move. It is also important that, intraoperatively and postoperatively, steps are taken to minimize coughing, vomiting, and other reflexes that can cause prolapse of the intraocular structures and wound dehiscence.

Some patients who have undergone intracapsular cataract surgery previously may elect to have an artificial lens implanted. This is known as a secondary intraocular lens implantation; it requires the opening and resuturing of the eye, as with a primary cataract procedure.

Corneal Surgery

When the existing cornea is damaged, scarred, chronically edematous, or misformed, corneal transplants are routinely performed to provide a new clear, refractive surface. Once the decision to transplant the cornea has been made, the patient is put on a waiting list to receive a donor cornea, as one becomes available. As with all organ transplants, the demand for donor tissue exceeds the supply. However, in the case of corneal transplantation, this disproportionality is somewhat mitigated by the fact that corneal donor tissue can be stored for a limited period of time.

Corneal transplantation is technically straightforward. The donor tissue is prepared and precisely cut, using a trephine, so that the size of the donor "button" corresponds to the diseased or damaged portion removed—roughly a circular piece of tissue from 7 to 9 mm in diameter. Under microscopic visualization, the donor tissue is carefully sewn into position. As with cataract surgery, care must be taken to ensure that, when the eye is opened, no pressure is exerted on the eye. Similarly, during the postoperative period, the delicate wound must be protected from inadvertent injury.

Glaucoma Surgery

Surgical treatment for open-angle glaucoma is usually reserved for patients who do not respond to maximal medical therapy or to the new technique of laser trabeculoplasty. Most glaucoma operations, such as trabeculoplasty, are designed to create a fistula to allow for the intraocular aqueous humor to bypass the normal drainage channels and pass out of the eye. Often these fistulas scar down, and repeat surgery may be required.

Sudden attacks of angle-closure glaucoma can often be treated by performing a peripheral iridectomy. In these operations, a small hole is made in the iris to allow for the direct passage of the aqueous humor to the drainage channels. A small corneoscleral incision is required to gain access to the iris. In many cases, laser photocoagulation can be used instead of surgery.

Vitreoretinal Surgery

A large number of different operative procedures have been developed to repair retinal detachments and their complications. Many retinal detachments, especially those without complicating factors, can be treated by scleral buckling procedures. The principles of treatment involve finding the retinal break causing the detachment, treating the break with cryotherapy (cold) or diathermy (heat), and buckling or indentation of the eye to eliminate intraocular tractional forces and to seal the retinal break.

Many different techniques and materials have been developed in order to produce the buckling effect. In general, shaped pieces of silicone are sutured to or imbedded into the sclera or white of the eye. Fluid that has accumulated beneath the retina is often drained.

Complicated retinal detachments and trauma involving the posterior pole of the eye often require intraocular surgical techniques. Instruments have been developed that allow for the intraocular manipulation of tissues. These tools, known as vitrectomy instruments, have revolutionized the treatment of retinal detachment and trauma. Also, a wide variety of microsurgical instruments, including intraocular lasers, have been developed. The use of intraocular gases and vitreous substitutes, such as silicone oil, is common in the management of complicated cases.

Surgery of the Orbit and Ocular Adnexa

Ophthalmic plastic surgical procedures most commonly involve the lids and lacrimal apparatus (nasolacrimal system). Cosmetic procedures on the lids (blepharoplasty) commonly involve the resection of redundant skin and prolapsed orbital fat tissue. Frequently, biopsy and resection of tumors of the eyelid are performed. The most common lid tumors are basal cell epithelioma and squamous carcinoma, which are usually resected. Depending upon the size and cell type of the tumor, reconstructive procedures are often necessary.

Access to the orbit is achieved through orbitomy. This access may be achieved through an anterior approach or through a lateral approach (Kronlein procedure), in which a piece of the bony lateral wall of the orbit is removed in order to gain access to the posterior aspect of the orbit. At the end of the procedure, the bony fragment is wired into place. Such procedures are performed under general anesthesia.

Obstruction of the tear drainage system, the nasolacrimal system, may be treated by means of lacrimal probing or, in more severe cases, by direct cannulation from the lacrimal sac (located along the bridge of the nose) through bone into the nose. This latter procedure is called dacryocystorhinostomy.

Surgical repair of ptosis (droopy eyelid) may involve a variety of procedures of varying anatomic complexity, depending upon the extent and nature of the defect and the degree of lid function still present. At one extreme, the total absence of lid function may require the construction of a sling from silicone or fascial material in order to support the lid. On the other hand, a slight ptosis with good lid function may be treated by a simple resection of the tissues under the eyelid (Fasanella-Servat procedure).

Strabismus Surgery

The surgical correction of ocular deviations is performed after a careful analysis of ocular motility. This involves careful identification of the abnormality and quantified adjustments to the insertions of the extraocular muscles. The muscles may be partially shortened (resected), or their insertions may be moved (recessed).

Depending upon the motility defect, a combination of muscles is usually operated upon. Strabismus surgery is usually performed on children, but adults may also have acquired defects of ocular motility that may be surgically repairable.

ANESTHETIC CONSIDERATIONS

Local Anesthesia

Local anesthesia is used for most eye surgery. Regional anesthesia of the eye and orbit is easily and, for the most part, safely achieved. The respiratory and circulatory side effects of general anesthesia are thus avoided, a particularly important consideration when dealing with patients with underlying medical problems, such as diabetes mellitus or cardiac disease. Another advantage of local anesthesia is that, after the surgery, there is a reduced risk of vomiting or coughing, actions that are particularly hazardous if the patient has undergone a procedure during which the eye has been opened, as in cataract extraction or corneal transplantation. Also, if the patient is awake at the end of the procedure, it will be much easier to position the patient as necessary following retinal detachment surgery.

Preoperative Medication

Most patients who undergo eye surgery under local anesthesia are given some form of preoperative sedation. Not only does such premedication reduce the anxiety of the patient, the effectiveness of the anesthetic agent is actually enhanced. Narcotics, such as meperidine (Demerol), are often given because of their analgesic effect. In addition, barbiturates are often prescribed because of the limited sedative effects of the narcotics and because it is believed that barbiturates reduce the frequency of toxic reactions to the local anesthetics themselves. Tranquilizers such as diazepam (Valium) are often used, but such drugs have the disadvantage of inducing hypotension in some patients.

Local Anesthetic Effects

Akinesia and anesthesia of the eye and orbit are achieved by regional infiltration to deaden the sensory nerves and paralyze the orbicularis muscle by blocking facial nerve function. A retrobulbar injection produces sensory anesthesia and completely immobilizes the eye. It should be noted that injection of an anesthetic into the retrobulbar space often causes a sensory block of the optic nerve. Local anesthetic agents commonly used in ophthalmic surgery include lidocaine (Xylocaine), mepivacaine (Carbocaine), and bupivacaine (Marcaine). The effect of lidocaine may be enhanced through the use of epinephrine in the injection solution.

Anesthetic effect is believed to be enhanced by vasospasm. Although the concentrations of epinephrine commonly used with lidocaine are low, its use should be avoided in patients with hypertension or cardiac disease and in those with a history of thyrotoxicosis. Hyaluronidase (Wydase) is often added to the injection mixture because it increases the permeability of the surrounding tissues to the anesthetic drug.

Complications of local anesthesia fall into two categories. First, some patients may experience toxic reactions to the drugs used. This may be the result of allergy or, more commonly, the result of systemic absorption of excessive amounts of the drug. An anesthetic drug may be inadvertently injected into the circulation during local infiltration. For this reason, the total amount of drug to be injected should be below the maximum dose for the patient.

Second, local anesthesia may be complicated by problems that develop as the result of the injections themselves. The most serious of such complications are inadvertent perforation of the eye during retrobulbar injection and the development of retrobulbar hemorrhage following injection.

General Anesthesia

Although general anesthesia is safe for most patients, its use may be hard to justify if the procedure can be performed just as easily under local anesthesia. Morbidity and mortality in general anesthesia is low, but primary anesthetic death can occur, albeit rarely. In some situations, there is no question that general anesthesia is preferable to local block. This may be the case with children or with potentially uncooperative patients or when a prolonged or extensive procedure is anticipated.

Modern anesthetic technique usually involves rapid intravenous induction, followed by maintenance with an inhalation agent. Smooth induction of anesthesia is particularly desirable when the patient has an open globe, as in the case of many injuries. In such instances, uncontrolled laryngospasm or coughing can dramatically elevate venous pressure, which can lead to prolapse of intraocular structures.

In inhalation anesthesia, gaseous anesthetic agents should not be used when intraocular gases are being used as part of the procedure (usually retinal detachment cases). Dangerous elevations of intraocular pressure may result if anesthetic gases are used in these situations.

Muscle relaxants are commonly used during anesthesia (the postanesthesia akinesia is limited, however, and some surgeons augment the general anesthesia with local orbicularis block in order to minimize squeezing). Succinylcholine (Anectine) should be used with care during an eye surgery because of the elevations of intraocular pressure associated with its use. It should not be used if the globe is open. Succinylcholine may not be effective if the patient has been using a cholinesterase inhibitor, such as echothiophate iodide (Phospholine), for the treatment of glaucoma. Succinylcholine (and some inhalation anesthetics) may in some rare cases trigger a familial metabolic disturbance, malignant hyperthermia, which requires prompt treatment and may be quite dangerous to the patient.

Cardiac arrest during anesthesia for eye surgery is rare, but when it occurs it may be associated with the oculocardiac reflex that manifests itself by bradycardia following traction on the extraocular muscles. The pathways of this reflex are poorly understood, and it is not clear whether such preventive measures as retrobulbar anesthesia or the use of intravenous atropine are effective.

POSTANESTHESIA CARE

General Considerations

Postanesthetic care of the patient who has undergone eye surgery depends on several factors. Foremost among these is the type of surgery performed. Patients who have undergone cataract extraction, repair of trauma to the anterior segment of the eye, corneal surgery, or glaucoma surgery all have delicate, finely sutured wounds. It is common practice after most ophthalmic surgical procedures for the eye to be dressed with eye pads and then protected with a metal or rigid plastic shield. It is very important that this shield be securely taped. If the patient has undergone general anesthesia, postoperative vomiting and coughing should be controlled to minimize the effects of sudden elevations of the venous pressure, which can cause wound dehiscence.

Head Positioning

Commonly, patients who have had retinal detachment surgery have to be positioned postoperatively. Careful positioning is usually done to enhance the absorption of subretinal fluid or to localize such fluid away from the fine vision area (macula). Such positioning may be critical to the patient's eventual visual recovery. In more complicated cases, where intraocular gases or vitreous substitutes, such as silicone, have been used, head positioning may also be very important. Intraocular gases are used to tamponade the detached retina; therefore, in such cases, proper positioning depends upon the location and extent of the detachment.

In general, patients on whom an intraocular gas has been used should avoid lying down with their face up. In this position, the gas bubble is in maximum contact with the lens (or cornea if the patient has had a cataract extraction), a situation that can damage the lens (or cornea). In the past, patients who had cataract surgery were strictly positioned and immobilized; this is no longer necessary. However, although many ocular surgical procedures, including cataract surgery, may now be performed on an outpatient basis, bending or heavy lifting should be avoided.

Postoperative Complications

Most eye operations are not particularly painful, and it is unusual for patients to require heavy analgesia after surgery. Thus, although some discomfort is to be expected after the anesthetic wears off, the development of severe pain should be promptly investigated. Pain accompanied by nausea is often a sign of elevated intraocular pressure. Transient elevations of pressure may occur after cataract surgery, especially when viscoelastic substances, such as sodium hyaluronate (Healon), are used. Intraocular pressure may in fact rise dramatically postoperatively if expanding intraocular gases are used during retinal detachment surgery. In these cases, prompt decompression of the eye, either through the use of osmotic diuretics or by actual venting of intraocular gas, may be necessary.

Another, fortunately rare, complication of cataract and glaucoma surgery that can cause severe postoperative pain is expulsive hemorrhage. Expulsive hemorrhages are caused by uncontrolled choroidal bleeding within the eye. These can occur during the operation or, more rarely, in the postoperative period. Such hemorrhages often severely impair vision and respond only poorly to subsequent surgical treatment.

BIBLIOGRAPHY

Adriani, J., Arens, J., and Anthony, S. "Postanesthetic Vomiting." *Journal of the American Medical Association* 175 (1961):666.

Atkinson, W.S. "The Development of Ophthalmic Anesthesia." *American Journal of Ophthalmology* 51 (1961):1.

Duane, T., ed. *Clinical Ophthalmology*. Philadelphia: Harper & Row, 1971.

Helveston, M. *Atlas of Strabismus Surgery*, St. Louis, Mo.: C.V. Mosby, 1973.

Jaffe, N.S. *Cataract Surgery and Its Complications*, 3d ed. Philadelphia: J.B. Lippincott, 1981.

Jones, L.T., and Wobig, J.L. *Surgery of the Eyelids and Lacrimal System.* New York: Aesculpaius, 1976.

Lewallen, W.M., and Hicks, B.L. "The Use of Succinylcholine in Ocular Surgery." *American Journal of Ophthalmology* 61 (1966):985.

Petruscak, S., Smith, R.B., and Breslin, P. "Mortality Related to Ophthalmological Surgery." *Archives of Ophthalmology* 89 (1973):106.

Pollack, F.M. *Corneal Transplantation.* New York: Grune & Stratton, 1977.

Chapter 5
Postanesthesia Care After Oral and Maxillofacial Surgery

David Behrman, D.M.D.

INTRODUCTION

Oral and maxillofacial surgery deals with the jaws, the maxilla and the mandible, and their associated soft tissues. Surgical procedures include the treatment of pathology, infection, trauma, and skeletal abnormalities. Orthognathic surgery (ortho meaning straight, gnathic meaning jaws) involves repositioning of the jaws, in whole or in part, for functional and aesthetic reasons. Almost all maxillofacial surgery is done via the oral route to avoid skin incisions. Early postoperative care of the patients can be a very difficult process. In this chapter we discuss the regimen used at one hospital where major oral and maxillofacial surgical procedures are performed on a weekly basis.

FACTORS INFLUENCING POSTOPERATIVE CARE

There are several aspects of oral and maxillofacial surgery that influence early postoperative care. The most important influencing factor is that all surgery is done in and through the patient's airway. The PACU nurse must be constantly aware of the significantly increased risk of airway compromise. Other influencing factors are:

- edema
- bleeding

- intermaxillary fixation
- secretions

Each of these areas is examined in the following sections. In each case, the common factor is the effect on the airway.

Edema

All surgical procedures in oral and maxillofacial surgery are performed on and around the face. Postoperative edema, which can develop quite rapidly and extensively, can affect the entire head—the eyes, cheeks, nose, lips, chin, and neck. Ice bags or cold packs are applied to the face as soon as possible and are maintained for 48 hours (see Figure 5-1). Chilled gauze pads are placed over the eyes. Many surgeons place their patients on steroid medications to minimize postoperative edema.

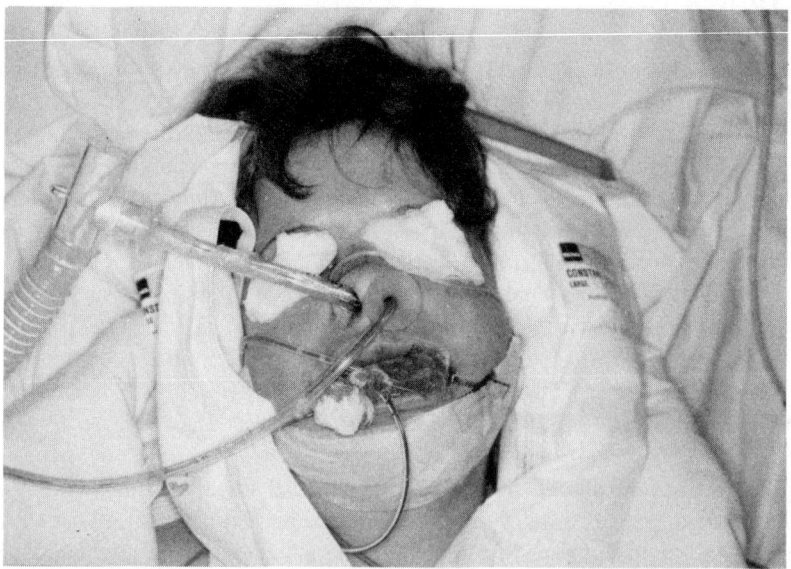

Note: Ice bags are placed around the face, and iced saline gauze pads are placed on the eyes. When the patient is extubated, the soft nasal airway placed in that nostril will be the only pathway for air exchange. The Jackson-Pratt drains and nasogastric tube should be taped to the patient's cheeks so that they do not rest on the lips, causing irritation.

Figure 5-1 A Patient with Postoperative Edema Shortly after Entering the PACU.

Bleeding

The bones of the face and their associated soft tissues are very vascular. Slight bleeding from the surgical sites is common during the first 24 hours after surgery. Small suction-type drainage catheters can be placed in each mandibular site to assist in controlling hematoma formation. Drainage of 5–20 mL per wound over the first 24 hours is usually within normal limits. Gauze packs are often placed between the cheeks and the teeth to provide a form of pressure tamponade. Extra-oral pressure dressings are seldom used.

Severe or life-threatening hemorrhage is a rare complication, but the potential exists, particularly with maxillary surgery such as LeFort I, II, or III. However, bleeding into the nasal and oral pharynx is possible and can be very difficult to detect. The PACU nurse should become concerned if the patient begins to cough up blood or if the nasogastric tube begins steadily to drain bright red blood.

Intermaxillary Fixation

A general principle of orthopedic surgery is that fractured bones must be approximated and immobilized to encourage healing. This applies as well to oral and maxillofacial surgery. Of course, a plaster cast cannot be placed on the face. Currently two methods of fixation and stabilization are used. Frequently, small metal plates and screws are used to approximate the bony segments to achieve rigid fixation and permit early postoperative movement. When rigid fixation is not acceptable or applicable, the jaws are secured together (held shut) to provide immobilization. This intermaxillary (between both jaws) fixation can be achieved with wire or rubber bands applied to special braces on the teeth (see Figure 5-2). Intermaxillary fixation prevents movement of the jaws during the healing period. Therefore, the patient will be unable to talk clearly, if at all, while in the PACU. The nurse must be particularly aware of this and try to anticipate the patient's questions and concerns. Frequent reassurance is very important to these patients.

Secretions

The average adult produces from 20 to 50 mL of saliva per hour while at rest. When a stimulus is introduced—surgery or appliances for example—salivary flow of 200 mL per hour is not uncommon. Irritation to the nasal mucosa from tubes or surgery will also cause increased mucous production. These increased secretions add to the patient's difficulty in swallowing because of the surgery. Sometimes

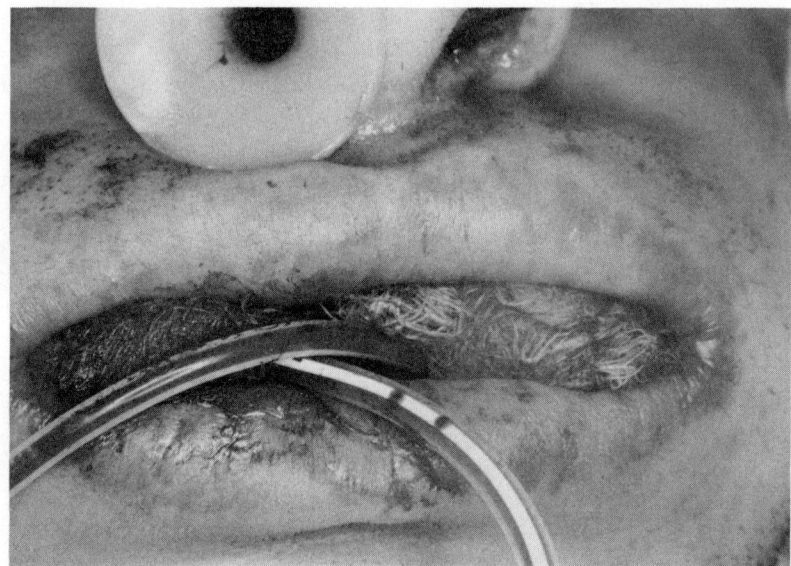

Note: While the gauze packs are in place, there is no oral space for breathing. The Jackson-Pratt drains should be taped to the patient's cheeks so that they do not rest on the lips.

Figure 5-2 Gauze Pressure Packing in a Patient with Rubber Band Intermaxillary Fixation and Two Jackson-Pratt Suction-Type Drains

---

patients feel "as if they are drowning." In such cases, the chance of aspiration is accordingly much greater.

A nasogastric tube is usually placed for 24 hours to keep the stomach empty and to minimize the danger of vomiting. Frequent suctioning of the oral and nasal pharynx is necessary. The patient can be kept in a slightly head-up, semi-Fowler position to make it easier to swallow.

The patient's lips will become irritated from surgical retraction. Therefore, the lips should be kept well-lubricated through frequent applications of surgical lubricant.

AIRWAY ASSESSMENT

While the patient is intubated, the airway is well-protected against possible compromise. However, when the patient is extubated, airway embarrassment is a very real concern. This could result from edema or, much more likely, from blockage with secretions or clotted blood. In such cases, certain basic precautions must be taken.

The best treatment is always prevention. Patients are allowed to awaken very slowly. In fact, they can be sedated in the PACU so that they remain intubated for two to six additional hours. This gradual awakening allows the patient to begin to accommodate to the intermaxillary fixation; it also gives the patient the best chance to maintain an adequate airway when extubated. Extubation is not attempted until the patient is fully awake. We have never had a postoperative airway problem when this routine has been followed.

Obviously, reintubating a patient whose face and respiratory passages are edematous and whose jaws are "wired shut" would be a very difficult procedure. In such cases, should reintubation become necessary, the appropriate process would be to remove the intermaxillary fixation and initially place an oral endotracheal tube. This could be changed to a nasal tube in the operating room under controlled conditions, at which time the jaws could be correctly repositioned. Scissors and a wire cutter should be kept at the patient's bedside in plain view. Rubber bands can be cut with a scissors or pulled off with a finger. Removal of wire intermaxillary fixation requires a wire cutter. As a precaution, a tracheostomy set should be kept at the bedside.

OTHER ASPECTS OF POSTANESTHESIA CARE

Temperature

Properly, a source of concern for PACU nurses is the elevated temperature of the oral and maxillofacial surgical patient. Any surgical procedure performed in the mouth will induce a transient bacteremia and consequent fever. After extensive surgical procedures, temperatures of 38.0 °C to 39.5 °C are very common during the first 24 hours. Our treatment regimen includes acetaminophen every 4 hours, as needed, for temperatures of 38.5 °C and higher. A hypothermia blanket is used for temperatures of 39.5 °C and higher. Shaking chills are almost never seen. Should they occur, it could be an indication of a potentially severe problem, such as an aspiration pneumonia, and would require immediate investigation. Patients other than those having dentoalveolar surgery are started on an antibiotic covering normal mouth flora, such as penicillin, at the time of surgery.

Hypotensive Anesthesia

Blood loss during oral and maxillofacial surgery ranges from less than 100 mL up to 1,000 mL for major procedures. Intraoperative replacement is with crystalloid fluids and blood products, frequently autologous. Postoperative fluid replacement is calculated in the standard fashion, based on fluid loss, replacement, and need.

Hypotensive anesthetic techniques, which lower the systolic blood pressure to 70–80 mm Hg, are frequently employed to minimize the surgical blood loss. In our institution, this is achieved through deep inhalation anesthesia, without use of nitroglycerin or nitroprusside (Nipride). There are a few side effects caused by this hypotensive period that the PACU nurse must be aware of. Kidney function will decrease during hypotensive anesthesia, while the body responds to a perceived hypovolemic state and attempts to maintain cerebral blood flow. Intraoperative urinary output will therefore decrease, despite adequate fluid load. Increased diuresis during the first 24 hours will occur as the body returns to its preoperative state. Occasionally, bladder tone is decreased during the hypotensive period. This can result in urine retention and bladder distention postoperatively. For shorter surgical procedures of two to three hours, treatment of bladder distention is single-use straight catheterization. If retention recurs, the patient could be catheterized for 24 hours to allow bladder tone to return. Patients undergoing longer surgical procedures are catheterized at the time of surgery and maintained for 24 hours postoperatively.

Occasionally, patients who have undergone hypotensive anesthesia experience a hypertensive rebound phenomenon during the initial 6–12 hours postoperatively. Blood pressures of 170–200/90–100, or higher, have occurred in previously normotensive individuals. No treatment is necessary for patients in this range unless other physiological parameters are significantly abnormal.

Systolic pressures of 210 or greater and diastolic pressures of 110 or greater have responded to incremental titration with hydralizine or other vasodilating or antihypertensive agents. In our experience, this rebound phenomenon has not lasted past 12 hours postsurgery. Similarly, patients who have undergone hypotensive anesthesia may be significantly tachycardic postoperatively, up to 140 beats per minute. It is not known whether this is a response to the elevated temperature or a perceived fluid imbalance or is another variation of rebound to the hypotensive anesthesia. Most likely all three factors contribute. In our experience, no treatment has been necessary, since such patients have remained clinically stable and are not uncomfortable. A gradual return to a normal heart rate occurs over the next 36 hours.

BIBLIOGRAPHY

Archer, W.H. *Oral and Maxillofacial Surgery,* vols. 1 and 2. Philadelphia: W.B. Saunders, 1975.
Bell, W.H., Proffit, W.R., and White, R.P. *Surgical Correction of Dentofacial Deformities,* vols. 1–3, Philadelphia: W.B. Saunders, 1980.

Bergman, S., Hoffman, W.E., Gans, B.J., Miletich, D.J., and Albrecht, R.E. "Blood Flow to Oral Tissues: A Comparative Study with Enflurane, Sodium Nitroprusside and Nitroglycerin." *Journal of Oral and Maxillofacial Surgery* 40 (1982):13.

Dingman, R.O., and Natvig, P. *Surgery of Facial Fractures*. Philadelphia: W.B. Saunders, 1964.

Dolwick, M.F., and Sanders, B. *TMJ Internal Derangement and Arthrosis*. St. Louis, Mo.: C.V. Mosby, 1985.

Fonseca, R.J., and Davis, W.H. *Reconstructive Preprosthetic Oral and Maxillofacial Surgery*. Philadelphia: W.B. Saunders, 1986.

Kinni, M.E., and Stout, M.M. "Aspiration Pneumonitis: Conditions and Prevention." *Journal of Oral and Maxillofacial Surgery* 44 (1986):378–384.

Topazian, R.G., and Goldberg, M.H. *Management of Infections of the Oral and Maxillofacial Regions*. Philadelphia: W.B. Saunders, 1981.

Chapter 6

Postanesthesia Care After Head and Neck Surgery

Robert F. Ward, M.D.

INTRODUCTION

The head and neck region covers a wide variety of organ systems and pathological processes that require operative intervention. Excluding the brain, eye, and major arterial vessels of the neck, the surgical procedures of the head and neck involve the ear, nose, oral cavity, pharynx, larynx, esophagus, and the soft tissue structures of the neck. The major disease processes requiring surgical intervention that are discussed in this chapter are in two main categories: (1) infectious processes and (2) neoplastic processes. Other problems, including congenital abnormalities (such as cleft lip and palate) and traumatic deformities, are not considered here; however, the same general principles of postoperative care apply as well to these conditions. In addition, the discussion focuses on those areas that involve the upper aerodigestive tract and deep neck structures, excluding pathological processes of the ear and scalp.

ANATOMY AND PHYSIOLOGY

The neck comprises only a small percentage of the total body surface, but it contains some of the most important structures of the body. It acts as a highway that connects the head with the rest of the body. In addition to carrying major blood vessels, lymphatics, and nerves that control most of the voluntary and involuntary activities of the body, the neck contains the upper aerodigestive tract. This tract can be divided into the digestive portion, including the oral cavity, pharynx, hypopharynx, and upper esophagus, and the airway portion, consisting of the larynx and upper trachea. Figure 6-1 presents a midsaggital section through the head and neck region and shows the close relationship of the various structures.[1] As can be seen, the laryngotracheal complex and the esophagus share a common opening, which consists of the oral cavity, pharynx, and hypopharynx. Since any surgery performed in this region can affect the upper airway, the area is of prime concern in any procedure or operation performed in the head and neck.

The larynx is a complex and sophisticated structure consisting of cartilage, muscles, nerves, and ligaments. The primary, and most primitive, function of the upper airway, and more specifically the larynx, is to act as a sphincter to prevent the entrance of anything except air into the lungs.[2] The larynx also acts as a connection between the oral cavity and the lungs. In the human, the sphincteric closure of the lyarynx serves other functions besides protection. These include coughing, straining or "valsalva" ability, and phonation. Although of great social and psychological importance in humans, the ability to phonate and talk remains a

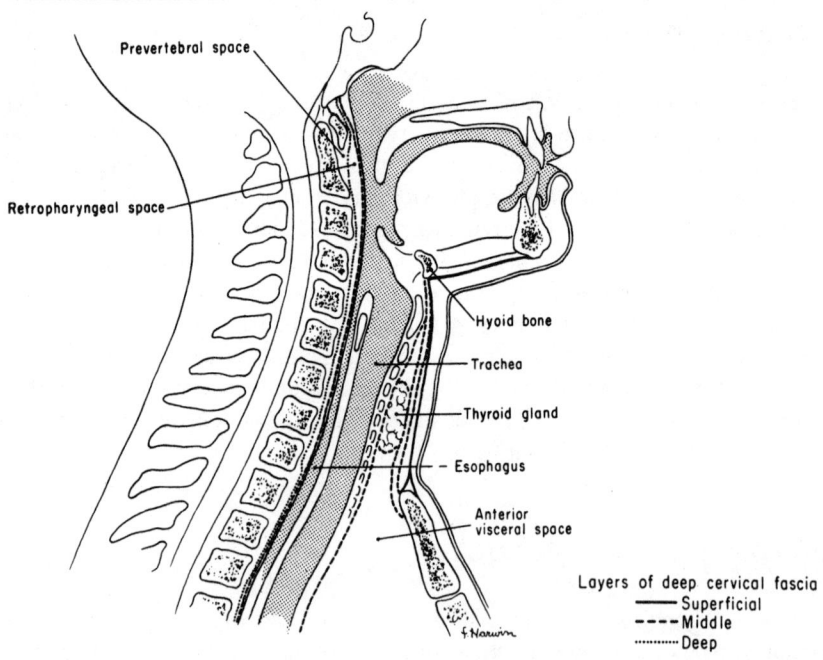

Figure 6-1 Midsaggital Section of Neck. *Source:* Reprinted from *Otolaryngology, Vol. 3* by M.M. Papparella and D.A. Shumrick (Eds.), p. 2312, with permission of W.B. Saunders Company, © 1980.

secondary function. The primary laryngeal role involves the protection of the airway and the transmission of air to the lower respiratory tract.

The esophagus is a tubular connection between the oral cavity (specifically, the pharynx) and the stomach. It is demarcated from these adjacent structures by sphincters or muscle groups, which are normally closed except during the passage of liquids or solids into the stomach.[3] The upper sphincter acts to prevent air from filling the esophagus during inspiration, and the lower sphincter prevents reflux of stomach contents into the esophagus. The principle function of the esophagus is the active transport of food substances into the stomach by peristaltic muscle activity.

SURGICAL PROCEDURES

In this section, we examine several common surgical procedures that are performed in the head and neck region. In each case, the discussion includes information on postanesthetic care procedures that are routinely performed in the PACU.

Tracheotomy

Tracheotomy has developed from a surgical technique used to relieve upper airway obstruction into a therapeutic modality for prolonged respiratory and ventilatory support.[4] It also provides improved pulmonary toilet and respiratory management. With the advances in surgical procedures for the management of upper aerodigestive cancers, tracheotomy is now frequently performed to ensure initially an adequate and safe airway following the trauma and edema caused by surgical intervention. Usually, in an elective situation the tracheotomy incision is made between the third and fourth cartilaginous rings of the trachea (see Figure 6-2).[5] This bypasses the larynx and prohibits the patient from phonating in the immediate postoperative period. In sum, the goal of tracheotomy is to provide an adequate airway either to bypass an obstruction or to allow for improved pulmonary toilet and assistance.

Endoscopy

Endoscopy is a surgical procedure performed for either diagnostic or therapeutic purposes. Endoscopy of the upper aerodigestive region can be divided into three procedures:

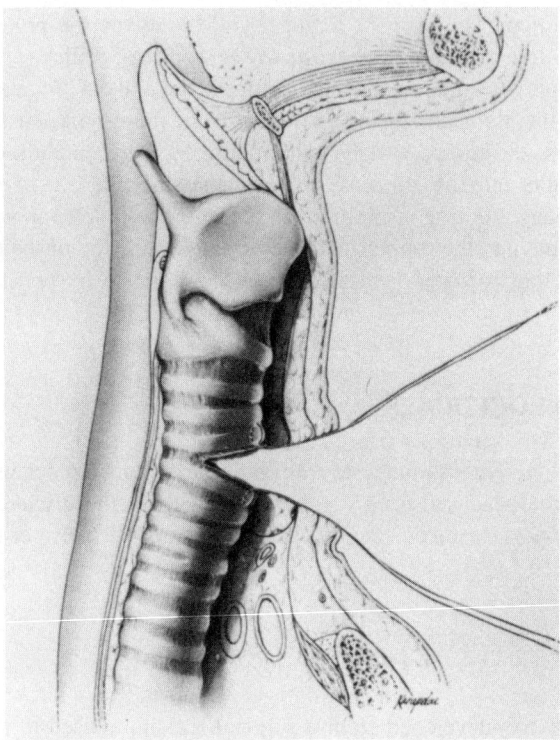

Figure 6-2 Location of Tracheotomy through the Third and Fourth Cartilaginous Rings. *Source:* Reprinted from *Complications of Head and Neck Surgery* by J. Conley, p. 276, with permission of W.B. Saunders Company, © 1979.

1. laryngoscopy, the examination of the larynx and related structures
2. bronchoscopy, the examination of the trachea and the right and left main bronchus
3. esophagoscopy, the examination of the esophagus

In terms of diagnostic evaluation, endoscopy is frequently performed to evaluate a suspected neoplasm of the upper respiratory or digestive tract. It provides information as to the exact location, size, and nature of the lesion. A biopsy is taken at the time of endoscopy to identify the exact pathology of the lesion. This helps to determine the therapeutic modality used to treat the specific disease.

Endoscopy is also carried out for removal of foreign bodies lodged in the pharynx, esophagus, or respiratory tract. After identification, these foreign objects can be removed by use of specifically designed instruments that can be manipulated through the various endoscopes.

Neck Mass Biopsy

Frequently a patient will present with a mass in the region of the neck. Based on a careful history and physical examination and evaluation by various laboratory tests, a biopsy of the mass may be necessary. Because of the depth of most of the nodal groups in the cervical region, it is frequently necessary to perform the biopsy under general anesthesia. Pathology can range from reactive hyperplastic adenopathy as the result of an infection to any of a variety of hematopoietic tumors, such as lymphoma. In some cases, an acute infectious process can lead to a suppuration of any of the nodes in the neck. This condition will not resolve on antibiotic therapy alone and requires an incision and drainage of the abscess collection. This type of deep neck infection can be quite serious, since the purulent material can spread along various fascial planes that lead to the mediastinum, great vessels of the neck, the paratracheal area, or even the abdominal cavity.[6]

Tonsillectomy and Adenoidectomy

In the past, tonsillectomy and adenoidectomy were among the most frequently performed surgical procedures. Today, they are performed less frequently, but they still remain among the top ten operations performed in the United States.[7] Although considered by many to be minor operations, these procedures carry a significant risk in both the child and the adult.

The two most common indications for removal of the tonsils are airway obstruction and inflammatory disease. Patients with inflammatory or infectious disease processes of the tonsils have either a history of repeated acute infections or a chronic infection that is not responding completely to appropriate antibiotic therapy. On occasion, patients will develop a peritonsillar abscess in the region around the tonsillar fossa, which requires incision and drainage. In the adult patient, this can frequently be performed under local anesthesia; but in the pediatric age group, it is usually done under general anesthesia.

Thyroidectomy

The thyroid gland is situated in close proximity to the trachea and esophagus. Enlargement of the gland or the development of an intraglandular tumor may restrict respiration and/or swallowing. Enlargement of the gland may be diffuse or nodular. Diffuse enlargement is usually representative of functional or inflammatory conditions. In the past, this was probably the most common indication for thyroidectomy. Today, with advances in the medical management of thyroid disease, the main indication for partial or total thyroidectomy is the presence of a suspicious solitary nodule in the gland.[8]

Salivary Gland

The majority of surgical procedures performed on the salivary glands involve either the parotid or submandibular (submaxillary) gland. Typically, the patient undergoing parotid surgery presents with a totally asymptomatic lump in the region of the gland. Approximately 20 percent of these asymptomatic masses will be cancerous; the remaining 80 percent will be benign tumors.[9] On rare occasions, the parotid gland is removed for treatment of chronic sialadenitis, that is, a chronic, recurrent parotid gland infection. In contrast, surgery of the submandibular gland is performed primarily for salivary stones (calculi), which cause obstruction of the salivary duct (also known as sialolithiasis). On rare occasions, tumors of the submandibular gland will develop; in such cases, there is about a 50-percent incidence of malignancy. Occasionally, chronic infectious processes, such as atypical mycobacterium, may cause salivary gland enlargement, with the development of cutaneous fistual tracts. This is best treated by surgical excision of the involved gland and overlying skin.

Neoplastic Disease of the Head and Neck

The vast majority of head and neck tumors are malignant squamous cell lesions. Of the total number of estimated cases of cancers in the U.S. population in a 1984 census numbering 870,000, approximately 53,650 were estimated to be cancers of the head and neck. This represents about 3.5 percent of all cancer deaths.[10] Table 6-1 lists the various sites of squamous cell carcinoma and the respective incidence of the disease. By far the most common site is the larynx, with 11,100 new cases, or 25 percent of all head and neck cancers, each year (see Table 6-2).[11]

Lesions of the head and neck are categorized in stages according to the standard TNM classification, that is, in terms of tumor size, cervical node involvement, and metastatic disease.[12] The majority of early-stage cancers, namely Stages I and II, are frequently treated with radiation therapy (RT) alone. Advanced-stage diseases are now usually treated with surgical therapy followed by radiation therapy. This protocol has led to an overall increase in the survival rate of patients with head and neck squamous cell cancers (except for the esophagus). Early-stage lesions usually require only a biopsy and are then treated by RT. The procedures for

Table 6-1 Numbers of Head and Neck Cancers and Frequency of Death in 1984.

Site	Estimated New Cancer Cases	Estimated No. of Cancer Deaths
Lip	4,900	175
Tongue	4,900	2,050
Salivary gland		700
Floor of mouth	9,800	525
Other oral sites		1,600
Pharynx	7,900	4,300
Larynx	11,100	3,750
Thyroid	10,300	1,100
Head/neck melanoma	3,500†	1,200†
Head/neck bone and soft tissue	1,250†	500†
Total	53,650	15,900 (3.5% of cancer deaths)
Total cancers in U.S. population, 1984, all sites‡	870,000	450,000 (20.6% of all U.S. deaths)

*From Silverberg.[10] Reproduced by permission.
†Estimated allocation to head and neck area.
‡Does not include carcinoma in situ and nonmelanoma skin cancers.

Source: Adapted from CA, Vol. 34, No. 1, pp. 14 and 15, with permission of American Cancer Society, © 1984.

treating advance-stage disease involve ablative surgery, which often sacrifices vital structures of the upper aerodigestive tract. This frequently involves portions of the tongue, mandible, or larynx. Regional disease in the nodal groups of the neck is treated at the time of resection of the primary tumor, usually by a radical neck dissection. This involves sacrifice of the sternocleidomastoid muscle, the internal jugular vein, the 11th cranial nerve (also known as the spinal accessory nerve), and the lymph nodes on the involved side.

Advanced cancers of the larynx usually require total removal of the voice box, that is, a total laryngectomy. In this procedure, the larynx and supraglottic structures, including the hyoid bone and the epiglottis, are removed; and a stoma or permanent connection between the skin and the trachea is created (see Figure 6-3). The surgical creation of this connection is called a tracheostomy. The connection is located just above the suprasternal notch and functions as the patient's new upper airway. The patient can no longer speak using the larynx and must learn an alternative mode of speaking, called alaryngeal speech. This form of

Table 6-2 Incidence of Head and Neck Cancer by Primary Site

Site	Rate/100,000	% of Head/Neck Cancers	% of All Cancers
Lip	1.9	12	0.6
Tongue	2.1	13	0.7
Other oral:	2.8	20	0.9
Floor of mouth	(1.0)	(7)	(0.3)
Buccal	(0.7)	(5)	(0.2)
Gingival	(0.7)	(5)	(0.2)
Palate	(0.4)	(3)	(0.1)
Salivary gland	1.1	7	0.4
Total oral	7.9	52	2.6
Nasopharynx	0.6	4	0.2
Other pharynx	2.4	15	0.8
Larynx	4.2	25	1.4
Nose and Paranasal sinus	0.7	4	2
Cervical esophagus	0.35	15	0.8
Ear	0.15	1	0.1
Unknown primary	0.35	2	0.2
Total head/Neck	16.12	100	5.5
Expanded Head and Neck			
Thyroid	3.6		1.2
Soft tissue and bone (H/N)	0.5		.2
Melanoma (H/N)	1.3		.4
Total expanded	21.5		7.3

Some subcategories do not add precisely due to rounding errors.

Source: Reprinted from *Clinical Decisions and Management Principles for Head and Neck Cancer:* (NIH Publication No. 80), p. 2037, U.S. Department of Health, Education and Welfare, September, 1979.

---

speech can be esophageal speech, mechanical speech performed with an electrolarynx, or speech performed by a tracheoesophageal puncture.

Recent advances have allowed for conservation and preservation surgery of the larynx, in which only a part of the larynx is removed.[13-15] Depending on the exact location of the primary tumor, this surgery can be either (1) a vertical hemilaryngectomy (a supraglottic laryngectomy), in which the superior portion of the laryngeal structures is removed, or (2) a horizontal hemilaryngectomy, in which one side of the endolarynx is surgically excised (see Figures 6-4 and 6-5). Both

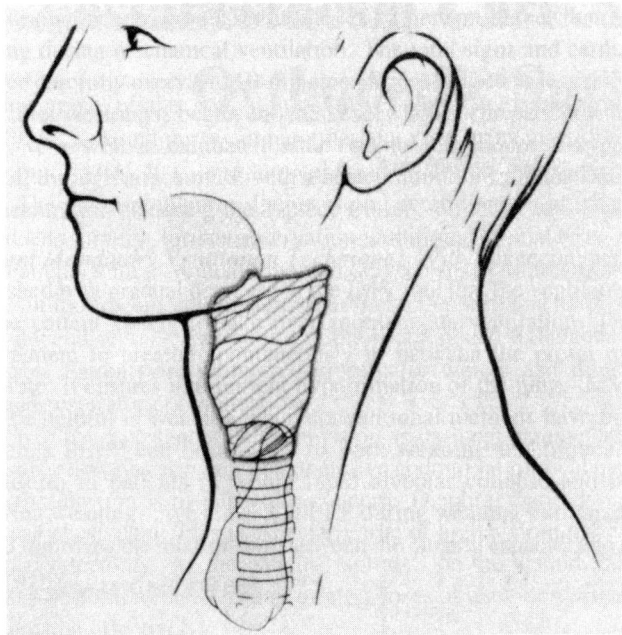

Figure 6-3 Schematic Representation of Total Laryngectomy. *Source:* Reprinted from *Head and Neck Surgery: Indications, Techniques and Pitfalls,* Vol. 4, by H.H. Naumann (Ed.), p. 209, with permission of Georg Thieme Verlag, © 1984.

procedures require placement of a tracheotomy tube below the surgical site to protect the airway in the immediate postoperative period. Usually this tube can be removed after one to two weeks.

Cancers of the oral cavity or oropharynx frequently require excision of part of the tongue, pharynx, and mandible. In the past, if the remaining tissues were closed primarily, this created a significant functional and cosmetic deformity for the patient. Since the introduction of myocutaneous flaps, however, the role of reconstructive surgery following ablative cancer surgery has thrived. Patients are now able to achieve markedly improved functional and cosmetic results. Today, use of the pectoralis major myocutaneous flap as the workhorse of the reconstructive effort in the head and neck region is well-established (see Figure 6-6).[16]

INTRAOPERATIVE AND ANESTHETIC CONSIDERATIONS

General Problems

More than 95 percent of patients who enter the operating room for diseases of the head and neck undergo surgery without any serious immediate or late

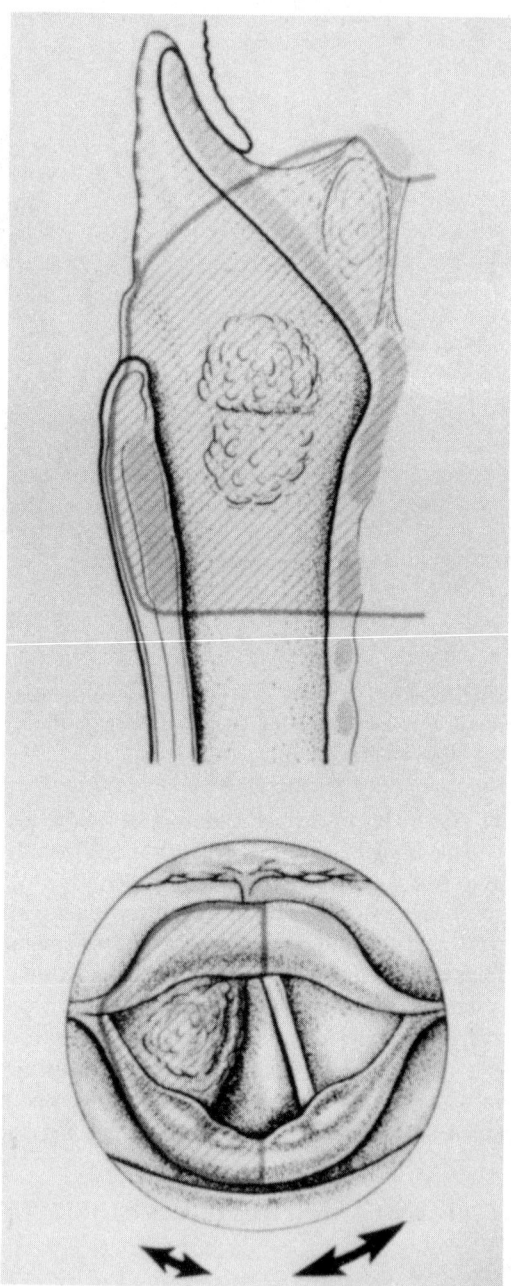

Figure 6-4 Vertical Hemilaryngectomy in which the Upper Portion of the Larynx Including the Epiglottis and False Vocal Cords is Removed. *Source:* Reprinted from *Head and Neck Surgery: Indications, Techniques and Pitfalls,* Vol. 4, by H.H. Naumann (Ed.), p. 186, with permission of Georg Thieme Verlag, © 1984.

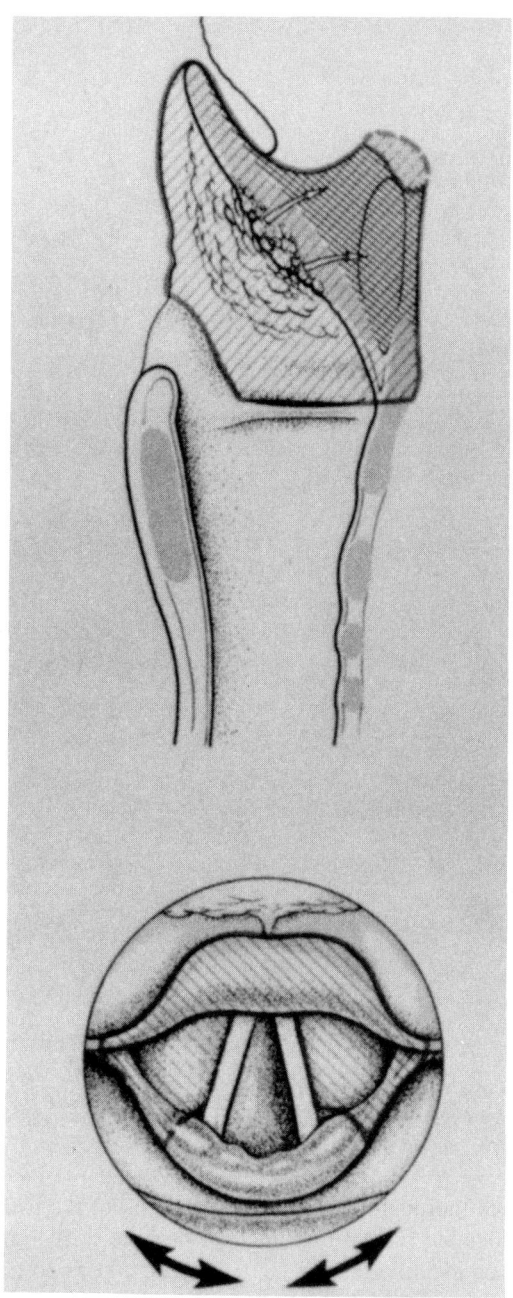

Figure 6-5 Horizontal Hemilaryngectomy in which One Side of the Larynx is Removed Sacrificing both True and False Vocal Cord. *Source:* Reprinted from *Head and Neck Surgery: Indications, Techniques and Pitfalls*, Vol. 4, by H.H. Naumann (Ed.), p. 199, with permission of Georg Thieme Verlag, © 1984.

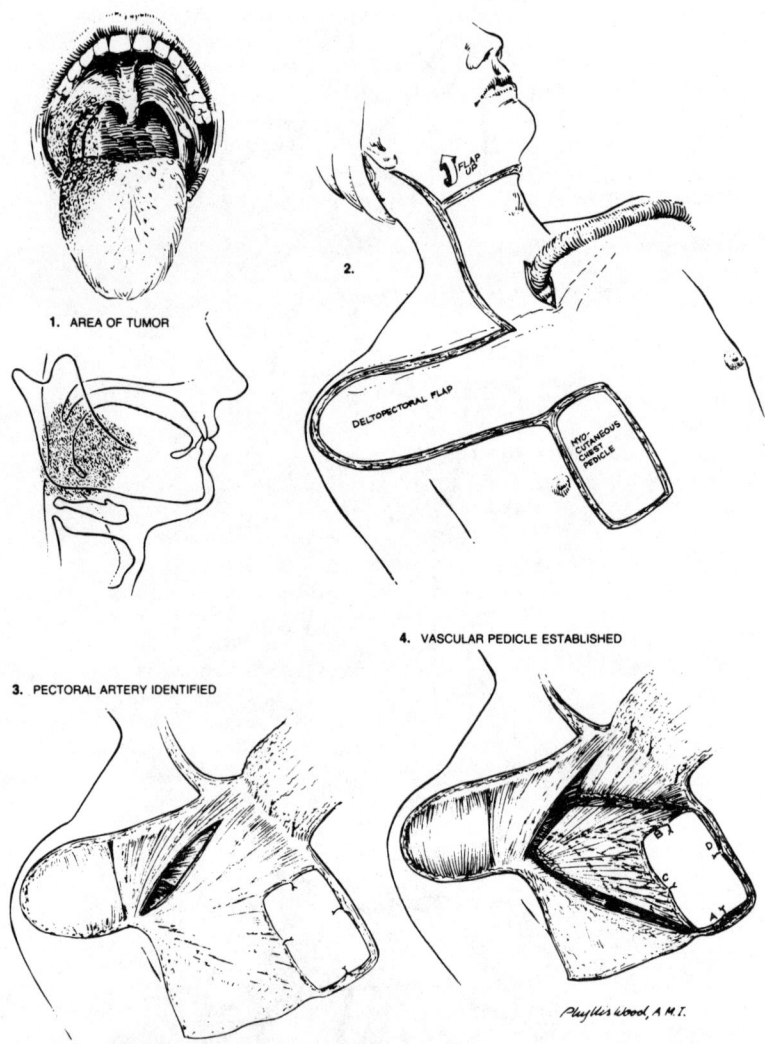

Figure 6-6 Example of a Composite Resection and Reconstruction Using a Myocutaneous Flap. *Source:* Reprinted from *Otolaryngologic Clinics of North America*, Vol. 16, No. 2, pp. 333–335, with permission of W.B. Saunders Company, © 1983.

---

complications.[17] A thorough preoperative evaluation of the patient will help to identify any predictable factors that might contribute to the development of a complication. Once identified, these factors can be addressed to help avoid any difficulties in the operative period.

Since the vast majority of operations in the head and neck area are done under general anesthesia, the anesthesiologist is the surgeon's most important collab-

Head and Neck Surgery 63

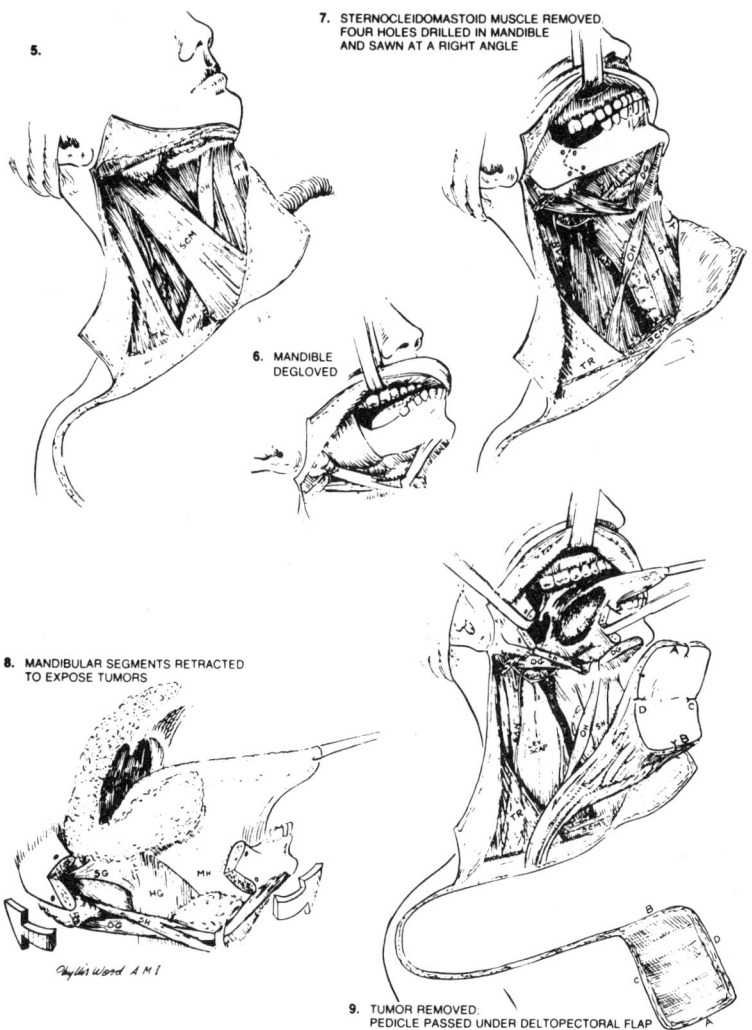

Figure 6-6 continued

---

orator. It has been said that the anesthesia may actually represent the most dangerous aspect of surgery in the head and neck.[18]

Perhaps the most important fact to remember is that the airway must be shared at the same time by the surgeon and the anesthesiologist. Thus, close cooperation and communication between the two is essential. Should the surgeon require a momentary displacement of the endotracheal or anode tube in order to facilitate the procedure, it is imperative that that requirement be immediately made known to

64   HANDBOOK OF POSTANESTHESIA NURSING

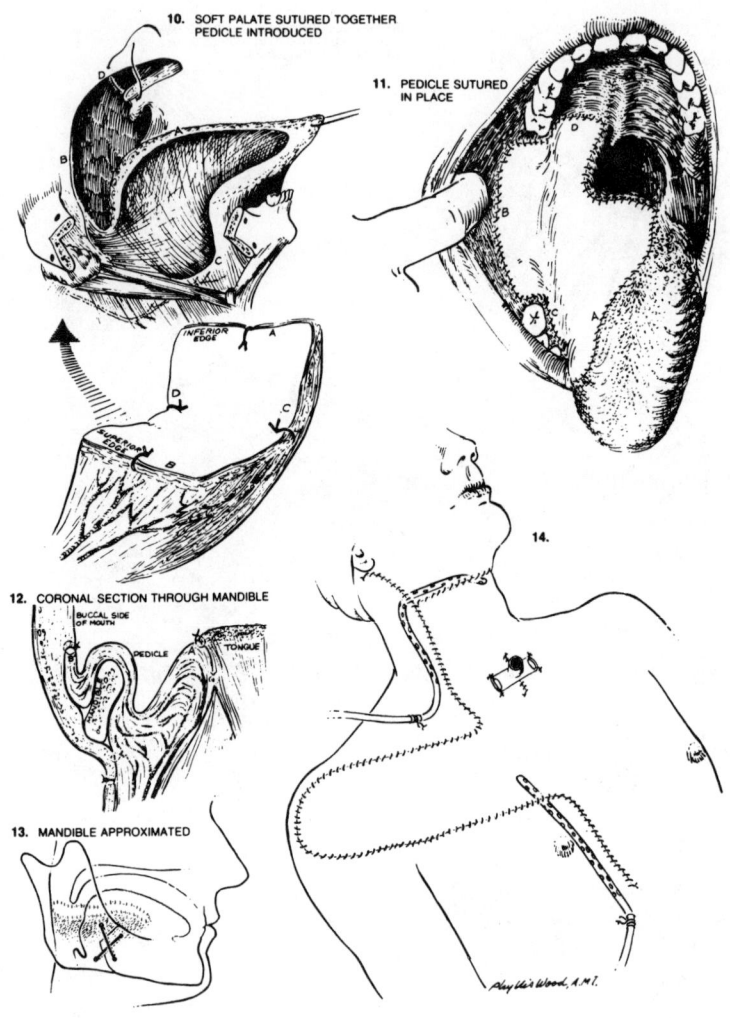

Figure 6-6 continued

the anesthesiologist, who must then decide whether the patient can withstand interruption of ventilation and, if so, for exactly how long. Any indication by cardiac monitoring or oximeter of deterioration or other abnormality must be attended to instantly. This may even mean interruption of the surgical procedure and adjustment of the airway. Also, during various head and neck procedures, it is necessary to manipulate the head, with the possibility of dislodging the endotracheal tube. It is therefore necessary either to have the endotracheal tube continuously visualized or to allow the anesthesiologist access to the tube.

Complications in the operating room during head and neck surgery include some that are common to any surgical procedure and some that are unique to this area. Commonly shared complications revolve around blood loss and the achievement of adequate hemostasis. This is particularly important in cases in which the airway has been somehow violated or entered in order to avoid the entry of significant amounts of blood into the trachea and lower airway.

Special Problems

Besides the obvious concern for the maintenance of a stable airway, intraoperative problems that are unique to the head and neck region include the following.[19]

Carotid Sinus Reflex

The carotid sinus is a pressoreceptor. It is focused at the proximal segment of the internal carotid artery just above the bifurcation of the common carotid artery. Stimulation of this sinus causes slowing of the pulse and a commensurate decline in blood pressure. The sinus can be stimulated during surgery by direct or indirect pressure, twisting, touching, or manipulation of the great vessels. It is more sensitive in the older patient and in those with atheromatous disease.

The anesthesiologist should be alerted when the surgeon is working in the regioin of the carotid bulb. It is estimated that about 15 percent of patients having a radical neck dissection will manifest a carotid sinus reflex to some degree. When the surgeon is alerted by the anesthesiologist to an abrupt drop in blood pressure or to the development of bradycardia or an arrhythmia, the surgeon should stop stimulating the carotid sinus. The reflex can be controlled either by the use of intravenous atropine or by local infiltration of lidocaine into the adventitia around the carotid sinus.

Air Embolus

During surgery in the neck, unnoticed open venous vessels can draw in unwanted air. Owing to the negative pressure in the veins, there is a potential for air to pass directly through the open lumen into the main venous collecting channels. If this air is in sufficient quantities, it can lead to an air embolus. A large air embolus of 50–60 cc or the accumulation of smaller bubbles in the right atrium may be sufficient to interfere with normal cardiac function. Also, central nervous system damage may result if sufficient air passes through the cardiac circulation into the cerebral circulation.

Fortunately, an air embolus in quantities sufficient to lead to a serious complication in head and neck surgery is extremely rare. This does not eliminate the possibility of its occurrence, however, and one should be prepared for immediate action. Treatment consists of placing the patient with the left side down and the head in the Trendelenburg position; 100-percent oxygen should be administered, and the right atrium should be aspirated through the chest.

Pneumomediastinum and Pneumothorax

Operations in the base or root of the neck often cause tears and openings in the deep cervical fascia. A valve-like effect at the tear can occur, causing sucking of air into the deep fascial planes with inspiration. As respiration continues, the air moves into the mediastinum, and also into the subcutaneous spaces. On rare occasions, it can eventually rupture the pleura and cause the development of a tension pneumothorax.

A more common cause of the development of a pneumothorax intraoperatively is the creation of a small tear in the parietal pleura in the root of the neck while dissecting the tissues in the supraclavicular region. A small pleural leak intraoperatively can often be treated by inflating the lungs mechanically to expand the visceral pleura and lung and thus eliminate the trapped air. However, a large pleural leak can lead to a tension pneumothorax, which is truly a surgical emergency. In such cases, it is quickly apparent that there is respiratory embarrassment, and shortly thereafter there is circulatory collapse. In severe circumstances, immediate aspiration with a large bore needle in the upper thoracic space will confirm the diagnosis and improve the patient's clinical picture. The definitive treatment is thoracentesis and chest tube drainage.

POSTANESTHESIA CARE

Postoperative Monitoring

Postoperative complications broadly fall into two main categories: (1) those that specifically relate to the surgical procedure performed and (2) those related to the general physiological condition of the patient. The goal is to avoid those complications that are preventable by diligence and thoroughness, but still to ensure early recognition of other potentially serious complications in order to avert their serious consequences.

The physiological alterations that may exist and lead to perioperative complications include cardiovascular disease, including arrhythmia, ischemic heart disease, or congestive heart failure; pulmonary disorders most commonly related to chronic obstructive lung disease; metabolic disorders, such as diabetes, renal failure, alcoholism, or fluid and electrolyte abnormalities; liver disease; and blood dyscrasias.[20] The primary task in the perioperative period is to be aware of any of these potential physiological alterations and then to be able to make the necessary adjustments to prevent any complications that might arise from them.

Dr. John Conley has noted that where there is surgery, there are complications, and that often there is no single explanation for an unexpected and unwanted development.[21] In certain cases, the calculated risk is evident from the beginning, for example, in the patient with severe chronic obstructive lung disease who develops advanced laryngeal cancer requiring a laryngectomy. In other cases, an ideal operation may be performed on an ideal patient under ideal circumstances, and a serious complication may still occur. This is exemplified in the development of a wound infection or breakdown after major ablative surgery for head and neck cancer.

There are, however, certain fundamental principles of procedure and care of the surgical patient that are inviolable. Any breach of these principles may have untoward results. The principles and rules governing hemostasis, wound closure, gentle tissue handling, and proper suture technique all point to a successful surgical procedure; yet, they are no guarantee.

In particular, the attitude of attentiveness and diligence must be carried over to the postoperative period, particularly in the PACU. Obviously, first and foremost, the vital functions of the surgical patient must be continuously monitored in the immediate postoperative period until there is full recovery of all vital functions and physiological stability is attained. The main areas of concern are the maintenance of an adequate airway and close observation of the wounds to prevent the formation of a hematoma.

Care of the Airway

Since a majority of patients undergoing head and neck surgery have some manipulation of their airway, it is critical to ensure its patency and stability.

For patients who have had less extensive operations, such as tonsillectomy or endoscopy, it is important to realize that edema can develop around the laryngeal region. If severe enough, this can cause significant airway obstruction and compromise. The most consistent sign of airway edema at the level of the larynx is stridor. There are various types of stridor, and each can give clues as to the exact location of the surgical edema. Inspiratory stridor associated with a muffled voice or cry usually signifies a lesion in the region of the supraglottic larynx. Biphasic stridor (both on inspiration and expiration) associated with a normal or slightly hoarse voice suggests edema in the region directly below the vocal cords at the level of the cricoid cartilage. This area is known as the subglottic larynx. Aphonia associated with inspiratory stridor and a slight expiratory component is more likely to place the edema at the glottic level.[22] These various levels of laryngeal edema are usually best treated with high humidity given with oxygen and topical mucosal vasoconstrictors, such as racemic-epinephrine. For anticipated extensive and marked airway edema, a bolus of intravenous steroids, usually dexamethasone (Decadron), given intraoperatively can greatly aid in controlling the soft tissue swelling.

In addition to stridor, the signs of upper airway obstruction include increasing restlessness, a desire of the patient to get out of bed, and an increase in the respiratory and heart rates. There also can be seen retractions of the accessory muscles of respiration suprasternally, substernally, and in the intercostal area. This is particularly true in infants and young children. As the airway obstruction continues and worsens, the late signs that are seen are cyanosis, somnolence, and difficulty in arousing the patient. Again, treatment must be directed at maintaining an adequate airway by medical therapies, humidification, and gentle suctioning of the oral pharynx. If the condition is severe enough, the patient may require reintubation.

Patients who undergo extensive ablative surgery of the head and neck will usually be provided with an in-dwelling tracheotomy tube, which will bypass any edema at the operative site. Meticulous tracheotomy care and suctioning are necessary to keep the airway clear of secretions and blood. Usually, the tracheotomy tube has an inflatable cuff, which should be kept inflated for the first 24 hours postoperatively. Patients who have undergone a total laryngectomy have a permanent tracheostoma in the lower neck called a tracheostomy. This, like the tracheotomy tube, must be kept clean and free of any secretions. Since this stoma represents a fresh wound, care must be taken when suctioning and cleaning around it so as not to disrupt the suture line. It is extremely important to maintain a high level of humidity at the site to prevent crusting and drying of the mucosa.

Care of Wounds

After care of the airway, the next most important postoperative consideration is care of the wounds. In smaller procedures, such as cervical lymph node biopsy or incision and drainage of an abscess, wounds are usually drained by Penrose drains. These drains permit accumulated blood, serum, or pus to move along the channel created by the drain and thus exit in a dependent manner. The Penrose drain will not precipitate bleeding, and it will not prevent the formation of a hematoma if bleeding is excessive. Thus, care must be taken to inspect the area operated on to make sure there is no hematoma formation. If a small hematoma has developed under the skin, it can often be evacuated by "milking" the skin over the hematoma. If a large hematoma forms, it usually is necessary to return the patient to the operating room for exploration of the wound to identify the bleeding site.

In major head and neck procedures, the Penrose drain has been replaced in most cases by the hemovac drain, that is, by suction drainage. Hemovac drains represent a significant advance in the control of healing wounds in the region of the head and neck. They assist in the coaptation of the tissues in the wound, reduce the incidence of hematoma formation, and decrease the likelihood of internal and external contamination of the wound. Their system of internal suction reduces the importance of the external pressure dressing that is necessary with the use of the Penrose drain. Hemovac drains allow direct inspection of the wounds and can therefore alert one to any problem of hematoma formation that may arise in the PACU. However, though they can prevent or clear small hematomas, they will not prevent a hematoma if there is excess bleeding. Also, they will not prevent the development of a blood collection if they are malpositioned in the wound or if they are nonfunctional.

Although nothing can be done in the PACU about excess bleeding or malposition of the drains, one can ensure proper functioning of the hemovacs. Because of the large raw surface area and skin incisions in major ablative head and neck surgery, often a water-tight skin closure is not possible. Therefore, it is extremely important that the hemovac drains be placed to continuous wall suction immediately in the PACU. If the drains are allowed to clot from stasis early in the postoperative period, they will fail to function properly. The principal complication of wound drainage is failure of the drains to function; and this, in most instances, is due to a failure on the part of the supervising attendant.

With the greater use of myocutaneous flaps for reconstruction after head and neck surgery, care must be taken in the PACU not to compromise the arterial or venous blood supply that runs in the pedicle of the flap. This means that care must be taken to avoid any compression or pressure at the pedicle (see Figure 6-5). Typically, tracheotomy ties that are secured too tightly around the neck will compromise blood flow to the flap. For this reason, some head and neck surgeons avoid the use of tracheostomy ties and suture the tracheotomy tube directly to the skin of the neck. Even a tracheotomy collar used to provide oxygen and humidity to the patient can cause damage to the myocutaneous flap if it is fastened too tightly. When the patient arrives in the PACU or ICU, the surgeon should communicate to the nursing staff exactly where the pedicle lies and thus enable the staff to help in avoiding injury to it.

Ligation of the Internal Jugular Vein

A further complication that should be addressed at this point concerns the ligation of the internal jugular vein during radical neck dissection.[23] Typically, as part of the standard radical neck dissection, the internal jugular vein on the side of the lesion is ligated. This usually causes a postoperative finding that is more frightening than it is serious. After ligation of the internal jugular vein, the patient's head becomes edematous and appears cyanotic. This usually is not due to poor oxygenation, but rather results from venous engorgement and plethora. Postoperatively, such patients should have the head of the bed elevated approximately 30 to 45 degrees. Rarely does any other intervention need to be considered.

If, however, the patient undergoes ligation of the second internal jugular vein, one must carefully follow the patient for signs of cerebral edema and concomitant increased intracranial pressure. Such patients should be positioned with the head at a 45-degree angle and should not be permitted to move their head from side to side. Any sudden temperature elevation within the first 12 hours after surgery may signal the development of serious cerebral edema and attendant cerebral anoxia. This can be initially treated with the use of diuretics, such as Mannitol, and by fluid restriction and head elevation. Rarely, cerebral spinal fluid decompression will be necessary. This can be done by placing an in-dwelling subarachnoid catheter or a neurosurgically placed Richmond's cranial screw.

CONCLUSION

Unlike patients who have major surgery involving the abdomen or skeletal system, those who undergo major head and neck surgery have a relatively small amount of pain. This is in large part due to the fact that the cervical sensory nerves are sacrificed in the radical neck dissection, thus destroying the pain pathways of the neck. The patient does experience a significant degree of discomfort, which is related primarily to the various alterations in the normal physiological functions that have occurred with the interruption of the basic anatomical structures of the upper aerodigestive tract.

Similarly, the ability to cough and breathe deeply should not be greatly restricted, since there is no insult to the thoracic cavity or the abdominal wall. Patients should be encouraged to participate in their own pulmonary toilet once they have begun to recover from the effects of the general anesthetic.

Based on a full understanding of the basic anatomy and physiology of the head and neck, as well as thorough comprehension of the various surgical procedures performed in this region of the body, the postanesthetic care of the patient can be optimal, and the amount and degree of the various complications can be significantly reduced.

NOTES

1. G.W. Levitt, "Cervical Fascia and Deep Neck Infection," *Laryngoscope* 80 (1970):409.

2. S. Meller, "Functional Anatomy of the Larynx," in *Symposium on the Larynx, Otolaryngologic Clinics of North America*, ed. M. Fried (Philadelphia: W.B. Saunders, 1984), 3–12.

3. M.W. Donne, "Physiology of the Esophagus," in *Otolaryngology*, vol. 1 (Philadelphia: W.B. Saunders, 1980), 345–353.

4. J. Conley, "Complications of Tracheotomy," in *Complications of Head and Neck Surgery*, ed. John Conley (Philadelphia: W.B. Saunders, 1979), 274–289.

5. Ibid., 276.

6. D.D. Rabuzzi and J.T. Johnson, *Diagnosis and Management of Deep Neck Infections*. (Washington, D.C.: American Academy of Otolaryngology and Head and Neck Surgery, 1978), 12. (self-instructional package).

7. D. DeWeese and W.H. Saunders, *Textbook of Otolaryngology*, 6th ed. (St Louis, Mo.: C.V. Mosby, 1982), 65–76.

8. N. Thompson et al., "The Continuing Development of the Technique of Thyroidectomy," *Surgery* 73 (1973):913–927.

9. J. Batsakis, *Tumors of the Head and Neck: Clinical and Pathological Considerations*, 2nd ed. (Baltimore: Williams & Wilkins, 1979), 1–75.

10. E. Silverberg, "Cancer Statistics," *Cancer* 34 (1984):7–23.

11. U.S. Department of Health, Education, and Welfare, *Management Guidelines for Head and Neck Cancer*, USDHEW NIH publication No. 80–2037 (Bethesda, Md.: 1979).

12. American Joint Committee on Cancer, *Staging of Cancer of the Head and Neck and of Melanoma* (Author, 1980).

13. J.H. Ogura, "Supraglottic Subtotal Laryngectomy and Radical Neck Dissection for Carcinoma of the Epiglottis," *Laryngoscope* 68 (June 1958):983–1003.

14. J.J. Pressman, "Cancer of the Larynx: Laryngoplasty to Avoid Laryngectomy," *Archives of Otolaryngology* 59 (April 1954):395–412.

15. B.J. Bailey, "Glottic Reconstruction After Hemilaryngectomy: Bipedicle Muscle Flap Laryngoplasty," *Laryngoscope* 85 (June, 1975):960–977.

16. C. Cummings and C.T. Yarrington, "Reconstruction Following Composite Resection," in *Symposium on Reconstruction in Head and Neck Surgery, Otolaryngologic Clinics of North America*, ed. C. Cummings (Philadelphia, P.A.: WB Saunders, 1983), 331–341.

17. J. Conley, ed., *Complications of Head and Neck Surgery* (Philadelphia: W.B. Saunders, 1979), 3.

18. R. Hicks, "Anesthesia Complications in Head and Neck Surgery," in *Complications of Head and Neck Surgery*, ed. John Conley (Philadelphia, PA: W.B. Saunders, 1979), 13–24.

19. J. Conley, "Intraoperative Complications in Head and Neck Surgery," in *Complications of Head and Neck Surgery*, ed. John Conley (Philadelphia, PA: W.B. Saunders, 1979), 25–39.

20. J. Angus and A. Angus, "Management of the Medical Complications of Head and Neck Surgery," in *Complications of Head and Neck Surgery*, ed. John Conley (Philadelphia, PA: W.B. Saunders, 1979), 40–62.

21. J. Conley, ed., *Complications*, 1.
22. G.B. Healy, "Neoplasia of the Pediatric Larynx," in *Symposium on the Larynx, Otolaryngologic Clinics of North America*, ed. Marvin Fried (Philadelphia, PA: W.B. Saunders, 1984), 69–70.
23. R. Hicks, "Anesthesia Complications in Head and Neck Surgery," in *Complications of Head and Neck Surgery*, ed. John Conley (Philadelphia, PA: WB Saunders, 1979), 13–24.

BIBLIOGRAPHY

Cummings, C., and Yarrington, C.T., eds. *Symposium on Reconstruction in Head and Neck Surgery, Otolaryngologic Clinics of North America*. Philadelphia, PA: W.B. Saunders, 1983.

Fried, M., ed. *Symposium on the Larynx, Otolaryngologic Clinics of North America*. Philadelphia, PA: W.B. Saunders, 1984.

McQuarrie, D., ed. *Head and Neck Cancer: Clinical Decisions and Management Principles*. Chicago, IL: Year Book Publishers, 1986.

Montgomery, W.W. *Surgery of the Upper Respiratory System*. Vols. 1 and 2. Philadelphia, PA: Lea and Febiger, 1973.

Paparella, M.M., and Schumrick, D.A., eds. *Otolaryngology*. Vols. 1–3. Philadelphia: W.B. Saunders, 1980.

Shapshay, S., and Ossoff, R., eds. *Symposium on Squamous Cell Cancer of the Head and Neck, Otolaryngologic Clinics of North America*. Philadelphia, PA: W.B. Saunders, 1985.

Sigler, B.A. "Nursing Care for Head and Neck Tumor Patients." In *Comprehensive Management of Head and Neck Tumors*, edited by C. Cummings and C.T. Yarrington. Vol. 1, 79–99. Philadelphia: W.B. Saunders, 1987.

Chapter 7

Postanesthesia Care After Cardiac Surgery

Fun-Sun F. Yao, M.D.

INTRODUCTION

There are three types of cardiac disease: congenital, ischemic, and valvular. Postanesthesia care of cardiac patients depends on a thorough knowledge of the pathophysiology of the patient's cardiac lesion, the surgical intervention, and the anesthetic management.

CARDIAC SURGICAL INTERVENTION AND ANESTHETIC MANAGEMENT

In this first section, we review the pathophysiology, surgical procedures, and anesthetic considerations of major cardiac problems.

Coronary Artery Disease

Coronary artery disease (CAD) is the most serious medical problem in the United States today. It is the leading cause of death, accounting for nearly a third of all deaths of persons 35 to 65 years of age. Approximately 1.3 million Americans suffer myocardial infarction each year, and at least 4.0 million Americans have clinically evident CAD. Coronary artery bypass grafting (CABG) is the most common heart operation performed in the United States. Each year nearly 200,000 patients have CABGs.

About 250 mL of blood (5 percent of cardiac output) supply the coronary circulation. Seventy percent of coronary blood flow is provided during the diastolic phase of the cardiac cycle. The branches of the coronary arteries are shown in Figure 7-1. The sinus node is supplied by the right coronary artery (RCA) in about 55 percent of human beings and by the circumflex artery (CFX) in the remaining 45 percent. The atrioventricular (A-V) node is provided by the RCA in 90 percent of human beings and by the CFX in the remaining 10 percent. Therefore, complete A-V block usually accompanies diaphragmatic myocardial infarction, which is caused by occlusion of the RCA. The most common arteries for coronary artery bypass grafting are the left anterior descending (LAD), the obtuse marginal (OM), and the posterior descending (PDA) arteries.

Pathophysiology

Acute myocardial ischemia can be caused either by increased oxygen demand or decreased oxygen supply to the myocardium. The primary task of the coronary circulation is to provide adequate amounts of oxygen and substrates for the myocardium and to remove the end products of cardiac metabolism. When the oxygen supply cannot meet the myocardial oxygen demand, myocardial ischemia ensues.

The following equations are relevant:

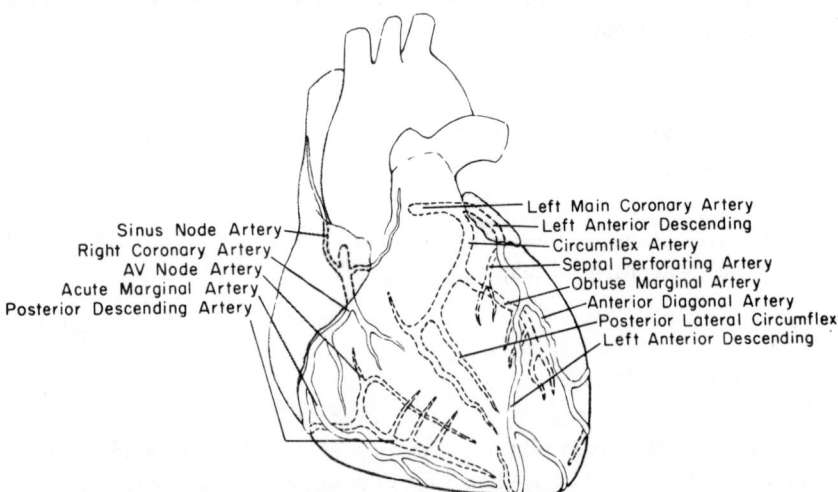

Figure 7-1 Branches of Coronary Arteries. *Source:* Reprinted from *Anesthesiology: Problem Oriented Patient Management* by F.S. Yao and J.F. Artusio, Jr. (Eds.), p. 92, with permission of J.B. Lippincott Company, © 1983.

- Myocardial oxygen supply = coronary blood flow × arterial oxygen content
- Coronary blood flow = coronary perfusion pressure/resistance
- Coronary perfusion pressure = aortic diastolic pressure − left ventricular end diastolic pressure (LVEDP)

Coronary vascular resistance depends on the patency of the coronary arteries. Coronary arteries become flow-limiting in two circumstances: (1) with intraluminal obstruction, as in atherosclerosis; and (2) with coronary spasm.

Arterial oxygen content is determined by the following equation: $CaO_2 = 1.34 \times Hb\ g\% \times O_2$ saturation $+ 0.0031 \times PaO_2$. Therefore, myocardial oxygen supply can be decreased by the following situations: aortic hypotension, increased left ventricular end diastolic pressure, coronary atherosclerosis, coronary spasm, hypoxemia, and anemia.

The three major determinants of myocardial oxygen demand are myocardial wall tension, contractility, and heart rate. Myocardial wall tension is clinically measured by:

- preload—LVEDP, left atrial pressure, or pulmonary capillary wedge pressure (PCWP)
- afterload—systolic ventricular pressure or systolic blood pressure

Contractility is measured by:

- invasive technique—maximal velocity of contraction (Vmax), dp/dt (pressure time indexes of ventricle)
- noninvasive technique—preejection period (PEP)/left ventricular ejection time (LVET); myocardial wall motion and systolic wall thickening by echocardiography

Therefore, myocardial oxygen demand can be increased by increased preload, such as fluid overloading or congestive heart failure; hypertension; aortic stenosis; increased myocardial contractility from inotropic agents; or tachycardia.

Surgical Procedures

Five indications for coronary artery bypass grafting are:

1. chronic stable angina pectoris with disabling symptoms, despite maximal medical therapy
2. unstable angina pectoris or episodes of prolonged myocardial ischemia

3. repeated episodes of myocardial ischemia following myocardial infarction
4. Prinzmetal's angina (variant angina) with coronary obstruction
5. high-grade left main coronary artery obstruction, triple- or double-vessel obstruction, or proximal left anterior descending artery obstruction

Coronary artery bypass grafting is the most common heart operation performed in the United States. Each year approximately 200,000 patients undergo CABGs. The concept is simple. A segment of saphenous vein taken from the legs is anastomosed to the aorta and to a point on a coronary artery beyond a stenotic lesion; this bypasses the blockage. Recently, internal mammary artery grafts have been used because their patency rate is superior to that of saphenous vein grafts (85–95 percent versus 38–45 percent at ten years).

Percutaneous transluminal coronary angioplasty (PTCA) has developed rapidly since its introduction by Gruntzig in 1978. It is now an acceptable method of treating selected patients who have angina pectoris. This technique involves the passage of a small (3F) catheter selectively into the involved coronary artery and through the stenosis. With the balloon portion of the catheter straddling the stenosis, inflations are performed that result in enlargement of the stenotic lumen. The luminal widening is achieved by a controlled injury involving, to varying degrees, plaque compression, intimal fissures, and medial stretching.

Anesthetic Considerations

A smooth induction is essential to prevent hypertension, hypotension, and tachycardia. Different techniques may be used to achieve a smooth induction. We prefer to use fentanyl 5 mcg/kg and a hypnotic dose of sodium thiopental, 1 to 2 mg/kg, to attenuate the hemodynamic changes induced by endotracheal intubation. Anesthesia may be maintained with moderate-dose fentanyl with nitrous oxide, high-dose fentanyl, or low-dose fentanyl with low concentrations of enflurane or isoflurane. The choice of anesthetic agents is still debatable. Both inhalational and intravenous agents have been used successfully. They both have advantages and disadvantages. An understanding of the cardiovascular effects of each anesthetic agent and careful titration of each drug will improve the balance between myocardial oxygen demand and supply.

Early detection and appropriate control of the major determinants of myocardial oxygen demand (BP, HR, PCWP) are mandatory if myocardial ischemia is to be avoided. Monitoring is essential. Transesophageal echocardiography is the most sensitive means of monitoring segmental wall motion abnormalities. ST-segment depression in Lead V5 of the ECG is the most practical sign in diagnosing ischemia. If there are no precordial leads in the ECG machine, a modified V5, CM5 or CB5 may be used. For CM5, place the right arm (RA) electrode on the

Cardiac Surgery 77

middle part of the manubrium, the left leg (LL) electrode on the V5 position (anterior axillar line at the 5th intercostal space), and the left arm (LA) electrode on the left arm or on any part of the body, and monitor Lead II (RA to LL). For CB5, place the RA electrode over the center of the right scapula and the LL electrode over the V5 position and monitor Lead II.

Valvular Heart Disease

Aortic Stenosis

Isolated aortic stenosis (AS) is the most common cardiac valvular abnormality. It may be congenital or acquired. In the absence of other valvular disease, AS is almost always congenital in origin, with rheumatic disease accounting for less than three percent of cases. Bicuspid valve is the most common type of congenital AS. Calcific AS is the most common form of acquired valvular aortic stenosis.

Pathophysiology. The anatomical obstruction to left ventricular ejection imposed by the stenotic aortic valve produces a chronic pressure overload of the left ventricle. To overcome the pressure overload, the left ventricle becomes hypertrophic, resulting in decreased diastolic compliance. Patients with aortic stenosis are at risk for myocardial ischemia. Myocardial oxygen demand is markedly increased because of a massively hypertrophied myocardium produced by the stenotic aortic valve. Myocardial oxygen supply is decreased because of a decreased time for diastolic coronary perfusion, a decreased coronary perfusion pressure due to turbulent blood flow and an increased LVEDP, and coexisting coronary artery disease. Tachycardia is the hazard most likely to precipitate an imbalance between myocardial oxygen demand and supply.

Surgical Procedures. The indications for surgical correction of AS are as follows:

- Patients are symptomatic, including the triad of dyspnea, angina, and syncope.
- The calculated aortic valve area is less than 0.8 cm^2 per m^2 (Normal: 1.5 to 2.0 cm^2 per m^2).
- The transvalvular pressure gradient is greater than 50 mm Hg.

Aortic stenosis is most commonly corrected by aortic valve replacement, utilizing cardiopulmonary bypass and a combination of topical profound hypothermia, moderate systemic hypothermia, and cardioplegic arrest.

Prosthetic Heart Valves. Prosthetic cardiac valve substitutes are of three basic types. The original design was the ball poppet within a cage. The Starr-Edwards, Braunwald-Cutter, Smeloff-Cutter, and Magovern valves are examples of this type. The second basic configuration is the disk occluder within a cage, where the disk moves parallel to the plane of the sewing ring. The Beall, Kay-Shiley, and Starr-Edwards disk valves are of this type. The third basic type is the tilting or pivoting disk valve, in which the disk occluder pivots from a closed position parallel to the sewing ring to an open position approximately perpendicular to the sewing ring and annulus. Examples of this type are the Bjork-Shiley and Lillehei-Kaster prostheses. All prosthetic valves currently in use require life-long anticoagulation, usually with sodium warfarin (Coumadin) therapy. Despite this therapy, there remains a 5 percent incidence per patient year of thromboembolism, to which must be added a 5 percent risk per patient year of hemorrhage, usually manifested as a cerebrovascular accident.

Tissue Valves. The porcine heterograft valve has been in widespread clinical use since the early 1970s. The major advantages of the tissue valves are the simulation of normal flow characteristics and the use of natural or biological materials with a reduced propensity for thrombosis and embolization. Therefore, anticoagulation therapy is not required. The disadvantages of tissue valves are that they are less durable and have relatively smaller effective valve orifices, compared with mechanical prosthetic valves.

Aortic Insufficiency

Aortic insufficiency (AI) may be congenital or acquired. The more common causes of acquired AI are rheumatic heart disease and endocarditis. AI also occurs commonly in association with aortic root dissection.

Pathophysiology. In acute AI, a left ventricle (LV) of normal size and compliance is suddenly presented with severe diastolic overload from regurgitation. This produces an increase in left ventricular diastolic pressures, resulting in premature closure of the mitral valve. Therefore, stroke volume and cardiac output decrease. Blood pressure is maintained by an increased heart rate and peripheral resistance. In chronic AI, left ventricular volume overloading increases LV end-diastolic wall tension with resultant eccentric hypertrophy (increase in *both* chamber size and wall thickness). This is in contrast to the elevated systolic wall tension characteristic of aortic stenosis, which produces concentric hypertrophy (increase in wall thickness, no change in chamber size). Usually, high-diastolic compliance is the hallmark of the eccentrically hypertrophied ventricle. Therefore, the large end-diastolic volumes are accommodated with only minor increases in LV end-diastolic pressure. Myocardial contractility is usually preserved until late in the course of the disease.

Surgical Procedures. Aortic insufficiency is an insidious disease; by the time symptoms of congestive heart failure are clinically evident, an advanced degree of LV decompensation is found. The indications for aortic valve replacement include the following:

- progressive enlargement of heart size seen on chest roentgenograms or echocardiography
- a low aortic diastolic pressure, less than 50 mm Hg
- cardiac catheterization documentation of increased pulmonary artery or LV filling pressures in the presence of aortic regurgitation

Anesthetic Considerations. The hemodynamic goal is to avoid increases in regurgitation that occur in the diastolic phase. Maintenance of low systemic vascular resistance promotes forward flow and reduces the regurgitation fraction. A slightly increased heart rate decreases regurgitant flow because the diastolic time decreases during tachycardia.

A variety of general anesthetic agents are acceptable for patients with good LV function. These patients tolerate the inhalation agents quite well. Isoflurane is the agent of choice because it not only decreases peripheral vascular resistance but also causes mild tachycardia, resulting in decreased aortic regurgitation. Balanced or narcotic-based techniques should be considered for patients with known LV dysfunction. Afterload reduction may be achieved by using vasodilators.

Mitral Stenosis

Rheumatic fever is the most common cause of mitral stenosis (MS). Less common etiologies include congenital MS in infants and children and stenotic fibrous plaques in association with the carcinoid syndrome.

Pathophysiology. With progressive stenosis at the mitral valve, the left ventricle is chronically volume-underloaded, while the left atrium and structures behind it face both pressure and volume overloading.

Left ventricular function is usually normal in mitral stenosis; LVEDP is in the normal range. There is pressure gradient across the mitral valve during diastole. Tachycardia decreases cardiac output because of decreased diastolic filling time. Left atrial dilatation develops because of both pressure and volume overloading. Pulmonary hypertension develops in patients with long-standing mitral stenosis, due to elevated left atrial pressure and, later, pulmonary arteriolar hyperplasia. With severe chronic pulmonary hypertension, right heart failure with functional pulmonic and/or tricuspid regurgitation may occur.

Surgical Procedures. Surgical corrections for MS include closed transatrial commissurotomy without cardiopulmonary bypass, open commissurotomy, or mitral valve replacement with cardiopulmonary bypass. The normal mitral valve area is 4.0 to 6.0 cm^2. Patients usually do not become symptomatic until the mitral area is decreased to between 2.0 and 2.5 cm^2 (correlated with NYHA Functional Class I). When the valve area decreases to approximately 1.0 cm^2, patients are usually symptomatic with minimal exertion, correlated with NYHA Functional Class III. Any patient with significant functional limitation of life style because of mitral stenosis should be considered a candidate for surgical correction.

Anesthetic Considerations. The hemodynamic principles are avoiding tachycardia, keeping intravascular volume adequately full, and avoiding exacerbation of pulmonary hypertension. Fentanyl–N_2O-O_2 techniques are ideal in patients with severe pulmonary hypertension, with or without right heart failure. Inhalation anesthetics may be used in patients who have good ventricular function. Isoflurane, pancuronium, and gallamine may not be the agents of choice because they produce tachycardia.

Mitral Regurgitation

Rheumatic endocarditis is the most common cause of mitral regurgitation (MR) or mitral insufficiency. Bacterial endocarditis can cause severe acute mitral insufficiency from valvular destruction and rupture of the chordae tendineae. Up to 15 percent of patients with mitral valve prolapse syndrome develop varying degrees of MR. Ischemic heart disease, especially posterior inferior myocardial infarction, causes papillary muscle dysfunction or rupture, resulting in MR. Other lesions of the valve itself are less frequent; they include congenital abnormalities, connective tissue disorders, mitral valve ring calcification, and trauma, for example, from steering wheel injury.

Pathophysiology. In acute MR, the smaller and less distensible atrium does not absorb the regurgitant flow, as in chronic MR. Therefore, left ventricular end-diastolic pressure, left atrial V-wave pressure, and pulmonary venous and arterial pressures are higher in acute MR than in chronic MR.

In chronic MR, the left atrium is enlarged and more distensible; therefore, little pressure is reflected in the pulmonary circulation. The left ventricle is dilated and hypertrophic in chronic MR; this condition results in higher left ventricular end-systolic and end-diastolic volumes. In chronic MR, atrial fibrillation is the most common rhythm. The presence of normal sinus rhythm suggests acute MR rather than chronic MR.

Surgical Procedures. Mitral valve replacement is the most common procedure for mitral insufficiency. However, mitral valvuloplasty and annuloplasty can be done if the valvular structure itself is not severely destroyed or deformed. Symptomatic patients with significant mitral regurgitation (3 to 4 plus) in ventriculogram are candidates for surgery.

Anesthetic Considerations. The anesthetic considerations for MR are similar to those for patients with aortic insufficiency. A mild tachycardia decreases mitral regurgitation because the regurgitant orifice area may decline in the faster, smaller heart. Patients with mitral valve prolapse are exceptions to this principle, because prolapse of redundant mitral leaflets is minimized by increases in ventricular volume. Decreasing systemic vascular resistance will promote forward ejection and reduce mitral regurgitation. In addition, peripheral venodilation will further decrease preload and heart size, resulting in less regurgitation.

POSTOPERATIVE CARE

Immediate PACU or ICU Care

Upon arrival in the PACU or ICU, the following items should receive immediate attention:

- ECG monitoring is switched from transport monitor to unit monitor, with digital display of rate and ability to print out strips of the ECG for closer examination.
- Pressure monitoring is switched from transport monitor to unit monitor; leveling of transducers and checking of calibration are done as quickly as possible; all pressure monitoring systems should be connected to automatic flushing systems containing 1 unit/mL of heparin.
- Sphygmomanometer and cuff are applied, and manual blood pressure is checked to correlate with transduced pressure.
- Ventilator is checked to see that appropriate tidal volume, rate, and inspired oxygen concentration are set and that it is operating correctly. The ventilator is attached to the endotracheal tube; the thorax is observed to rise and fall with ventilator breaths and both sides of the chest are auscultated to determine the presence and equality of breath sounds.
- Chest tubes should be stripped and attached to underwater seal drainage with -20 cm of water suction; initial volume of blood in drainage bottle is noted and marked.
- The patient is examined. The heart is auscultated for murmurs, rubs, or gallops. Skin color and temperature and peripheral pulse indicate adequacy of

peripheral perfusion. Lungs are auscultated for character of breath sounds and presence of wheezes or rales. Central nervous system status is assessed by level of consciousness, ability to move extremities, and pupillary size, equality, and light-responsiveness.

Many or all of the above steps may be done simultaneously, depending on the number of people available to help. Once these initial steps are completed, the team should move to complete the admission procedure, which includes the following:

- Intravenous lines are sorted out, and levels of fluids are noted and marked. All subsequent measurements of fluids should be taken from these baselines.
- Urinary catheter drainage is noted and marked. Urinary output should be recorded on an hourly basis.
- Rectal probe is inserted for continuous measurement of temperature. If continuous measurement is not available; rectal temperature should be measured every 30 minutes to one hour until it is stable.
- Head of bed may be elevated 20° to 30° if the cardiovascular status is stable. This will help drainage of chest tubes.
- Pacemaker function, if present, should be checked.
- Endotracheal tube cuff is deflated completely and refilled with the minimal amount of air, which will stop any air leak around the tube. The volume of air injected and the intracuff pressure is recorded.
- Arterial blood gases are drawn, and initial ventilation settings are adjusted as needed.
- Blood is sent to the laboratory for rapid determination of hemoglobin levels; hematocrit values; electrolyte, creatinine, and glucose levels; prothrombin time; partial thromboplastin time; and platelet count.
- A portable chest x-ray is taken.
- Twelve-lead ECG is recorded.

The anesthesiologist should communicate to the unit team (both nursing and physician staff) as much information about the patient as possible. This should include:

- operative procedure and complications
- anesthetic technique and complications
- total fluids and blood given during surgery and whether volume replacement was a continuing requirement

- urinary output and estimated blood loss during the operation
- coagulation factors given during surgery (for example, platelets or fresh frozen plasma)
- associated medical conditions (for example, asthma, diabetes, or glaucoma)

Patients are often hypothermic on arrival in the PACU or ICU. Heating lights, a warmed blanket, heated water mattresses, warmed humidified inspired gases, and warming intravenous fluids should be ready to facilitate maintenance of body temperature. Administration of small doses of chlorpromazine, 0.5 to 2.0 mg, prevents shivering, which may increase oxygen consumption 4 to 5 times the normal rate.

The main goal is to achieve circulatory stability during the immediate postoperative period. This includes:

- securing a favorable balance between myocardial oxygen supply and demand
- ensuring an adequate cardiac output
- preventing cardiac arrhythmias
- maintaining hemostasis

Common Postoperative Problems

Hypertension

Hypertension is a common consequence of peripheral vasoconstriction and emergency from anesthesia in the early postoperative period, particularly following a coronary artery bypass operation. This increase in afterload raises myocardial oxygen demand and limits cardiac output. Also, the high central pressure places additional stress on the aortic and coronary suture lines and tends to increase blood loss through the chest tubes. For these reasons, it is important to control the blood pressure within relatively narrow limits during the early postoperative period. Mean arterial pressure is usually maintained between 70 and 90 mm Hg unless specific indications for a higher pressure exist. Treatment is aimed at pain relief and vasodilatation. Initial therapy should ensure adequate analgesia (for example, morphine sulfate, 2–5 mg, intravenous doses) before turning to vasodilator therapy.

Among the vasodilators, sodium nitroprusside (Nipride) is probably the most commonly used. Its rapid onset of action and evanescent effect allow titration as necessary during a period in which cardiovascular changes can occur rapidly. It is commonly mixed in concentrations of 200 $\mu g/mL$ (50 mg/250 mL), and the usual dosage range is 0.5–3.0 μg/kg/min. Although cyanide toxicity with this drug is rare, the development of tachyphylaxis or a requirement for doses above the usual range should alert one to the possibility of toxicity. Cyanide toxicity should be suspected if nitroprusside is required for a prolonged period or unexplained metabolic acidosis occurs. Nitroprusside may cause myocardial ischemia from the "intracoronary steal" phenomenon. In addition, nitroprusside increases intrapulmonary shunting and causes hypoxemia, because it inhibits the "hypoxic pulmonary vasoconstriction."

Nitroglycerin infusion may be used to control hypertension in the postoperative period. Nitroglycerin exerts some specific, beneficial antiischemic effect on left ventricular function in patients after myocardial revascularization. It produces more venodilation than arteriolar dilation. Nitroglycerin, 20 to 500 μg/min, may be needed to control hypertension. Nitroglycerin is usually mixed in a concentration of 60 μg/mL (15 mg/250 mL). An infusion rate of 1 mL/hr delivers 1 μg/min.

Chloropromazine (Thorazine) (1–2 mg), trimethaphan (Arfonad) (1 mg/mL infusion titrated to effect), and phentolamine (Regitine) (0.5–1.0 mg/mL infusion titrated to effect) have also been used to control hypertension. Recently labetolol, an alpha and beta adrenergic antagonist, has been investigated to control postoperative hypertension.

Arrhythmias

Disturbances in cardiac rhythm in the early postoperative period are common and may be multifactorial in origin. The underlying cardiac disease, electrolyte abnormalities, the effects of manipulation of the heart during surgery, and acid-base disturbances may all contribute to the development of arrhythmias.

Conduction defects are the most common rhythm disturbances in the immediate postbypass period. These may be caused by hyperkalemia or residual cold from cardioplegic solutions. Direct surgical trauma or associated myocardial edema may be implicated after operations performed adjacent to the conductive tissues themselves. Regardless of the underlying cause, the defects are usually transient. Bradycardia can be corrected by a temporary pacemaker. Atrial pacing is preferred if the arteriovenous (AV) node is intact. Ventricular pacing is necessary when there is second- or third-degree AV block. When ventricular pacing is associated with hypotension or low cardiac output, AV sequential pacing is indicated, because "atrial kick" increases cardiac output by 25 to 30 percent.

Premature ventricular contractions (PVCs) are also a common arrhythmia in the early postoperative period. They are most often due to hypokalemia. Aggressive potassium replacement may be necessary for several hours to keep pace with urinary potassium excretion. Hyperventilation must be avoided, since a respiratory alkalosis will exacerbate the serum potassium deficit. All PVCs are potentially serious because they can initiate ventricular tachycardia or fibrillation. PVCs should be distinguished from aberrantly conducted PACs. On the ECG, PVCs produce a wide, slurred, and bizarre QRS complex followed by inverted T waves. The diagnostic features of PVCs include fully compensatory pause after beat, LBBB pattern of QRS complex, and fixed coupling interval. When PVCs are frequent (more than 6/min), multifocal, occurring in three or more consecutive beats, or occurring in a vulnerable period (R on T wave), immediate therapy is required.

Premature ventricular contractions are usually associated with hypoxia, pain, fluid overload hypokalemia, or ischemia. When these factors have been controlled, PVCs can usually be controlled by lidocaine (Xylocaine), 1.0–1.5 mg/kg, given as an intravenous bolus. If successful, it should be followed by a continuous infusion, 1–4 mg/min, which can be tapered over several hours if the PVCs do not recur. If lidocaine is unsuccessful in controlling ventricular irritability, intermittent doses of propranolol, 0.25–1.00 mg, or procainamide, 75–150 mg, may be given intravenously. However, these drugs must be used with caution in patients whose myocardial function is already compromised. Bretylium tosylate (Bretylol), 3 to 5 mg/kg intravenous bolus, may be useful for controlling refractory, recurrent ventricular tachycardia or fibrillation.

Ectopic beats of atrial or ventricular origin may be of an escape or competitive nature if the underlying sinus rhythm (or ventricular response) is slow. Pharmacological suppression of the competing atrial or ventricular focus is contraindicated since atrial, ventricular, or A-V sequential pacing at a rate faster than the competing focus may be all that is necessary.

Supraventricular tachycardias result from cardiac causes, infection, electrolyte abnormalities, medications, and hypoxia. Noncardiac causes should be eliminated if possible before treatment, or they should be treated concurrently. The presence of P waves in Leads II or CB_5 or in an esophageal lead can be used to differentiate supraventricular rhythms. Carotid massage, Valsalva's maneuver, or other measures to enhance vagal tone may slow the rate if paroxysmal atrial tachycardia is present. Digitalis, propranolol (Inderal), or verapamil (Calan) may be used to control paroxysmal supraventricular tachycardia. However, if digitalis toxicity is a likely cause, digoxin should not be given. Drug therapy may require as long as 30 minutes or more for results. Cardioversion may be helpful if significant hemodynamic impairment is present.

Hypotension

Hypotension is one of the most common problems in the postoperative period. It is usually associated with low cardiac output syndrome, which includes hypotension, oliguria, acidosis, low mixed venous oxygen tension, and mental obtundation. The following equations help to understand the causes of hypotension.

$$\text{Blood pressure} = \text{cardiac output} \times \text{systemic vascular resistance}$$
$$\text{Cardiac output} = \text{heart rate} \times \text{stroke volume}$$

Stroke volume depends on the preload and contractility. Therefore, blood pressure is determined by preload, contractility, heart rate, and systemic vascular resistance. Hypotension is usually caused by hypovolemia, heart failure, arrhythmia, or peripheral vasodilation.

Hypovolemia is extremely common in the immediate postoperative period, due either to bleeding or inadequate replacement. The diagnosis is easily confirmed by a low central venous pressure (CVP), pulmonary capillary wedge pressure (PCWP), or left atrial pressure (LAP). Lactated Ringer's solution or five-percent Albumin may be used to correct hypovolemia. Blood transfusion is indicated when the hematocrit is below 30 percent. Meanwhile, the patient should be put in a head-down position to improve venous return.

Peripheral vasodilation usually accompanies rewarming of the patient. This contributes to decreased systemic vascular resistance and peripheral pooling of blood, with resultant central hypovolemia. Cardiac output should be measured, and systemic peripheral resistance can be calculated to confirm the diagnosis. Treatment includes fluid replacement and increasing vascular resistance by the infusion of phenylephrine (Neosynephrine), 20 mg/250 mL, or metaraminol (Aramine), 200 mg/250 mL, titrated to effect.

Arrhythmias cause hypotension because they decrease cardiac output. Postoperatively, left ventricular compliance is often decreased, and the stroke volume is fixed. Therefore, bradycardia produces low cardiac output and hypotension. Atrial or ventricular premature contractions interfere with ventricular filling, resulting in decreased stroke volume and cardiac output.

Heart failure is the second most common cause of hypotension following cardiac surgery (hypovolemia is the most common cause). Ventricular dysfunction develops frequently after prolonged surgical manipulation and aortic cross-clamping. The diagnosis is confirmed by hypotension with an elevated PCWP or LAP. Inotropic support is indicated for heart failure.

Calcium chloride, 500 to 1,000 mg, may be given to improve contractility, since calcium levels are usually low postoperatively. Dobutamine (Dobutrex), 5–15 µg/kg/min, is the preferred adrenergic agonist for cardiac failure in the setting of acute ischemia because it may have a specific effect to increase coronary collateral flow while simultaneously enhancing contractility of ischemic myocardium. Dobutamine drips, 15 mg times body weight diluted in 250 mL of five-percent dextrose solution, given at a rate of 1 mL/hr, deliver 1 µg/kg/min.

Dopamine is commonly used as an inotropic agent postoperatively because it specifically increases the renal blood flow in the dose range of 1 to 3 µg/kg/min. Positive inotropic and chronotropic effects predominate at infusion rates of less than 10 µg/kg/min. Dopamine causes more tachycardia than dobutamine does at the same dosage. Dobutamine may be combined with a renal dose of dopamine to increase the inotropic effect without increasing tachycardia and peripheral resistance. Epinephrine, 2 mg/250 mL, given at 2 to 8 µg/min, is also used alone or in combination with dobutamine or dopamine to increase contractility.

Vasodilators may be added to the inotropic support if low cardiac output persists and high peripheral resistance develops. Vasodilators decrease peripheral resistance and thus increase stroke volume in patients with myocardial dysfunction. Nitroprusside, 50 mg/250 mL, at a rate of 0.2 to 8.0 µg/kg/min, may be titrated to effect.

An intraaortic balloon pump (IABP) is indicated when low cardiac output and high ventricular filling pressures persist despite maximal therapy with inotropic agents and vasodilators. IABP counterpulsation is designed to increase the myocardial oxygen supply during diastole and to decrease myocardial oxygen demand during systole. The balloon is inflated during diastole to increase the diastolic aortic pressure, resulting in increased coronary blood flow. The balloon is deflated just prior to the next systole to decrease the intraaortic pressure and afterload, resulting in decreased myocardial oxygen consumption. The cardiac output is increased because of increased coronary perfusion and decreased resistance.

Postoperative Respiratory Care

Such preoperative conditions as cardiac failure, chronic lung disease, history of heavy smoking, pulmonary hypertension, severe obesity, and advanced age predispose the cardiac patient to postoperative respiratory problems. Ventilation/perfusion (V/Q) abnormalities and increased dead space/tidal volume ratios (V_D/V_T) are common findings for chronic cardiac patients, especially with mitral stenosis. Pulmonary function is significantly compromised by cardiac operative procedures. Invasion of the thorax causes deleterious changes in respiratory mechanics, and cardiopulmonary bypass is associated with parenchymal lung changes. These changes, along with cardiovascular and metabolic alterations in the postoperative period, combine to impair gas exchange and increase respiratory work. Careful monitoring and support of pulmonary function is necessary to avoid serious respiratory problems.

Initial Ventilator Settings

It is most important to set tidal volume, respiratory rate, inspiratory flow rate and FIo_2. Normal tidal volume is 7 mL per kilogram of body weight. For postoperative cardiac patients, the tidal volume is usually set at 10 to 12 mL per kilogram of body weight because of increased physiological dead space (V_D/V_T). Respiratory rate is usually set at 8 to 10 per minute. Inspiratory flow rate is usually set at 30 to 40 liters per minute. Slow inspiratory flow rate allows more even distribution of inspired gas, but it may compromise venous return because of prolonged inspiratory phase. FIO_2 is set at 50 to 60 percent oxygen. The settings are changed according to blood gases. Periodic sighs have been replaced by the use of large tidal volumes because of a lack of demonstrated clinical efficacy and frequent intolerance by awake patients. When tidal volume is more than 10 mL/kg, it is not necessary to set sigh volume. Normal tidal volume, 7 mL/kg, needs occasional sighs to prevent atelectasis. Sigh volume is usually set at twice the tidal volume and three to six per hour. The high airway pressure limit is set at 10 to 20 cm H_2O above the patient's normal peak airway pressure to prevent barotrauma due to sudden increase in resistance. The safety alarm system can be set by low inspiratory airway pressure and/or low exhaled tidal volume to detect leak or disconnection of ventilator. Usually, the low limit of exhaled tidal volume is set at 100 to 200 mL below the preselected tidal volume; the low limit of inspiratory pressure is set at 10 to 15 cm below the patient's usual peak inspiratory pressure.

General Airway Care

The patient's head should be kept in a neutral position to avoid kinking or undue pressure of the endotracheal tube. Endotracheal tubes with low pressure cuffs should be utilized to prevent tracheal damage. Endotracheal suction and instillation of sterile saline followed by suctioning will clear secretions. Hyperinflation after suctioning should be routinely performed. Suctioning is performed every two hours, or more if necessary. Systematic turning of the patient reduces the incidence of postoperative fever, as well as preventing skin changes from prolonged pressure.

Effects of Intermittent Positive Pressure Ventilation

The initiation of intermittent positive pressure ventilation (IPPV) is associated with a decrease in cardiac output and arterial blood pressure in patients without significant lung consolidation. Cardiac output and stroke volume decrease as the peak airway pressure increases. There is also a fall in cardiac output with increasing inspiratory-to-expiratory ratios. IPPV increases intrathoracic pressure, resulting in decreased venous return and cardiac output. Patients with normal lungs behave differently from patients with significant cardiopulmonary disease. When pulmonary compliance decreases, the transmission of airway pressure to intrathoracic pressure decreases. Patients with more rigid lungs can tolerate higher airway pressures.

IPPV decreases transmural pulmonary artery pressure, as well. There is no change in pulmonary vascular resistance. The systemic vascular resistance increases slightly when IPPV is begun. The fall in cardiac output during IPPV is rarely of any clinical significance because it is compensated by an increase in peripheral vascular resistance in nonanesthetized patients. When patients are hypovolemic, the decrease in blood pressure can be significant.

Complications of Mechanical Ventilation

The physiological complications of mechanical ventilation include:

- decreased cardiac output due to increased intrathoracic pressure
- respiratory alkalosis from hyperventilation
- increased venous admixture (QS/QT) from prolonged low tidal volume ventilation

The pulmonary complications of mechanical ventilation include:

- infection
- barotrauma-pneumothorax, mediastinal, interstitial, and subcutaneous emphysema in 10 to 15 percent of adults
- oxygen toxicity if the inspired oxygen concentration is more than 60 percent
- atelectasis due to immobilization, ineffective humidification, and low tidal volume ventilation

Complications from endotracheal intubation include the following:

- problems with tubes: bronchial intubation, kinking or obstruction, leaking cuffs
- nasal intubation: nose bleeding, fractured turbinates, septal perforation, partial loss of alae nasae, nasal synechiae
- laryngeal damage: edema, vocal cord paresis and granulomata, laryngotracheal membranes, subglottic fibrotic stenosis
- tracheal damage: tracheal erosion, tracheoesophageal fistula, tracheomalacia, tracheal stenosis

Hyperventilation causes hypocapnia during mechanical ventilation of cardiac patients and is especially deleterious. It reduces cardiac output, cerebral and coronary blood flow, and release of oxygen to the tissues. Alkalosis may alter myocardial sensitivity to circulating catecholamines and cause arrhythmias. The arrhythmias are usually supraventricular and include atrial tachycardia, nodal tachycardia, and AV or junctional dissociation with or without tachycardia. Hypocapnia also prolongs AV nodal conduction and functional refractory period, promoting reentrant arrhythmias. Alkalosis may cause tissue hypoxia, due to a shift in the oxyhemoglobin dissociation curve to the left, resulting in hemoglobin being more saturated with oxygen and its release to tissues being inhibited. Alkalosis also decreases serum potassium levels. Hypocapnia during mechanical ventilation can be corrected by decreasing the rate and/or tidal volume of the ventilator, using intermittent mandatory ventilation (IMV), using sedation, adding mechanical dead space to the respirator tubing, or adding one- to three-percent carbon dioxide to the inhaled gas.

Weaning from Respirator

The disadvantages of prolonged mechanical ventilation, including the increased requirement of sedatives and narcotics, and the complications of prolonged intubation are well known. It is not necessary to keep the cardiac patients mechanically ventilated overnight. Early extubation is a well-accepted practice when the criteria for extubation are met.

Five criteria for discontinuance of mechanical ventilation are:

1. clear consciousness with adequate gag and cough reflex
2. cardiovascular stability
3. stable metabolic state without hypothermia, hyperpyrexia, metabolic acidosis, or alkalosis
4. normal coagulation studies and chest tube drainage less than 150 mL/hr
5. adequate pulmonary function:
    - Mechanics: (1) a vital capacity of more than 10 mL per kilogram or more than twice the normal tidal volume, (2) a maximum inspiratory force of at least -20 to -30 cm H_2O
    - Oxygenation: (1) Pa_{O_2} more than 80 mm Hg with FI_{O_2} 0.4, (2) A-aDO_2 less than 300 mm Hg with FI_{O_2} 1.0, (3) QS/QT less than 15 percent
    - Ventilation: (1) Pa_{CO_2} less than 45 mm Hg, (2) V_D/V_T less than 0.6

There are two methods for weaning the patient from the respirator: (1) the conventional T-piece technique and (2) the intermittent mandatory ventilation technique.

Conventional T-Piece Technique. When the patient meets the criteria for weaning, a T-piece adaptor and heated humidifier are connected to the patient's endotracheal tube. The patient should be in a semisitting or sitting position. The inspired oxygen concentration is set at a level 10 percent higher than the patient was receiving during mechanical ventilation. The vital signs and cardiac rhythm are monitored carefully every 5 to 10 minutes. Arterial blood gases are determined 15 minutes after weaning is begun and then every hour. The patient who tolerates the T-piece very well is extubated after two to four hours. Oxygen is then administered, through a face mask with a heated humidifier, at the same inspired oxygen concentration as during the T-piece trial.

Intermittent Mandatory Ventilation Technique. With this technique, weaning is accomplished by a gradual decrease in the IMV rate that the ventilator delivers, allowing the patient slowly to take over spontaneous ventilation. This system allows the patient to breathe spontaneously in between the preset mechanical ventilatory rate. It ensures intermittent hyperinflation of the lung. IMV has been reported to be helpful in weaning when conventional methods have failed.

Spontaneous PEEP can be applied to both weaning techniques. PEEP is especially useful in patients in whom rapid alveolar collapse and hypoxemia develop during weaning. Five cm H_2O PEEP during weaning minimizes alveolar collapse and improves the relationship between the closing capacity and functional residual capacity.

Postextubation Respiratory Care

After extubation, patients should receive nothing by mouth until it is ascertained that normal glottic reactivity has returned, usually within six to eight hours. Oxygen therapy should be given to all cardiac patients after extubation. Oxygen may be administered through a face mask, face hood, face tent, nasal cannula, or nasal prongs. The FIo_2 depends on the patient's inspiratory flow rate and the flow rate and concentration of delivered oxygen. The inspiratory flow rate is usually 30 to 40 liters/min. If the delivered flow rate is lower than inspiratory flow rate, air will be breathed in to mix the delivered oxygen and the FIo_2 will be lowered. To ensure adequate FIo_2, oxygen at 10 to 15 liters per minute should be run through a venturi humidifier to deliver 50-percent oxygen with mist to the patient. It is important to specify a high oxygen flow rate to satisfy the patient's inspiratory flow rate.

Postoperative Respiratory Maneuvers

After extubation, the following are recommended: chest physiotherapy, including incentive spirometry, deep breathing, and encouragement to cough; mobilization of secretions; early ambulation; and proper pain control.

We recommend incentive spirometry instead of IPPB for postoperative cardiac patients. The ideal respiratory maneuver is one in which a high alveolar-inflating pressure is sustained for a relatively long period of time, and this can be achieved only with a large inhaled volume. A high inhaled volume can be achieved passively by proper IPPB or actively by incentive spirometry. Recently, IPPB has lost its popularity because, as usually performed, the inflating volume is not measured and the tidal volume is limited by the peak airway pressure. In addition, the use of IPPB may lead to cross-contamination from the equipment, pneumothorax, and decreased cardiac output by decreasing the venous return to the heart. Moreover, the cost of using IPPB is ten times that of using incentive spirometry.

Postoperative Respiratory Complications

Postoperative respiratory complications include atelectasis, pulmonary congestion and edema, pneumonia, pneumothorax, pleural effusion, and ARDS. Persistent atelectasis may require fiberoptic bronchoscopy to clear the bronchus if such conventional measures as humidity, postural drainage, chest physiotherapy, and suctioning fail. Pulmonary edema may be the first manifestation of inadequate left ventricular function. It may be present even with normal left atrial or pulmonary wedge pressures. The treatment of significant pulmonary congestion includes use of high tidal volumes, via an endotracheal tube, positive end-expiratory pressure, high FIo_2, and efforts to improve cardiac function. Diuretics and vasodilator therapy, particularly venodilator therapy with nitroglycerin and morphine, often produce marked improvement.

ARDS results from diffuse injury to the alveolar capillary membranes. It encompasses a clinical syndrome that was previously called "post-traumatic pulmonary insufficiency," "pump lung," "postperfusion lung," "shock lung," or "congestive atelectasis." It can follow almost any injury. Although the onset may be acute, there is usually a latent period of hours or days during which respiratory damage is minimal or slowly progressing. Then, progressive, severe respiratory failure develops, and it usually advances rapidly to the point of requiring tracheal intubation, mechanical ventilation, and use of PEEP. The physiological changes are characterized by hypoxemia, reduced functional residual capacity and compliance, increased intrapulmonary shunting; radiologically, they are characterized by pulmonary interstitial infiltrate.

Application of Positive End-Expiratory Pressure

The first step in the application of PEEP to improve hypoxemia is to increase FIo_2. However, prolonged exposure to high concentrations of oxygen may cause oxygen toxicity. Oxygen toxicity is governed by the oxygen partial pressure during exposure, the duration of exposure, and the susceptibility of the individual to pulmonary oxygen injury. The degree of toxicity is related to the partial pressure, but not to the percentage of oxygen inspired, as shown by toleration of 100-percent oxygen for two to four weeks at a tension of 250 mm Hg during U.S. space flights. Systemic oxygen toxicity is related to arterial oxygen tension, whereas pulmonary oxygen toxicity depends on alveolar oxygen tension. Retrolental fibroplasia in the premature neonate has been reported after exposure to Pao_2 of more than 150 mm Hg for a few hours. Pulmonary toxicity can develop after prolonged exposure to oxygen at concentrations of between 0.5 and 1.0 atmospheres. It must be emphasized that, generally, the adult patient can tolerate one atmosphere of oxygen partial pressure for at least 24 hours.

In order to avoid oxygen toxicity, PEEP is applied to improve oxygenation and lower the Flo_2 to acceptable levels. When Pao_2 is less than 60 mm Hg with Flo_2 of 0.5 or more, PEEP is indicated. The mechanism of improving oxygenation by PEEP is related to an increase in the functional residual capacity (FRC). The FRC expands linearly with increase in the end-expiratory pressure, usually at a rate of 400 cc or more for each 5 cm H_2O end-expiratory pressure. This increase in FRC represents alveoli that remain open and available for gas exchange during all phases of the respiratory cycle. The increase in FRC improves the relationship between FRC and closing capacity and therefore decreases intrapulmonary shunt or venous admixture.

Respiration may be categorized by the following three types: (1) spontaneous breathing (SB), (2) mechanical ventilation (MV), and (3) intermittent mandatory ventilation (IMV), which is the combination of SB and MV.

Mechanical ventilation with inspiratory positive airway pressure (IPAP) and zero end-expiratory pressure (ZEEP) is called intermittent positive pressure ventilation (IPPV). Mechanical ventilation with PEEP is equal to continuous positive pressure ventilation (CPPV). Therefore, CPPV = IPPV + PEEP. Both CPPV and continuous positive airway pressure (CPAP) have positive airway pressure during both inspiratory and expiratory phases, that is, both IPAP and expiratory positive airway pressure (EPAP). CPPV is usually used with mechanical ventilation, whereas CPAP is usually used with spontaneous breathing.

PEEP is often referred to as CPPV. However, "spontaneous PEEP" has been used to describe a different respiratory pattern. In spontaneous PEEP, the inspiratory airway pressure can be positive, zero, or negative, depending on the inspiratory efforts and the level of PEEP. When PEEP is low and inspiratory effort is strong, the inspiratory airway pressure tends to reach levels below zero. PEEP or EPAP describe only the airway pressure during expiration and is not equivalent to CPAP or CPPV. The different airway pressure patterns are shown in Figure 7-2.

Ranges of PEEP. The ranges of PEEP can be divided into the following three groups:

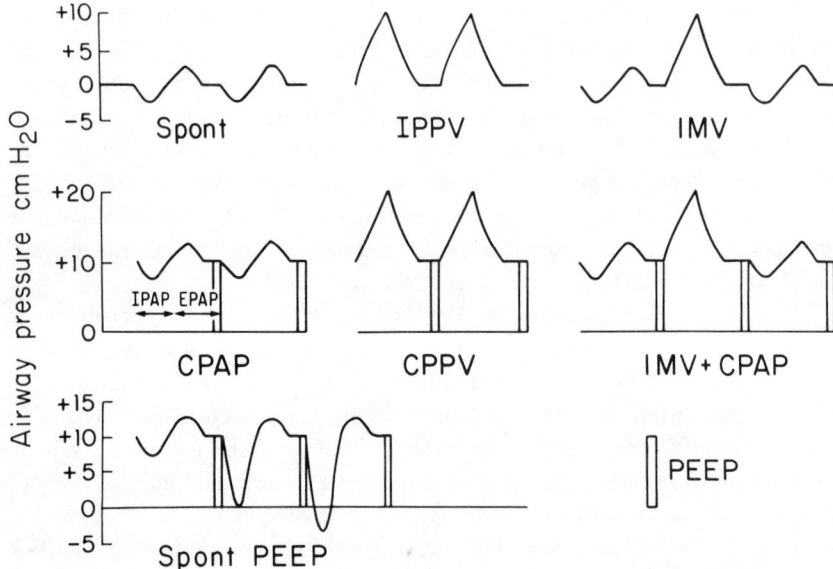

Figure 7-2 Airway Pressure Curves of Different Respiratory Patterns. *Source:* Adapted from *New England Journal of Medicine*, Vol. 292, No. 6, pp. 286 and 287, with permission of New England Journal of Medicine, © 1975.

1. prophylactic PEEP: 1 to 5 cm H_2O, used to increase FRC to more than closing capacity, to prevent atelectasis, and to decrease shunting
2. conventional PEEP: 6 to 20 cm H_2O, indicated if Pao_2 is less than 60 torr with FIo_2 more than 50 percent
3. high PEEP: more than 20 cm H_2O, used in extreme hypoxemia when there is no response to conventional PEEP

Best conventional PEEP was described by Suter and associates in 1975.[1] It is defined as the level of PEEP with the highest oxygen transport, which is the product of cardiac output and oxygen content. Best conventional PEEP correlates with the highest total respiratory compliance, the highest mixed venous oxygen tension, and the lowest V_D/V_T (see Figure 7-3). Arterial oxygen tension and intrapulmonary shunt are not good indicators of the best conventional PEEP; they continue to improve even after this level has been reached. Oxygen transport decreases after the best PEEP is reached because the cardiac output decreases.

Optimal high PEEP was described by Kirby, Civetta, and associates in 1975.[2] It is defined as the level of PEEP with the lowest intrapulmonary shunt and without compromising cardiac output. This PEEP, also called super PEEP, is more than 25 cm H_2O, while the best conventional PEEP of Suter and associates ranges from 5 to 20 cm H_2O.

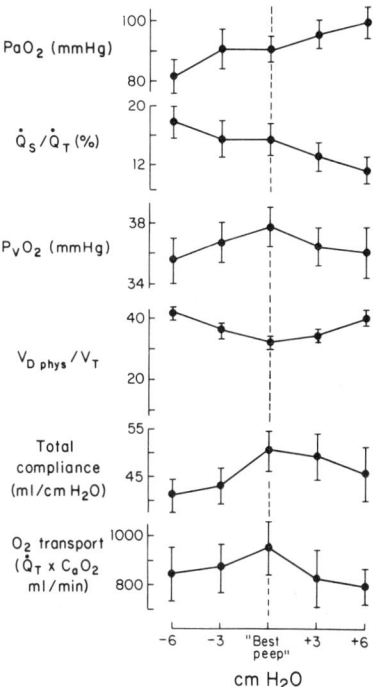

Figure 7-3 Best Conventional PEEP

The level of PEEP needed depends on the severity of the pulmonary injury and the response of the individual patient. It is important to titrate the levels of PEEP individually to maximize oxygen transport without compromising cardiac output. When low levels of PEEP (less than 10 cm H_2O) are used, Pao_2, total respiratory compliance, $P\bar{v}o_2$, $Aado_2$, and QS/QT have to be monitored. When high levels of PEEP are used, cardiac output measurement is necessary because excessive PEEP decreases cardiac output.

Cardiovascular Effects of PEEP. The cardiovascular effects of PEEP depend on the severity of respiratory failure, the level of PEEP, the intravascular volume, the contractility of the heart, and the pulmonary vasculature. In normal subjects without respiratory failure, PEEP decreases cardiac output mainly because of increased intrathoracic pressure resulting in decreased venous return. In persons with respiratory failure, PEEP, up to optimal levels, usually increases or does not change cardiac output because of an increase in oxygenation with resultant improvement of cardiac performance. Cardiac output falls when PEEP exceeds the individual's optimal PEEP. Hypovolemia increases hypotension during PEEP therapy. If hypotension develops during mechanical ventilation with PEEP, hypovolemia has to be corrected first. When the patient is normovolemic, hypotension and low cardiac output from PEEP may be corrected either by expansion of the blood volume or by infusion of dopamine (Intropin). When there is some degree of cardiac failure, hypervolemia can be dangerous. Therefore, dopamine (Intropin) is preferred in cardiac patients, although it produces a substantial increase in pulmonary shunt.

Intermittent Mandatory Ventilation

IMV comprises breaths controlled by the ventilator, as well as breaths supplied spontaneously by the patient, as shown in Figure 7-2. Although IMV was originally introduced as a weaning technique, it is now used by some groups as a primary means of ventilatory support, especially in combination with high levels of PEEP, throughout the course of a patient's illness. Because the ventilator cycles are independent of the patient's breathing phase, airway and intrapleural pressure may increase when IMV inflations come at the end of spontaneous inhalation.

The advantages of IMV over controlled or assisted ventilation are several:

- It allows selective application of mechanical support in accord with the individual patient's need.
- It is more comfortable for the patient; there is less need for sedatives or narcotics.
- It has a higher cardiac output because of lower intrathoracic pressure.
- It results in decreased incidence of barotrauma because of lower airway pressure.
- It produces less discoordination on spontaneous breathing because the respiratory center is activated and the patient uses the respiratory muscles.
- It reduces psychological dependence on the ventilator.

NOTES

1. Suter, P.M., Failey, H.B., and Isenberg, M.D., "Optimum End Expiratory Airway Pressure in Patients with Acute Respiratory Failure," *New England Journal of Medicine* 292, No. 6 (1975):286.

2. Kirby, R.R., Civetta, J.M., Modell, J.H., Dannemiller, F.J., Klein, E.F. and Hodges, M. "High Level Positive and Expiratory Pressure (PEEP) in Acute Respiratory Insufficiency." *Chest* 67, (1975):161.

BIBLIOGRAPHY

Barash, Paul G. "Monitoring Myocardial Oxygen Balance: Physiological Basis and Clinical Application." In *ASA Refresher Courses in Anesthesiology*, vol. 13, 21–32. Park Ridge, Ill.: American Society of Anesthesiologists, 1985.

Conahan III, Thomas J., ed. *Cardiac Anesthesia*, 304–328. Menlo Park, Calif.: Addison-Wesley, 1982.

Ream, Allen K., and Fogdall, Richard P., eds. *Acute Cardiovascular Management, Anesthesia and Intensive Care*, 481–548. Philadelphia: J.B. Lippincott, 1982.

Stevenson, Robert L., and Rogers, Mark C. "Diagnosis of Cardiac Dysrhythmias." In *ASA Refresher Courses in Anesthesiology*, vol. 14, 217–236. Park Ridge, Ill.: American Society of Anesthesiologists, 1986.

Sharpiro, Barry A., Cane, Roy D., and Harrison, Ronald A. "Positive End-Expiratory Pressure Therapy in Adults With Special Reference to Acute Lung Injury: A Review of the Literature and Suggested Clinical Correlations." *Critical Care Medicine* 12 (1984):127–141.

Tarhan, Sait, ed. *Anesthesia and Coronary Artery Surgery*, 308–358. Chicago: Year Book Medical Publisher, 1986.

Thomas, Stephen J., ed. *Manual of Cardiac Anesthesia*, 173–204, 231–258, 419–456. New York: Churchill Livingstone, 1984.

Yao, Fun-Sun F. "Aspiration Pneumonitis and Acute Respiratory Failure." In *Anesthesiology, Problem Oriented Patient Management*, edited by Fun-Sun F. Yao, and J.F. Artusio, Jr. Philadelphia: J.B. Lippincott, 1987.

Yao, Fun-Sun F. "Ischemic Heart Disease and Coronary Artery Bypass Graft." In *Anesthesiology, Problem Oriented Patient Management*, edited by Fun-Sun F. Yao, and J.F. Artusio, Jr. Philadelphia: J.B. Lippincott, 1987.

Chapter 8

Postanesthesia Care After Thoracic Surgery

John A. Lundberg, M.D.

GENERAL CONSIDERATIONS

Thoracic surgery patients require differing types of care and vigilance, depending upon various factors, including:

- the patient's preoperative pulmonary and cardiac function
- the nature of the operative procedure
- the type of incision made
- the type of monitors placed
- types of drains or chest tubes placed

Often thoracic operations are associated with prolonged stays in the ICU, multiple chest tubes, multiple invasive catheters, and considerable pain. Nurses in the PACU should realize thoracic surgery patients deserve a compassionate explanation about monitoring techniques, invasive catheters, and chest tubes.

Measurements of Pulmonary Function

Specific measurements of pulmonary function that are of greatest value in the preoperative evaluation of the thoracic surgery patient include tests for arterial blood gases, lung volumes, and the mechanics of breathing. Together, these are termed pulmonary function tests; their normal values are detailed in Table 8-1.

No single test provides an overall evaluation of pulmonary function, but the preoperative tests considered to be most predictive are those for forced vital capacity, FEV/FVC, maximum midexpiratory flow, maximum voluntary ventilation, and arterial blood gases. If these values are within 80 percent of the expected values, the patient has a higher probability of having an uncomplicated postoperative course. Tests for the mechanics of breathing may be difficult to interpret because they depend on a cooperative patient and are related to the effort the patient is willing to expend; thus, they may underestimate pulmonary function.

Thoracotomy Incisions

Three standard thoracotomy incisions are in widespread use:

1. anterolateral
2. posterolateral
3. median sternotomy

A thoracoabdominal incision is an inferior posterolateral thoracotomy combined with an abdominal incision. The posterolateral thoracotomy is used in the majority of pulmonary resections (except lung biopsy), posterior mediastinal operations, esophageal operations, and approaches to the vertebral column. If the patient needs a bone graft or has a rigid thoracic cage and broad exposure is

Table 8-1 Normal Adult Male Pulmonary Function Tests

Mechanics of breathing	
Forced vital capacity (FVC)	4.75 liters
Forced expiratory volume in 1 Second (FEV1)	3.87 liters
Forced expiratory volume in 3 Seconds (FEV3)	4.41 liters
FEV1/FVC	83%
FEV3/FVC	97%
Total lung capacity	6.5 liters
Functional residual capacity	2.7 liters
Residual volume	1.8 liters
Arterial blood gases	
pH 7.40	
P_{CO_2} 40 mm Hg	
P_{O_2} 95 mm Hg	

needed, the posterior two-thirds of a rib at the incision might be removed. This may increase postoperative pain.

The anterolateral thoracotomy incision allows rapid entry into the thorax in trauma patients and in patients with unstable cardiovascular systems. Unlike the posterolateral thoracotomy, in which the patient must be in the lateral position for incision, the arterolateral incision may be made with the patient supine, a position that is better tolerated by the patient. This also gives the anesthesiologist maximum control over the airway and cardiovascular system.

Monitoring

General

The essential monitors for the thoracic surgery patient in the postanesthetic period are electrocardiogram, blood pressure, and temperature. Other optional monitors might include those for arterial cannulation, pulse oximetry, tidal CO_2, transcutaneous Po_2, transcutaneous CO_2, continuous pulmonary artery pressure, and mixed venous Po_2.

Atrial fibrillation is the most common arrhythmia in the postoperative period. This usually reverts to a normal sinus rhythm with little or no intervention. Atrial fibrillation can, however, cause an elevated heart rate and a serious decrease in blood pressure because the heart is unable to fill sufficiently during diastole. Elevated heart rates greater than 120/min that decrease blood pressure and cardiac output may be treated with calcium channel blockers, beta blockers, procainamide (Pronestyl), Digoxin, or electrical cardioversion.

Many surgeons and anesthesiologists insist on intraarterial cannulation (usually the radial, femoral, or axillary artery) for their thoracic surgery patients. This allows continuous monitoring of arterial blood pressure, as well as arterial access for blood gases. It is of utmost importance to check the arterial cannula pressure against a cuff pressure. The arterial monitoring tubing system should be scrutinized closely for air bubbles, and only special stiff, short, pressure monitoring tubing should be used. The arterial pulse contour should be examined closely for the dicrotic notch and evidence of clamping or resonance in the measuring system.

Pulse Oximetry

Pulse oximeters are commonly used intraoperatively for thoracic procedures because they give a continuous display of arterial hemoglobin saturation. It is likely that in the future pulse oximeters will become more common in the postanesthetic monitoring of all patients, especially thoracic surgery patients. Pulse oximeter sensors are placed on a toe, a finger, an earlobe, or the nose bridge; and a continuous readout of heart rate and arterial hemoglobin saturation is displayed. Small portable end tidal CO_2 monitors are now available and are commonly used intraoperatively. End tidal CO_2 is a very good estimation of arterial P_{CO_2} and gives the best indication of adequacy of ventilation.

Pulmonary Artery Catheters

Pulmonary artery catheters (Swan-Ganz catheters) are usually placed preoperatively in patients with limited cardiac or pulmonary reserve. Pulmonary artery pressure is monitored continuously. Cardiac output determinations can be made intermittently with this type of catheter, using the hemodilution method. A special type of catheter contains a fiberoptic cable and is capable of measuring continuous mixed venous hemoglobin saturation. Under most conditions, mixed venous hemoglobin saturation estimates cardiac output.

Transcutaneous Oxygen Monitoring

Transcutaneous oxygen monitoring involves the placement of a small dime-sized probe on the skin. Usually, the anterior thorax probe and underlying skin are heated to 44–45 °C, which causes vasodilation. Oxygen diffuses through the skin to a polarographic oxygen electrode where oxygen tension is measured. In a hemodynamically stable patient, this may give a good estimate of the arterial P_{O_2}, but the utility of these electrodes is limited by difficulties with electrode position, changing hemodynamic status, and damage to the underlying skin by heat. Electrode position should be changed every two to four hours to avoid damage to the skin. After placement, 15 to 30 minutes is necessary for heating of the skin before monitoring begins.

Postoperative Pain Considerations

Pain relief can be a major problem for patients with thoracic incisions. The act of breathing itself may be very painful; and coughing, which is necessary to clean secretions, may be excruciatingly painful. To minimize their pain, patients take shallow breaths and avoid coughing.

Analgesia may be provided by one or more of the following techniques:

- intravenous or intramuscular narcotics
- intraoperative intercostal block with local anesthetics

- epidural narcotics
- spinal (intrathecal) narcotics

Narcotics have for decades been the mainstay of postoperative pain relief. Intravenous administration provides rapid, efficient pain relief, but relative overdosage can be a problem in difficult-to-control patients. In general, the patient must be responsive to verbal commands and breathe at a rate of at least 14 breaths per minute. Intramuscular narcotics provide analgesia for a longer period but have less utility because of delayed onset of action.

Intercostal nerve block is done by injecting local anesthetic in the intercostal space below the appropriate ribs. This is done through the open thoracotomy before the incision is closed. Incision and rib pain are adequately blocked by this technique; but pleural pain, which can be a major component of pain, is not.

Epidural and intrathecal administration of narcotics delivers the narcotic directly to specific receptors in the spinal cord and thereby selectively blocks the transmission of pain impulses to the brain. Morphine is usually placed in the intrathecal or epidural space preoperatively by the anesthesiologist. Onset of analgesia is within 5 to 60 minutes. Duration of pain relief ranges from 6 to 24 hours, and sometimes even longer in cases of chronic pain.

Common side effects of epidural and intrathecal narcotics are respiratory depression, nausea, pruitis, and urinary retention. Side effects have been reported in as many as 70 percent of patients. Fortunately, these side effects can be reversed with nalaxone hydrochloride (Narcan). Because respiratory depression may be delayed as much as 24 hours, monitoring of respiratory rate must be vigilantly maintained.

Use of Chest Tubes

Chest tubes (thoracostomies) and their closed drainage systems serve three functions:

1. drainage of fluid from the pleural space
2. drainage of air from the pleural space
3. application of suction to aid in reexpansion of a collapsed lung

A closed chest tube drainage system may consist of one, two, or three bottles or chambers. In the disposable double-seal chest drainage unit, three chambers are combined in a single package (see Figure 8-1).

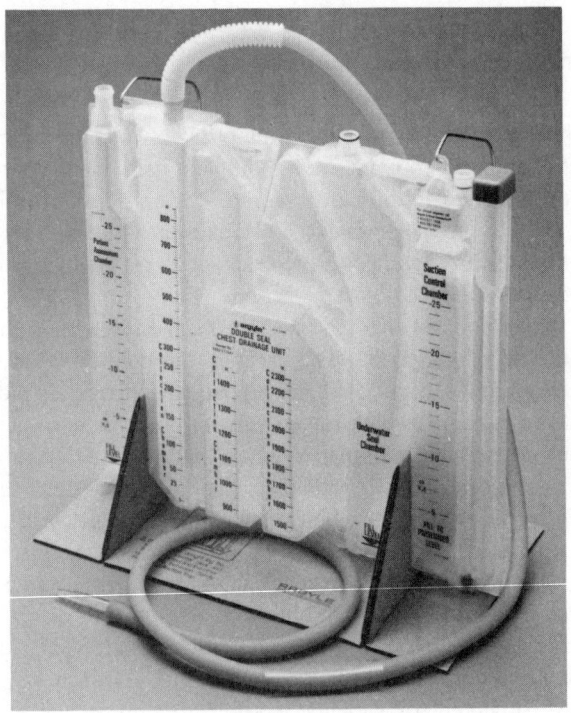

Figure 8-1 Double-Seal Chest Drainage Unit. *Source:* Courtesy of Sherwood Medical, St. Louis, Missouri.

The one-bottle water seal system uses a single bottle to provide a water seal and acts as a drainage bottle as well (see Figures 8-2, 8-3, and 8-4). If large amounts of drainage are expected, it is best to segregate the water seal bottle from the drainage by adding the second bottle. Constant pressure may be applied to the water seal bottle by adding a third pressure-regulator bottle that maintains a negative pressure of 0–25 cm of water. If a reliable suction motor that is capable of maintaining a stable negative pressure from 0–25 cm of water is available, this may be used in a two-bottle system, with suction being applied directly to the water seal bottle.

The water seal bottle should be examined carefully at least as often as vital signs are taken. During inspiration the water level should rise up the indicator tube, and during expiration it should fall. If an air leak into the pleural cavity is present, either through the incision or through the lung, air bubbles will exit through the indicator tube during expiration. A stable fluid level during inspiration and expiration may be due to a kinked or clogged tube.

Thoracic Surgery 105

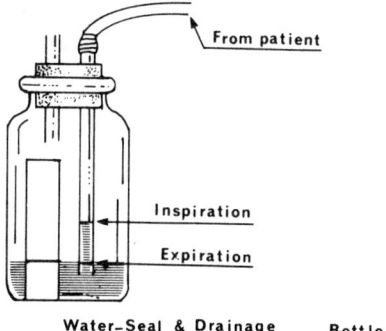

Note: Closed thoracic drainage of the gravity type. In this underwater-seal bottle, the level of water or saline in the indicator tube rises and falls in direct response to expansions and contractions of the chest muscles and inflation and deflation of the lungs.

Figure 8-2 One-Bottle Water Seal System. *Source:* Reprinted from *Closed Drainage of the Chest: A Programmed Course for Nurses,* U.S. Department of Health and Human Services, Public Health Service, Division of Nursing, May 1965.

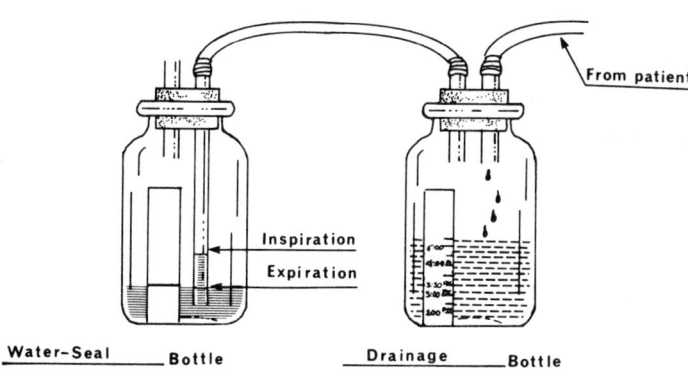

Note: Drainage of air and fluid from the chest without suction. Fluid from the chest drips into the empty bottle on the right.

Figure 8-3 Two-Bottle Water Seal System. *Source:* Reprinted from *Closed Drainage of the Chest: A Programmed Course for Nurses,* U.S. Department of Health and Human Services, Public Health Service, Division of Nursing, May 1965.

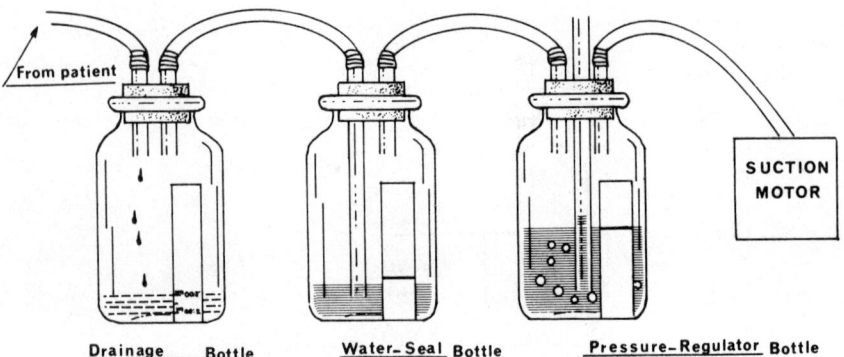

Note: Closed thoracic drainage of the mechanical suction type, showing the drainage of air and fluid. The depth of the tube under the water level regulates the suction vacuum.

Figure 8-4 Mechanical Suction System. *Source:* Reprinted from *Closed Drainage of the Chest: A Programmed Course for Nurses*, U.S. Department of Health and Human Services, Public Health Service, Division of Nursing, May 1965.

Mediastinal chest tubes (mediastinostomies) are placed in the mediastinum around the breast and are used in open-heart surgery patients. Their main function is to drain blood and fluid; seldom do they drain air. The rise and fall of the water level in the water seal indicator tube is usually much less pronounced than with thoracostomy chest tubes placed in the pleural space.

THORACIC PROCEDURES

Pneumonectomy

Pneumonectomy is usually reserved for patients who require removal of an entire lung and who can tolerate ventilation with one lung. The lung is removed at the hilum, and the evacuated thorax fills with fluid. Chest tubes are generally not used, since they cause overexpansion of the remaining lung and traction on the large thoracic vessels.

Central venous pressure monitoring lines are usually placed preoperatively to monitor function of the right heart. Pulmonary artery pressure monitoring lines may be placed preoperatively for patients with heart or lung disease. The right heart is especially stressed postpneumonectomy because it pumps the same amount of blood through half the pulmonary vascular bed. Immediately postpneumonectomy, central venous and pulmonary artery pressures are elevated. With time, the pulmonary vascular bed dilates, allowing more flow at lower pressures.

Until these vessels dilate, fluid restriction is necessary to prevent right-sided heart failure.

Lobectomy

Resection of a lobe or segment of lung is usually done for patients who have tumors within the removed portion of lung. Besides the obvious problem of pain control, these patients may have intrathoracic bleeding or air leaks, causing a hemothorax or pneumothorax. In resecting the lobe, the surgeon oversews airway and pulmonary vessels. These surgical closures may break down, creating a surgical emergency. Breakdown of a pulmonary vessel may cause bleeding through the chest tube at a rate greater than 200 cc per hour.

Breakdown of a bronchus or smaller airway can cause an air leak, which can easily be seen in the indicator tube of the water seal bottle. Small air leaks can be expected and will usually seal spontaneously. Large air leaks may cause major problems with the patient's ventilation if a pneumothorax results. Application of suction to the water seal bottle usually aids in lung reexpansion; if it does not, the patient must be taken back to the operating room where the communicating airway can be surgically closed.

Lung biopsy is usually done through a small incision to obtain a small amount of lung tissue for microscopic diagnosis by the pathologist. A chest tube is usually placed postoperatively. A small air leak is expected; this usually seals within a few days postoperatively.

Bronchoscopy

Rigid or flexible bronchoscopes may be used in the diagnosis and treatment of lung disease to visualize lung structures or obtain lung tissue for microscopic pathological diagnosis. A rigid bronchoscope is a tube with an internal light source that is placed in the mouth through the larynx to visualize the trachea and bronchi. Sites of bleeding can be cauterized and suspicious areas may be biopsied. Small amounts of bleeding may be expected postoperatively, and a mild sore throat is common.

Flexible bronchoscopy utilizes a fiberoptic cable with a light source that can be passed down into smaller airways to view their internal structure. Small tissue samples can be taken and fluid can be collected for pathological diagnosis. The procedure can be performed under local anesthesia with sedation or under general anesthesia.

Mediastinoscopy and Mediastinotomy

Mediastinal spread of thoracic neoplasms may be investigated with mediastinoscopy. A small transverse suprasternal notch incision is made; and the mediastinoscope, a short flat blade with a light source, is passed into the mediastinum. Mediastinal lymph nodes or tumors may be visualized and biopsied.

Mediastinotomy is performed through the second costal cartilage, and sometimes the third costal cartilage is removed as well for wider exposure. Lymph nodes of the pulmonary may be biopsied. Bleeding of large vessels may cause a hemomediastinum. A tear in the lung could result in pneumomediastinum or pneumothorax.

Mediastinoscopy and mediastinotomy are usually uneventful, and patients require minimal pain medication. Patients can often be discharged from the hospital within 24 to 48 hours if they require no further in-hospital procedures.

Thymectomy

Myasthenia gravis is an autoimmune disease characterized by destruction of acetylcholine receptors at the neuromuscular junction. Generalized weakness and fatigue result. Thymectomy may alter the patients' immune response and result in remission of symptoms. Perioperatively, patients are very sensitive to sedatives and muscle relaxants. Postoperative intubation may be necessary if ventilation is compromised.

A mediansternotomy is usually used; but, alternatively, a neck incision above the sternal notch may be used. Chest tubes are usually not used but may be placed to drain blood or fluid. Anticholinesterase medication is used in the treatment of myasthenia gravis to increase available acetylcholine at the neuromuscular junction. The dosage must be titrated carefully, since overdosage may result in cholinergic crisis with excessive lacrimation, salivation, secretions, bradycardia, and muscle weakness.

Pericardial Window

Accumulation of fluid in pericardium around the heart may impair filling of the heart and necessitate drainage of the pericardium. As ventricular filling is impaired, pulse pressure narrows, central venous pressure rises, and heart sounds are muffled. These three signs are known as Beck's triad of cardiac tamponade. To relieve the tamponade on the heart, a small piece of pericardium is removed to create a pericardial window. The window continues to drain fluid and decompresses the heart. Chronic renal failure, autoimmune-collagen vascular disease, infection, and tumor are pathological conditions associated with pericardial effusion and cardiac tamponade.

POSTANESTHESIA CARE

In the postanesthesia setting, care of patients undergoing thoracic surgery entails:

- maintaining chest tube drainage systems
- observing and recording drainage every hour
- reporting any sudden increase in drainage to the surgeon

Thoracic procedures are painful, and they can compromise adequate ventilation due to the anatomical site of the incision. Chest therapy must be instituted as soon as the patient is alert and able to follow commands. In the presence of pain, coughing, deep breathing, and change of position are difficult to achieve. Small titrated doses of narcotics ensure adequate pain control while preserving suitable ventilation.

Oxygen should be administered via a face tent to provide humidification to thin secretions. Suctioning may be necessary if the patient cannot expectorate effectively. IV fluids can also assist in thinning secretions, but urinary output must be monitored carefully to avoid fluid overload. Finally, breath sounds must be auscultated regularly, and any adventitious sounds should be reported.

The basic principles of PACU management—such as maintaining a patent airway along with coughing and deep breathing exercises—can help patients greatly in avoiding postoperative respiratory complications.

BIBLIOGRAPHY

Gustafsson, L.L., Schildt, B., and Jacobsen, K. "Adverse Effects of Extradural and Intrathecal Opiates: Report of a Nationwide Survey in Sweden." *British Journal of Anaesthesia* 54 (1982):479.

McDonald, D.A., Konchoukos, N.T., Shepard, L.C., and Kirkland, J.W. "Estimation of Stroke Volume and Cardiac Output from Central Arterial Pulse Contour in Postoperative Patients." *Circulation* 38, suppl 6 (1968):118.

Olsen, G.N., Block, A.J., Swenson, E.W., Castle, J.R., and Wynne, J.W. "Pulmonary Function Evaluation of the Lung Resection Candidate. A Prospective Study." *American Review of Respiratory Disease* 111 (1975):379.

Petty, T.L. *Pulmonary Diagnostic Techniques.* Philadelphia: Lea & Febiger, 1975.

Shulman, M., et al. "Postthoracotomy Pain and Pulmonary Function Following Epidural and Systemic Morphine." *Anesthesiology* 61 (1984):569.

Chapter 9

Postanesthesia Care After Abdominal Surgery

Eugene Nowak, M.D.
Douglas E. Paull, M.D.

GENERAL CONSIDERATIONS

The proper diagnosis and treatment of the patient with acute abdominal pain remains one of the greatest challenges facing surgeons and nurses. This chapter reviews the overall assessment of the acute abdomen and considers in some detail three of the more common intraabdominal crises: appendicitis, perforated ulcer, and diverticulitis.

In many ways, the evaluation of a patient with abdominal pain is similar to that for any other patient; it consists of a history, physical examination, and laboratory and radiologic procedures. The goal of the evaluation is to establish which patients require a surgical procedure and which do not. Those stable patients for which the diagnosis is unclear may at times benefit from serial physical exams and laboratory studies. One can appreciate the dilemma this poses by considering all of the possible extensive differential diagnoses involved (see Exhibit 9-1). All of these various conditions may cause pain by one of several mechanisms: perforation, obstruction, ischemia, inflammation, or hemorrhage. Treatment will vary considerably depending on the working diagnosis. The sooner correct treatment is rendered, the better the patient's prognosis. Error in judgment can lead to serious morbidity and even death.

PATHOPHYSIOLOGY AND SURGICAL PROCEDURES

Diagnosis

The character and location of abdominal pain offer important clues to the diagnosis (see Figure 9-1). Flank pain radiating to the groin, associated with

Exhibit 9-1 Causes of the Acute Abdomen

Aortic aneurysm	Lymphadenitis
Appendicitis	Mesenteric infarction
Bowel obstruction	Ovarian cyst
Cholecystitis	Pancreatitis
Diverticulitis	Pelvic inflammatory disease
Ectopic pregnancy	Peptic ulcer
Endometriosis	Pneumonia
Gastroenteritis	Pyelonephritis
Hepatitis	Renal stone
Inflammatory bowel disease	Sickle cell crisis

microscopic hematuria, suggests a renal stone. Epigastric pain radiating to the back in a heavy drinker indicates a strong possibility of acute pancreatitis. Small bowel obstruction leads to crampy abdominal pain associated with vomiting. Right upper abdominal pain after fatty meals suggests cholelithiasis.

Other symptoms may aid in the diagnosis. Gastroenteritis is characterized by watery diarrhea. Vomiting would be especially prominent in small bowel obstruc-

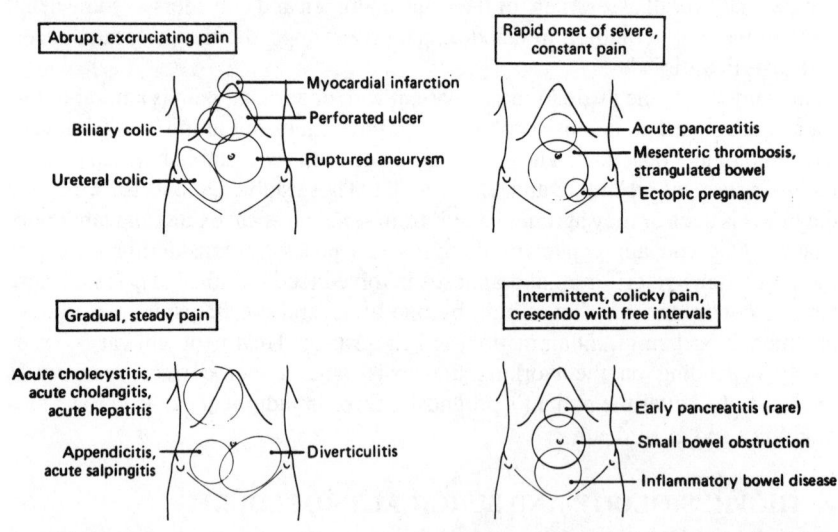

Figure 9-1 Location and Character of Pain and Causes of the Acute Abdomen. *Source:* Reprinted from *Current Surgical Diagnosis and Treatment* by L.W. Way (Ed.), p. 393, with permission of Lange Medical Publications, © 1985.

tion. Jaundice alerts the physician to biliary obstruction. Abnormal menstrual history may accompany an ectopic pregnancy. The patient's previous medical history can also be revealing. The patient with a long history of atrial fibrillation with the acute onset of severe abdominal pain may be suffering from an embolus to the superior mesenteric artery. The constellation of symptoms and their relationship to one another allow the health professional to narrow down the diagnostic possibilities.

Physical examination is the cornerstone of accurate diagnosis in the acute abdomen. Simple observation of the patient may be helpful. The experienced nurse will appreciate the contrast between the constantly squirming patient with a renal stone and the perfectly motionless patient with a perforated ulcer. Tachycardia is an early sign and hypotension a late sign in patients with hypovolemia due to bleeding (ruptured aneurysm) or to sepsis (peritonitis due to a perforated viscus). Fever implies inflammation but is not specific.

Inspection of the abdomen may disclose distention, which may be due to bowel obstruction. The presence of old surgical scars may suggest one possible etiology of the obstruction: obstructing adhesive bands. One auscultates the abdomen for the presence and quality of bowel sounds. Absent bowel sounds are found in the paralytic ileus in peritonitis, while hyperactive bowel sounds are characteristic of early small bowel obstruction.

The presence and location of abdominal tenderness on palpation is the most important step in diagnosing a patient with a surgical problem. Well-localized point tenderness in the right lower quadrant is the key finding in appendicitis. Left lower quadrant tenderness is present in acute diverticulitis. Palpation may also disclose any abnormal masses or hernias. A palpable pulsatile mass in a patient with abdominal pain necessitates emergency surgery for a suspected ruptured aneurysm. Patients should have a rectal exam to assess for masses and occult blood. A pelvic exam for females is mandatory. Cervical motion tenderness is found in patients with an ectopic pregnancy or pelvic inflammatory disease.

Routine laboratory investigation of the patient with acute abdominal pain includes a white blood cell count and differential, hematocrit, electrolytes, amylase, and urinalysis. The white blood cell count will be elevated in inflammatory conditions, with the differential displaying immature forms, the "left shift." The amylase is elevated in acute pancreatitis. Microscopic hematuria on urinalysis may indicate a renal stone. Pyuria suggests a urinary tract infection. Special tests might include a spot urine pregnancy test in women of child-bearing age, which may be positive in ectopic pregnancy. An electrocardiogram is necessary, especially in patients with known cardiac disease and in virtually all patients who require general anesthesia.

A chest x-ray should be obtained in the majority of patients. When taken in the upright position, it may show free air or pneumoperitoneum, which is usually present in a perforated ulcer. An abdominal x-ray can show the dilated bowel of obstruction or abnormal calcifications, suggesting a gallstone, renal stone, or appendicolith. Other special radiographic studies are used when specific diagnoses are entertained. A positive HIDA scan is diagnostic of acute cholecystitis, and an intravenous pyelogram will conclusively demonstrate a renal stone.

The correct diagnosis is arrived at by careful consideration and synthesis of the history, exam, and laboratory findings. At times, this means repeating the exam and/or laboratory tests serially. Clinicians must constantly weigh the risk of extensive diagnostic tests that may cause a delay against the need for early treatment. A specific diagnosis is not necessary to perform exploratory surgery. The clinician need only ascertain the probability of a life-threatening surgical problem to justify exploratory laparotomy.

While the diagnosis is being established, and prior to operative intervention, the patient requires resuscitation. An intravenous catheter should be inserted and a crystalloid solution of Ringer's lactate, a balanced salt solution, should be infused to correct hypovolemia. A Foley catheter may be inserted to monitor urinary output, and a nasogastric tube may be inserted to decompress the stomach and bowel. Antibiotics are administered. Electrolyte abnormalities should be corrected. For instance, the vomiting patient with resultant hypokalemia should receive intravenous potassium supplementation once an adequate urine output is established. The diabetic patient with hyperglycemia may require additional insulin during this period of stress. After resuscitation and diagnostic maneuvers are completed, consent is obtained and the patient is ready for transport to the operating room.

Case Histories

Considerable insight into the diagnosis and management of the acute abdomen can be gleaned from the following real-life case histories.

Case 1

> L.M. is a 40-year-old woman who presented with a 16-hour history of abdominal pain. She described the pain as migrating from the periumbilical area to the right lower abdomen. She complained of anorexia and nausea but denied vomiting, diarrhea, or menstrual irregularity. She was uncomfortable, her temperature was 37.6 °C, and there was marked right lower quadrant tenderness. Pelvic exam was normal. White blood cell count was 20,000 with a left shift; urinalysis and urine pregnancy test were negative. She underwent exploration via a transverse right

lower quadrant incision. An acutely inflamed nonperforated appendix was removed. She received liquids by mouth on the second postoperative day, and she was discharged from the hospital on postoperative Day 4.

Acute appendicitis is the most common condition of the abdomen requiring emergency surgical intervention. Though it is primarily a disease of young adults, it may occur at any age. The pathogenesis begins with obstruction of the narrow lumen of the appendix. Mucosal secretion persists, leading to appendiceal distention, inflammation, wall ischemia, and eventually perforation with abscess formation or peritonitis. Pain is characteristically periumbilical at first, later localizing to the right lower quadrant. Anorexia is almost always a constant feature of appendicitis. Vomiting, when it occurs, characteristically follows the onset of the pain, in contrast to gastroenteritis, where vomiting precedes the pain. Signs include mildly increased temperature and, most important, tenderness in the right lower quadrant at "McBurney's point," defined as a point one-third along the length of a line connecting the right iliac crest to the umbilicus. Laboratory studies include an elevated white blood cell count.

The primary complication of acute appendicitis is rupture, which accounts for at least half the mortality of the disease. The overall perforation rate is 15 to 30 percent, but it increases markedly to between 59 and 90 percent in the very young and the elderly, due to delay in diagnosis. Perforation leads to contamination of the peritoneal cavity by bacteria. The host may wall off this process with formation of an abscess, or the perforation may lead to generalized peritonitis, sepsis, and death. Clinicians must make the diagnosis early to prevent perforation.

Unfortunately, liberal use of exploration in all patients with vague symptoms or signs may lead to surgery in patients with a normal appendix and some other, nonsurgical, cause for their pain. A negative exploration carries a complication rate of 20 percent and is by no means inconsequential. On the other hand, studies in which the negative exploration rate is extremely low often show the highest perforation rates. This suggests that clinicians operating only on patients with obvious signs and symptoms may miss early cases of nonperforated appendicitis. Most surgeons would agree that a diagnostic accuracy rate of 80 percent is appropriate. The most common errors in diagnosis are mesenteric adenitis, pelvic inflammatory disease, ovarian cyst, and gastroenteritis. Appendicitis occurs in one of 2,000 pregnancies, and the point of maximal tenderness rises with the gestational period. The diagnosis may be difficult because of the normal leukocytosis found in pregnancy.

A particular diagnostic problem occurs in young adult females, where the negative laparotomy rate may increase to 45 percent, primarily because of the prevalence of ovarian cysts and pelvic inflammatory disease in this population.

Several clues may help the clinician make the correct diagnosis in this situation, especially in differentiating pelvic inflammatory disease from appendicitis. Pelvic inflammatory disease is associated with a longer duration of symptoms, often occurs within seven days of the menstrual period, and is characterized by cervical motion and bilateral adnexal tenderness. In contrast, appendicitis is commonly manifest by isolated right lower quadrant tenderness.

Prior to exploration, the patient is treated with intravenous fluids and an antibiotic that is effective against gram negative aerobic and anaerobic bacilli. Prospective studies have shown a decrease in wound infection rates when antibiotics are utilized.

After general anesthesia is established, the appendix is exposed through a transverse or oblique right lower quadrant incision centered on McBurney's point (see Figure 9-2). The appendix is removed by clamping and transecting it at its base and then closing the cecum by inverting the appendiceal stump with a purse-string suture. If a normal appendix is found, the pelvis is examined for other pathology. The small bowel is examined for an inflamed Meckel's diverticulum or Crohn's disease. An appendiceal abscess is drained with catheters. If the appendix was ruptured, the skin and subcutaneous tissues are packed open with saline-soaked gauze after closing the peritoneum and fascia. This helps prevent postoperative wound infection. The wound will heal by secondary intention, or a delayed primary closure can be carried out at the bedside.

The mortality of appendicitis is 0.1 percent overall, 3.0 percent when rupture is present, and 15.0 percent in an elderly patient. Death is usually due to sepsis. The higher mortality in the elderly patient is due to the higher perforation rate and associated medical problems. Wound infection occurs in 9 percent of patients. Postoperatively, a patient who has responded well without complications will become afebrile, have the return of normal bowel function with improvement in appetite, and have a well-healing, nondraining wound. In the case of an uncomplicated nonperforated appendicitis, the patient will be hospitalized for only several days. A major postoperative concern is the prompt diagnosis of wound infection or intraabdominal abscess requiring drainage and antibiotics. In the elderly patient, cardiac and respiratory status must be monitored closely for myocardial infarction, pneumonia, or pulmonary embolus.

Case 2

> E.R. is a 40-year-old female who developed severe abdominal pain six days after hip surgery for rheumatoid arthritis. At the time of consultation, she complained of a 24-hour history of severe abdominal pain, nausea, and vomiting. She had received nonsteroidal antiinflammatory medications for her arthritis. She was an ill-appearing female, with

Abdominal Surgery 117

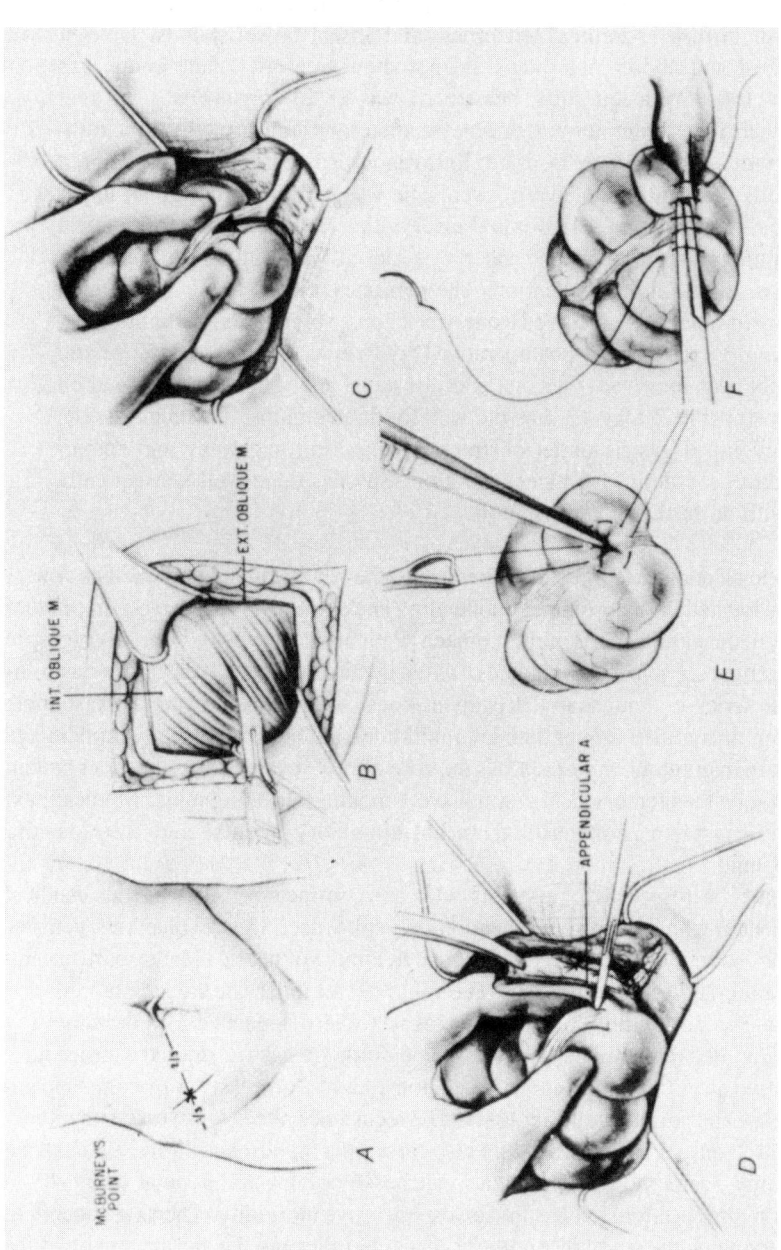

Figure 9-2 Appendectomy. *Source:* Reprinted from *Principles of Surgery* by S.I. Schwartz (Ed.), p. 1253, with permission of McGraw-Hill Book Company, © 1984.

blood pressure 100/70, pulse 108, and a temperature of 38.8 °C. There was diffuse abdominal tenderness and absent bowel sounds. Upright chest and abdominal x-rays did not show free air. White count was 14,100 with a left shift, hematocrit was 28.2, amylase was 50, and electrolytes were normal. A Foley catheter, nasogastric tube, and intravenous catheter were inserted. Intravenous Ringer's lactate, packed red cells, and antibiotics were given. She was explored through an upper midline incision. A perforated ulcer with a large volume of peritoneal spillage was found. The ulcer was closed with sutures bolstered by omentum, Graham plication. The peritoneal cavity was irrigated with warm saline. She received a one-week course of intravenous antibiotics. An ileus resolved by postoperative Day 8, at which time her nasogastric tube was removed. Her diet was advanced and she was discharged on postoperative Day 12. She did well for three months, at which time she developed gastric outlet obstruction, requiring vagotomy and antrectomy as a definitive ulcer operation. She has done well subsequently with no further ulcer symptoms.

Peptic ulcer disease affects two percent of the American population. The typical ulcer is located in the proximal duodenum. The etiology is excessive acid production from the parietal cells of the stomach. Patients usually have burning epigastric pain, relieved by food or antacids. After documentation by an upper gastrointestinal series or endoscopy, treatment consists of antacids and the histamine receptor antagonists cimetidine or ranitidine. Patients are usually middle-age adults; men outnumber women. As the case of E.R. exemplifies, the ulcer patient need not be the stereotypical compulsive, smoking, drinking male. Medications, including aspirin, nonsteroidal antiinflammatory agents, and steroids, are ulcerogenic.

Surgery is reserved for patients who are "refractory" to vigorous medical treatment or who develop complications of peptic ulcer disease: bleeding, perforation, or obstruction. The elective surgical treatment of peptic ulcer disease usually includes some form of vagotomy. The vagus nerves innervate the parietal cells and stimulate acid secretion. Since the vagus nerve also is needed for normal gastric emptying, its removal necessitates some form of gastric drainage procedure. Definitive ulcer operations include vagotomy and pyloroplasty, vagotomy and antrectomy, and parietal cell vagotomy. The recurrence rate is lowest after vagotomy and antrectomy, but this procedure also carries the highest morbidity. Parietal cell vagotomy—removal of only vagal branches supplying the parietal cells—has a higher recurrence rate but has the lowest operative morbidity. The exact operation will depend on the surgeon's preference and training and the age and health of the patient.

The perforated ulcer has a characteristic presentation. Patients can often give an exact time of onset of the abdominal pain. Half of the patients will have a prior history of ulcer symptoms. On examination, patients may show signs of volume depletion, such as tachycardia. This is due to sequestered fluid in the peritoneal cavity, inflamed by escaped duodenal chemical contents. Initially a sterile chemical peritonitis, this rapidly leads to bacterial peritonitis. The majority of patients will have diffuse abdominal tenderness and a "board-like" abdomen with absent bowel sounds. Nearly three-quarters of patients will have free air on an upright chest x-ray; hence, the correct diagnosis can often be made in the emergency department. The patient is resuscitated with intravenous fluids, and urine output is monitored to assess the adequacy of tissue perfusion. Broad spectrum antibiotics are administered.

There are two general surgical options: (1) simple closure, "Graham plication" of the duodenal perforation, or (2) the addition of one of the definitive ulcer operations discussed above (see Figure 9-3). The advantages of the Graham plication is its simplicity, especially when applied to the poor risk patient. The problem is recurrence of ulcer disease. The plication is a life-saving, temporary measure, but it does not treat the acid factor. Definitive surgery, such as vagotomy and antrectomy, has the advantage of a low recurrence rate, but it is a longer, technically more difficult, operation not undertaken lightly in a patient with gross contamination of the peritoneal cavity.

Studies of the natural history of the perforated ulcer patient after plication have clarified the above decision-making process. The majority of patients who develop a perforated ulcer with no previous history of ulcer disease and who undergo plication will remain asymptomatic in long-term follow-up. On the other hand, most patients with a previous ulcer history will have further ulcer disease if treated by plication alone. Thus, the surgical treatment of the perforated ulcer is plication when the patient has no prior ulcer history and a definitive ulcer procedure when a prior history is elicited. Other factors, such as the patient's age, associated illness, and degree of peritoneal contamination, must also be taken into consideration. The case of E.R. shows that simple plication, though life-saving, does not necessarily prevent further complications.

The overall mortality of a perforated ulcer is 7.4 percent, and the complication rate is 14.0 percent. Deaths and complications are due to peritonitis, bleeding, and pulmonary problems. Postoperatively, strict attention is paid to input/output and fluid balance and to aggressive pulmonary therapy. Patients usually receive a 7- to-10-day course of broad-spectrum antibiotics. Clinicians must remain alert to diagnose respiratory or intraabdominal septic complications early. Signs of improvement include normal temperature, a decreased fluid requirement with mobilization of administered resuscitative fluid, and resolution of the ileus. Patients are treated with antacids per nasogastric tube and intravenous histamine

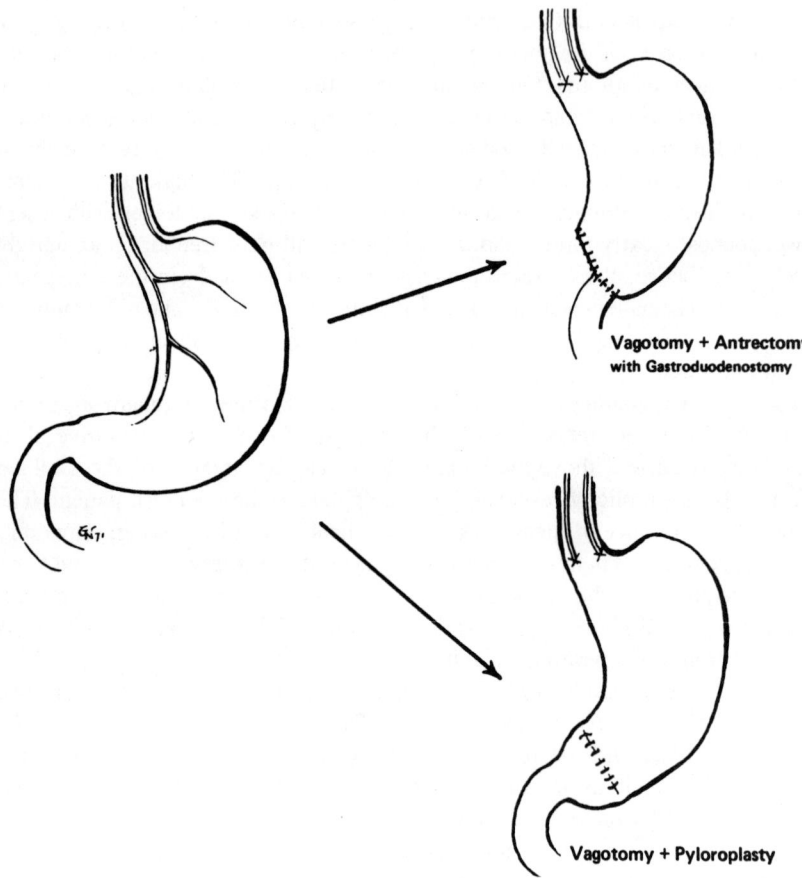

Figure 9-3 Operations for Duodenal Ulcer. *Source:* Reprinted from *Textbook of Surgery* by D.C. Sabiston (Ed.), p. 929, with permission of W.B. Saunders Company, © 1981.

---

blockers. Gastric pH can be measured and should be kept greater than 4 by titration with antacids. It is important to measure nasogastric output to ensure its proper replacement with an electrolyte solution. The nasogastric tube is removed when the patient passes flatus, has active bowel sounds, and has minimal amounts of drainage. After the nasogastric tube is removed, the diet can be gradually advanced. At the time of discharge, the patient should be afebrile off antibiotics, should be tolerating a regular diet, and have a well-healed wound.

Case 3

Z.R. is a 49-year-old female treated for diverticulitis with intravenous antibiotics twice in a two-year period. Diverticuli had been confirmed by barium enema. After the second episode, elective sigmoid resection was recommended. Unfortunately, four weeks before her scheduled elective sigmoid resection, she presented for the third time with left lower quadrant pain, fever, and chills. Temperature was 38.4 °C, and she had left lower quadrant tenderness and a palpable mass. Rectal exam was negative for occult blood. White count was 15,000 with a left shift, hematocrit was 38.6, and urinalysis was negative. She was started on intravenous antibiotics and a CT scan confirmed a sigmoid phlegmon. She underwent urgent sigmoid resection with creation of an end colostomy and mucus fistula for acute perforated diverticulitis. She did well postoperatively, becoming afebrile. Antibiotics were continued to complete a 10-day course. Liquids were given by mouth on postoperative Day 5. She was discharged on postoperative Day 12 on a regular diet with a well-functioning colostomy. Four months later, the colostomy was closed.

Diverticuli of the colon, usually located in the sigmoid colon, are outpouchings of the mucosal and submucosal layers through the muscular layers of the bowel. They are the result of increased intraluminal pressure and a weakness in the wall of the colon. One-third of Americans over the age of 60 have diverticuli. It is primarily a disease of Western society and is related to a diet with low fiber content. The majority of patients with diverticuli, however, are asymptomatic throughout life. A smaller group of patients will develop bleeding or inflammation, necessitating medical or surgical treatment.

Patients developing inflammation with left lower quadrant tenderness, fever, and leukocytosis have diverticulitis. The majority of patients with diverticulitis will respond to medical treatment consisting of antibiotics. However, one-third will either have persistent or recurrent attacks, abscess formation, peritonitis, fistula, or obstruction and will require surgery. Patients with recurrent attacks can often be scheduled for an elective sigmoid resection with preliminary bowel prep after the acute attack has subsided. This allows for primary resection and primary anastomosis in one operation, with relatively low morbidity and mortality.

The major problem is with those patients with unprepared acutely inflamed sigmoid colon who require immediate surgery. They may have peritonitis and an acute abdomen with the perforated diverticulitis found at laparotomy, or they may present with a phlegmon or abscess unresponsive to antibiotics. In this situation, primary resection and primary anastomosis are dangerous, with an increased risk of anastomotic leak, intraabdominal abscess, and sepsis. In this situation, most surgeons would prefer some form of "staged" procedure. One option is a two-stage procedure. In the first acute stage, the diseased sigmoid is resected, if technically possible; and, rather than a primary anastomosis, the proximal colon is brought out as an end colostomy and the distal end as a mucus fistula (see

Figure 9-4). The patient recovers and then, during a second elective hospitalization, the colostomy is closed.

Overall mortality for perforated acute diverticulitis is 11 percent. The patients are older (mean age 61) and often have associated illness. Postoperative complications include myocardial infarction, wound infection, intraabdominal sepsis, and pneumonia. Occasionally, young adults, aged less than 40, will develop diverticulitis. This population has been shown to be at high risk for further problems, with two-thirds eventually requiring colon resection.

Occasionally, patients may harbor a malignancy in the colon, as a cause of their symptoms or coexistent with diverticulitis. For this reason, patients who recover from an acute attack of "diverticulitis" should receive a barium enema and sigmoidoscopy to rule out carcinoma, in addition to establishing the diagnosis of diverticular disease. Fistulas may occur between the inflamed sigmoid colon and adjacent organs, most commonly the bladder. Patients usually have urinary symptoms, which may include pneumaturia. Diagnosis can be confirmed with cystoscopy, barium enema, and intravenous pyelogram. Surgery can often be done electively with the benefit of a bowel preparation. Sigmoid resection is performed with primary anastomosis, combined with bladder repair and drainage.

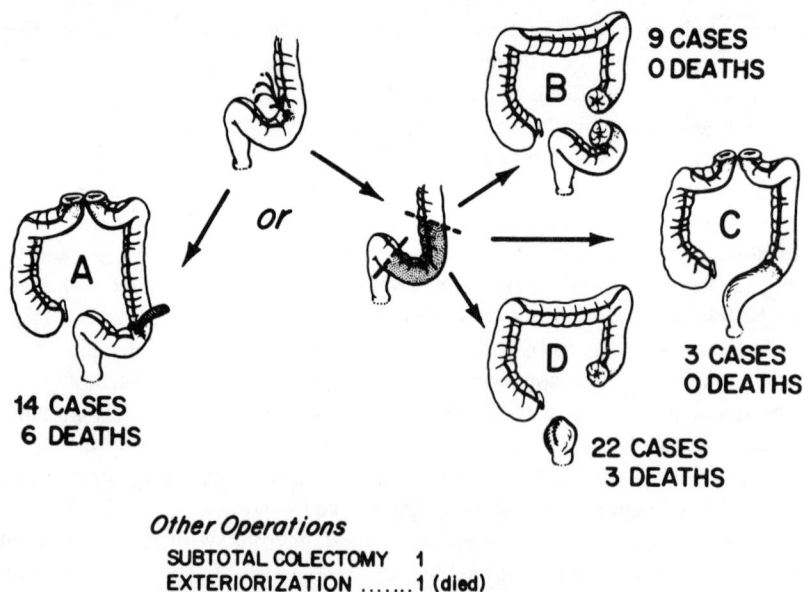

Figure 9-4 Operations for Perforated Diverticulitis. *Source:* Reprinted from *Annals of Surgery* Vol. 200, p. 472, with permission of J.B. Lippincott Company, © 1984.

POSTANESTHESIA CARE

The management of the patient with the acute abdomen requires a team approach. Physicians and nurses in the emergency department, radiology suite, operating room, PACU, ICU, and surgical floor will all be involved in the care of the patient. The initial problem is diagnosis and determination of whether or not the patient needs surgery, further observation, additional special tests, or medical treatment. Patients with a surgical illness undergo resuscitation with intravenous fluids, and antibiotics are administered. Surgery is prompt. The postoperative course will depend on the exact nature of the problem and the patient's age and other illnesses. Patients are monitored closely for wound and intraabdominal infections and respiratory complications.

In addition to basic postanesthesia admission assessment parameters, there are special considerations in caring for postoperative abdominal surgical patients. The location of the incision is of particular concern. Diaphragmatic descent during inspiration can cause pain. This is especially true of high abdominal procedures, such as cholecystectomy. As the patient "splints" on the wound, adequate air exchange may be compromised. Small titrated doses of narcotics will allow these patients to breathe effectively.

During each vital sign measurement the dressing should be checked, as well as the character of the abdomen. Hypotension coupled with a hard, rigid, and distended abdomen could mean intraabdominal bleeding and a return trip to the operating room. Nasogastric and Sump tubes will need to be monitored closely for patency as well as for the amount and type of drainage.

PACU nurses must also be aware of the fact that patients with preexisting cardiac disease require diligent vigilance. High abdominal procedures that have the potential for interfering with air exchange pose the danger of upsetting the balance between myocardial oxygen supply and demand. A situation such as this must be prevented, since it can lead to ischemia and possibly infarction. In all likelihood, these patients will have a Swan-Ganz catheter in place. Careful monitoring of pulmonary artery and capillary wedge pressures will quickly alert PACU nurses to any impending myocardial ischemia. Inadequate airway integrity, tachycardia, hypotension, fever, and physical or psychological distress call for cautious assessment and intervention, since all of these factors can increase myocardial oxygen demand.

Patients with associated risk factors for coronary artery disease (obesity, diabetes, hypertension, hyperlipidemia, and so on) who have never experienced angina pose a similar challenge. Given the stress of surgery and anesthesia, the development of ischemia is a potential danger for these individuals as well; thus, they will require the same postanesthesia care.

Despite the serious nature of diseases that affect the abdominal organs, the majority of patients do well, recover, and return to their premorbid health.

BIBLIOGRAPHY

Almy, F.P., and Howell, D.A. "Diverticular Disease of the Colon." *New England Journal of Medicine* 302(1980):324–331.

Auguste, L., Borrero, E., and Wise, L. "Surgical Management of Perforated Colonic Diverticulitis." *Archives of Surgery* 120(1985):450–452.

Berry, J., and Mait, R.A. "Appendicitis Near Its Centenary." *Annals of Surgery* 200(1984):567–575.

Boey, J., Lee, N.W., Koo, J., Lom, P.H.M., Wong, J., and Ong, G.B. "Immediate Definitive Surgery for Perforated Duodenal Ulcers." *Annals of Surgery* 196(1982):338–344.

Bongard, F., Landers, D.V., and Lewis, F. "Differential Diagnosis of Appendicitis and Pelvic Inflammatory Disease." *American Journal of Surgery* 150(1985):90–96.

Classen, J.N., Bonardi, R., O'Mara, C.S., Finney, D.C.W., and Sterioff, S. "Surgical Treatment of Acute Diverticulitis by Staged Procedures." *Annals of Surgery* 184(1976):582–586.

Diethelm, A.G. "The Acute Abdomen." In *Textbook of Surgery,* edited by D.C. Sabiston, Jr., 790–809. Philadelphia: W.B. Saunders, 1986.

Griffin, G.E., and Organ, C.H. "The Natural History of the Perforated Duodenal Ulcer Treated by Suture Plication." *Annals of Surgery* 183(1976):382–385.

Lewis, F.R., Holcroft, J.W., Boey, J., and Dunphy, E. "Appendicitis. A Critical Review of Diagnosis and Treatment in 1,000 Cases." *Archives of Surgery* 110(1975):677–684.

Owens, B.J., and Hamit, H.F. "Appendicitis in the Elderly." *Annals of Surgery* 187 (1978):392–396.

Sawyers, J.L., Herrington, L., Mulheris, J.L., Whitehead, W.A., Mody, B., and Marsh, J. "Acute Perforated Ulcer." *Archives of Surgery* 110(1975):527–536.

Schwartz, S.I., and Storer, E.H. "Manifestations of Gastrointestinal Disease." In *Principles of Surgery,* edited by S.I. Schwartz, 1021–1062. New York: McGraw-Hill Book Co., 1984.

Chapter 10

Postanesthesia Care After Vascular Surgery

Malcolm O. Perry, M.D.

INTRODUCTION

Arterial diseases rank among the most common illnesses of mankind and each year are responsible for an increasing number of deaths in the Western world.[1] Atherosclerosis, the most common of these arteriopathies, has been the subject of intensive study over the last decade. It is now clear that there is a strong hereditary predisposition to atherosclerosis and that certain groups of people have metabolic problems that lead to the more severe forms of the disease. These include patients with diabetes mellitis, obesity, or disorders of fat metabolism and some patients with diseases involving the connective tissues. Cigarette smoking has a particularly deleterious influence on the progression of peripheral arterial occlusive lesions. Cigarette smoking causes vasospasm and increases the tendency of the blood to clot. It has been clearly demonstrated that this is one of the most potent aggravating factors accounting for the increasing severity of arterial occlusive disease.

GENERAL CONSIDERATIONS

Several important morphological features have been delineated. Among these, the tendency of atherosclerosis to be segmentally accentuated rather than diffuse is particularly important.[2] This segmental nature produces disease that is primarily located where the vessels branch and curve, and thus preserve relatively normal proximal and distal arterial beds. This allows the vascular surgeon to "leap over the etiological wall" and effectively treat the patient, although the precise cause of the disease remains unknown.[3] Atherosclerotic plaques during their formative stages are eccentrically located within the arterial wall, sparing one side. This location allows bypass surgery to be applied. Studies have shown that, in some cases, the atherosclerotic lesions tend to become stable late in the course of the disease; thus, successful vascular reconstruction procedures are quite durable, especially if the known risk factors can be controlled.

The histologic features of atherosclerosis are consistent with the process beginning with the degeneration of smooth muscle cells in the arterial walls.[4] Changes in blood lipids, both in content and quality, exert undesirable influences upon the progression of the plaques. Prolonged hypertension has also been shown to accelerate the progression of the lesions. Although some atherosclerotic plaques may become stable late in the course of the disease, others are subject to sudden and increasing progression, particularly if intraplaque hemorrhage occurs. Hemorrhage within the wall of the artery is a particularly common finding in plaques that affect the bifurcation of the carotid arteries and may be responsible for sudden progression to occlusion and the emergence of severe symptoms.[5]

Other arteropathies, such as fibromuscular dysplasia, Marfan's disease, Erlos-Danlos disease, and other processes that destroy or modify the integrity of the arterial wall may contribute to progressive arterial disease. However, these processes occur less frequently and are poorly understood. Their etiology is obscure and the factors that affect their progress are unknown.[6]

Pathophysiology

Arterial occlusive disease that produces disturbances in blood flow will result in various clinical syndromes, depending on which target organ is subjected to ischemia. Interference with blood flow to the brain, for example, may produce small strokes or even frank strokes. Reduction in blood flow to the kidney may produce renovascular hypertension, and ischemia of the bowel can cause disturbances in absorptive and digestive functions. Although the basic problem remains the same—inadequate blood flow—the clinical syndromes are different and will be considered separately.

Cerebrovascular Occlusive Disease

The relationship between extracranial arterial occlusive disease and stroke was obscured for many years because of incomplete examination of the extracranial vessels; the standard pathological examination does not include direct visualization of the carotid and vertebral arteries in the neck. It is now apparent that segmental atherosclerosis and ulcerative plaques occur in the extracranial cerebral vessels as in other arteries.[7] The most common pattern of involvement is the presence of atherosclerotic plaques at the carotid bifurcation and the origins of the vertebral arteries. More than 50 percent of affected patients have multiple lesions. Since the circle of Willis, as depicted in the anatomy book, is intact in no more than half of the patients, many of these people will experience episodes of cerebrovascular insufficiency as a result of progressive occlusion of the extracranial cervical vessels.

Patients with cerebrovascular insufficiency are often divided into one of three groups, according to the type of symptoms. Some patients may have transient attacks of cerebral ischemia (TIA); these usually present with transient neurological dysfunction. In the territory of the carotid artery, this usually appears as numbness, paresthesias, and/or motor dysfunction of the contralateral extremity. Occasionally, it is associated with intermittent episodes of blindness in the ipsilateral eye. The pathological mechanisms causing these symptoms include the distal embolization of platelet, fibrin, or atheromatous debris from the atherosclerotic plaques at the bifurcation of the carotid artery. Such emboli may also come from lesions of the aortic arch, great vessels, and heart; but these are less frequent. In some cases, the multiple atherosclerotic plaques may reduce the overall cerebral blood flow to the extent that global symptoms of decreased profusion occur rather than focal temporary strokes. Patients occasionally are admitted with strokes in evolution (progressive strokes) with waxing and waning of their neurological symptoms. If untreated, these people usually proceed to the third category of frank strokes. They are admitted with a cerebral infarct; and, though they may be susceptible to measures that prevent further cerebrovascular disease, once brain injury occurs they are less likely to respond to either medical or surgical therapy.[8] It is clear that, in the treatment of cerebrovascular insufficiency from arterial occlusive disease, the identification of patients with carotid artery disease is an important concept, since only removal of the plaque can retard the progressive nature of the disease.

Acquired Diseases of the Aorta

Abdominal aortic diseases are usually divided into two groups: aneurysmal or obstructive. The abdominal infrarenal aorta is the most common location for aneurysms; 95 percent of aortic aneurysms occur here.[9] This is thought to be related to deficiencies in blood supply to the aortic wall, but there is also a strong hereditary predisposition for the disease. In families in which this tendency is evident, the disease occurs with equal frequency in men and women; otherwise, it is seen several times more commonly in men than in women. In one-third to one-half of patients, not only is the infrarenal abdominal aorta involved, but the iliac arteries also are affected. A diagnosis of aneurysm is made when the dilation exceeds twice the diameter of the normal aorta above and below; this usually means that an aneurysm of 4 cm or greater is considered to be significant and in most patients should be treated surgically. Associated aneurysms occur in these patients, most often in the popliteal arteries and the descending thoracic aorta and, occasionally, in the common femoral arteries.

Patients with aneurysmal disease rarely have symptoms unless the aneurysm becomes so large that it causes pressure problems by encroaching upon surrounding structures. More often, the disease remains silent until the aneurysm expands sufficiently and the wall becomes thin and rupture occurs. Therein lies the most severe problem in this disease: it may first be detected only because of rupture, hemorrhage, or shock. Noninvasive studies (ultrasound and computed tomography) have now permitted the diagnosis of these dangerous lesions prior to their becoming symptomatic, resulting in early effective treatment to prevent the often fatal outcome in patients with ruptured aneurysms.

Aortofemoral Occlusive Disease

Obstructive disease usually involves the aortoiliac and the femoral system, although in its early stages it may be confined to the aorta and the common iliac arteries.[10] Most patients have involvement of the aorta, common iliacs, and femoral arteries. In fact, over 90 percent of patients with the disease will have occlusive lesions affecting the superficial femoral artery at the adductor hiatus above the knee. These patients primarily seek assistance because of calf and hip claudication. In the usual pattern, because of narrowing of the aortoiliac system and severe narrowing or occlusion of the superficial femoral artery, calf claudication occurring after walking one to two blocks is the most common symptom. Calf claudication is a benign disease; in only 10 to 15 percent of patients will the disease be progressive and threaten viability of the limb. Selection of these patients for repair will depend on the extent of the obstructive disease and the severity of those symptoms that interfere with the patient's ability to earn a living. In most situations, operations are not recommended for claudication unless they fall into one of those two categories. When the disease is progressive, vascular reconstructive procedures are required to preserve the limbs.

Splanchnic Arteries

Obstructive disease involving the renal arteries has as its main manifestation the production of renovascular hypertension. In patients with severely progressive disease, viability of the kidneys may be threatened; and it is not uncommon for people with severe renovascular hypertension, if untreated, to progress to total occlusion and finally loss of kidney function. Identification of these patients requires an extensive evaluation, including arteriography and the detection and measurement of renin produced by the affected kidneys. In appropriate patients, either dilation of the renal artery or direct vascular reconstruction is often feasible, thus removing the stimulus for the production of renin and the associated hypertension and preserving kidney function.[11]

Visceral ischemic syndromes are rare, especially in their chronic form. They are most often due to mesenteric emboli that come from the heart and block the mesenteric artery, but they may be related to atherosclerotic lesions that involve the celiac and the superior mesenteric and inferior mesenteric arteries. The patient almost invariably has pain after eating and resulting weight loss, because of the fear of the pain that accompanies eating. There are no tests of value other than arteriography. Direct reconstructive procedures are available and, if applied before severe ischemia has caused gangrene, they are effective.

ANESTHETIC CONSIDERATIONS

Atherosclerotic disease involves the majority of the large and medium arteries throughout the body; but, as previously described, it tends to be segmentally accentuated in areas where vessels branch and curve. When patients with diffuse atherosclerosis are considered for operative procedures, the involvement of multiple arterial beds poses a serious problem in planning the operation. For example, patients with aortofemoral occlusive disease have a high incidence of associated hypertension (over 60 percent), and at least a third of these patients will have evidence of coronary occlusive disease.[12,13] Patients with cerebrovascular disease are even more inclined to have associated coronary artery disease. It has in fact been amply demonstrated by numerous investigators that an integral part of the evaluation and treatment of patients with abdominal aortic and carotid artery disease is a careful evaluation of their cardiac status. Many of these people require stress tests, radionuclide cardiac evaluations, and, in some instances, coronary arteriography and coronary artery bypass procedures prior to definitive treatment of arterial disease elsewhere.

The Anesthetic Agent

Although the type of anesthetic agent and the method of its administration will vary from patient to patient, depending on the severity of the cardiac disease, all such patients share a common problem: Agents that strongly depress myocardial function will tend to exert a deleterious effect during and immediately following the operation. Although conduction anesthesia and local anesthesia may be applied to patients with lesions in the carotid system, and occasionally to patients with occlusive problems in the femoral popliteal system, more often than not general anesthesia is chosen in order to maintain a satisfactory airway and oxygen delivery. In recent years, anesthesiologists have selected as their first choice the narcotic type of anesthesia used so successfully during cardiac operations in these very susceptible patients. A skillful blend of these agents, along with knowledge of those drugs that are used to modify cardiac preload and afterload, are essential in the successful management of the patient during the perioperative period.

Monitoring

Perioperative monitoring of patients is usually done with a Swan-Ganz catheter, which permits measurements of cardiac output as well as measurements of pressure. Changes in cardiac function are common, dictating the use of pharmacological therapy. In some cases, adjunctive measures, including the use of aortic balloon pumps, special cardiotonic drugs, and even on occasion emergency coronary artery bypass procedures, will be required.

Generally, patients are relatively unstable during the first few hours following major vascular procedures; however, instability is more of a problem in patients who have had cerebrovascular operations. Although poorly understood, it has been repeatedly observed that patients who have had carotid artery and vertebrobasilar artery operations tend to be hemodynamically unstable for 6 to 12 hours following the operation. Some investigators believe that this is a result of ischemia of the vasomotor centers in the brain stem during the course of the operation, while others suspect that it is caused by various changes in the elaboration of hormones (specifically brain renin and other neurotransmitters) as a result of alterations in cerebral blood flow. Whatever the cause, it is clear that these patients are particularly susceptible to any drug that has as a side effect the potential of changing vasomotor reactivity. This includes the opiates as well as antihypertensive medications, tranquilizers, and other agents with vasoactive properties. These drugs should be used extremely cautiously and in very limited dosages, if at all. When their use is necessary for the control of blood pressure, drugs such as nitroprusside (Nipride) are given, but they are carefully monitored with a continuous recording of blood pressure from an arterial line. In most situations, the unusual sensitivity to these drugs will resolve over the ensuing 12 hours or so, and by the first postoperative day the patient will return to the preoperative status. This is not invariably so, however, and the patients must be followed closely until it is evident that the problem no longer exists.

SURGICAL PROCEDURES

Endarterectomy

The operative management of arteriosclerosis is usually dictated by the nature of the lesion. Occlusive disease requires some type of disobliteration of the arterial tree or use of a bypass technique, and aneurysms are treated by grafting. The operative methods basically employ one of three techniques, or some combinations of them.

Thromboendarterectomy is a method of removing the diseased inner core of the atherosclerotic vessel. In this operation, the intima and almost all of the media are removed, leaving behind only the external elastic membrane and the adventitia. This rather thin wall is quite strong, and late aneurysmal dilation of such a repaired vessel is rare. The technique of endarterectomy is applied usually to localized areas of stenosis, and therefore is often used in treating plaques at the carotid bifuration and at the orifices of arteries in the aortofemoral tree. In such vessels, the disease is relatively limited, and there is a transition to normal intima distally. In more advanced disease, endarterectomy may not be possible because of the extensive nature of the lesion; in such situations, grafting is required. Carotid endarterectomy is the most common operation performed on the carotid bifurcation and rarely requires a graft; but, on occasion, patients with very small arteries who also require a long arteriotomy will require a patch graft closure in order to widen accurately the artery. Autogenous vein is usually chosen, although various forms of plastic prostheses are used as alternatives.

Arterial Grafts

The treatment of aortic aneurysmal disease requires a grafting procedure. Most commonly, the graft is sewn end-to-end to the normal abdominal aorta just below the renal arteries and is then attached to the common iliac, external iliac, or common femoral arteries, depending on the extent of involvement. The aneurysm is not totally resected, but the posterior wall and lateral walls are left intact in order not to disturb the adherent veins. A similar procedure is applied if the patient has popliteal or femoral aneurysms. Usually, in these situations the aneurysm is either removed or bypassed with a prosthetic Dacron graft; occasionally a polytetrafluorethylene graft is selected.

Patients who have occlusive disease of the aorta are treated in a similar fashion. Although endarterectomy was previously employed for localized lesions of the aorta and iliac system, more recently a bypass grafting technique is often utilized. The location of the bypass is dictated by the extent of the disease. For the most part, the technique is similar to that used in the treatment of aortic aneurysms. Grafts are sewed to the aorta just below the renal arteries and then attached distally at some accessible area of the large arteries beyond the diseased segments.

In patients who have occlusive disease involving the splanchnic vessels or the renal arteries, similar techniques are employed. Although endarterectomy may be used in certain cases where the disease is restricted to the orifice of the vessel, more commonly the obstructing lesions are bypassed with autogenous saphenous vein taken from the leg, with the hypogastric artery from the pelvis, or with a suitable tube graft made of Dacron or polytetrafluroethylene.

POSTANESTHESIA CARE

All patients who have atherosclerosis have common risk factors. Although certain groups of patients, such as those with cerebrovascular operations, appear to be more susceptible to alterations in hemodynamics during the postoperative period, all of these patients require careful monitoring to detect and treat the problems. High blood pressure and coronary artery disease are common in all of these groups; and, if these problems are not corrected prior to the elective vascular repair, they will require a great deal of attention in order to ensure a smooth convalescence.

It is common practice for the patient to be brought to the PACU with an arterial line in place, usually in a radial artery. Moreover, the patient will usually have a central line and/or a Swan-Ganz catheter in place. In patients who have full monitoring (an arterial line and a Swan-Ganz catheter), it is possible to obtain mixed venous blood samples that provide a great deal of information regarding the need for cardiopulmonary assistance.[14,15] Moreover, with a triple lumen catheter in place, it is possible, using cold bolus dilution techniques, to measure cardiac output and thus determine if the patient has adequate cardiac performance. In addition, the PACU nurse may make an assessment regarding the need for extra volume by measuring pressures in the pulmonary artery, pulmonary wedge pressures, and atrial pressures. Such assessments can provide valuable information regarding cardiopulmonary performance.

Most patients are transferred from the PACU and kept in the ICU for one to two days; when their cardiac and hemodynamic parameters are returned to a satisfactory position, they can go back to their private rooms. At this time, it is usual to return the patients to their preoperative medications, with the addition of whatever drugs are needed to maintain stable cardiopulmonary activity.

Among the problems that emerge in the immediate postoperative period, there is always the possibility of thrombosis of the repaired artery. This is more likely to occur if the patient experiences hypotension, such as might occur following antihypertensive medication. Extreme care is required in the treatment of these patients in order to prevent such hypotensive episodes. A fresh vascular reconstruction is particularly susceptible to thrombosis if blood pressure and blood flow fall for any reason. On occasion, patients who have reduced cardiac output may also suffer hypotension leading to graft thrombosis. In general, it is easy to detect this condition by routine examination of distal limb pulses and measurement of limb blood pressures, utilizing Doppler techniques or other noninvasive methods. A sudden change in blood pressure or a sudden alteration in distal blood flow is an indication for more specific studies, which may or may not include arteriography. In many instances, it is more expeditious and more fruitful to return the patient immediately to the operating room for removal of the clot. Of course, removal of the clot must be accompanied by correction of those factors that caused the hypotension.

It is also important to monitor such patients regarding their cerebrovascular status, since they frequently have combined system disease.[16] Recurrent neurological evaluation, as well as evaluation of distal pulses, is essential in the follow-up. If, following a carotid endarterectomy, the patient develops a neurological deficit as manifested by visual problems or paresthetic or motor dysfunction, one might suspect that the patient has either a thrombosis of the repaired carotid artery or a development of mural clots within the artery with thromboembolism to the brain. In these situations, an immediate noninvasive evaluation is required, perhaps followed by arteriography. If the patient develops an acute stroke (suggesting that the artery was occluded), it is usually best to return the patient immediately to the operating room to reopen the artery rather than to delay for studies—a delay that might permit the brain to enter the infarct phase.

All of these difficult problems require immediate attention and consultation among the various services. Their early detection and treatment is essential for a successful outcome in the patient.

NOTES

1. M.E. DeBakey, "Basic Concepts of Therapy in Arterial Disease," *Journal of the American Medical Association* 10(1963):484–498.
2. M.O. Perry, "Progress in Peripheral Vascular Surgery," *Western Journal of Medicine* 3(1976): 194–218.
3. DeBakey, "Basic Concepts," 484.

4. C.J. Schwartz, E.A. Sprague, and J.L. Kelley, "Atheroma: An Update," *Hospital Medicine* (December 1982):37–48.

5. R.J. Lusby et al., "Carotid Plaque Hemorrhage," *Archives of Surgery* 117(1982):1479–1488.

6. Perry, "Progress."

7. *Ibid.*

8. J.M. Giordano et al., "Timing of Carotid Endarterectomy After Stroke," *Journal of Vascular Surgery* 2(1985):250–254.

9. E.S. Crawford and C. Stowe, "True Aneurysms of the Aorta and Iliac Arteries," in *Vascular Surgery—A Comprehensive Review*, ed. W.S. Moore (New York, Grune & Stratton, 1983), 169–232.

10. Perry, "Progress."

11. *Ibid.*

12. *Ibid.*

13. Crawford and Stowe, "True Aneurysms," 432, 436, 438.

14. Crawford and Stowe, "True Aneurysms," 432, 433.

15. N.R. Hertzer and R. Arison, "Cumulative Stroke and Survival Ten Years After Carotid Endarterectomy," *Journal of Vascular Surgery* 2(1985):661–668.

16. *Ibid.*

Chapter 11
Postanesthesia Care After Burn Surgery

Michael Marano, M.D.
Joseph M. Thomas, M.D.

GENERAL CONSIDERATIONS

Burns are a common injury in the United States. They occur in people of all ages, in all sizes and distributions, at work or play, and they are not limited to certain geographic, social, racial, or economic groups. Most people who have sustained small burns recognize the pain and loss of function involved. The common kitchen accident causing a small fingertip injury involves a surface area of only a fraction of 1 percent. By comparison, burns requiring admission to an acute care facility frequently involve a surface area of 15 percent or more. Burns requiring hospitalization in a specialized burn treatment facility include third-degree burns (more than 10 percent of body surface), second-degree burns (more than 25 percent of body surface in adults), and smaller burns with such complicating features as extremes of age, preexisting disease, associated trauma, child abuse, or inhalation injury.

Try to imagine the potential for disability and suffering that an auto mechanic or a firefighter must endure when admitted to a burn center. Unlike cancer or heart disease patients, burn victims are generally younger and, if they survive the injury, have the potential for a long and productive life. Although the injury occurs in only a few seconds, the transformation from health to severe disability may last many years. Therefore, major thermal injuries requiring treatment at regional burn centers are major life stresses with life-long consequences.

It is useful to view the burned individual as a "chronic" trauma patient, that is, as a person who will likely require repeated operations and long intensive care unit exposure and who may suffer a number of medical complications on the way to recovery. The trauma may continue for years as social isolation, disability, impairment, and economic loss. Nevertheless, with the team approach, acute accident victims may still lead productive and meaningful lives. The burn team consists of physicians, nurses, occupational therapists, social workers, nutritionists, hospital administration personnel, and burn center employees.

Types of Burn Injuries

There are a number of important factors that must be considered in order to understand the thermally injured patient. First, one should remember that the skin consists of the epidermis and dermis with skin appendages (see Figure 11-1). Partial-thickness injuries affect both the epidermis and part of the dermis, although epithelization is still possible because viable tissue remains. Full-thickness injuries destroy the entire skin, creating a thick insensate leathery eschar that tenaciously adheres to the subcutaneous tissue and impairs wound closure. The eschar must be excised or allowed to separate on its own prior to skin grafting or to secondary healing.

The skin serves three major functions:

1. maintaining normal body temperature
2. preventing fluid loss by forming a barrier impermeable to water
3. preventing infectious organisms from gaining access to the host

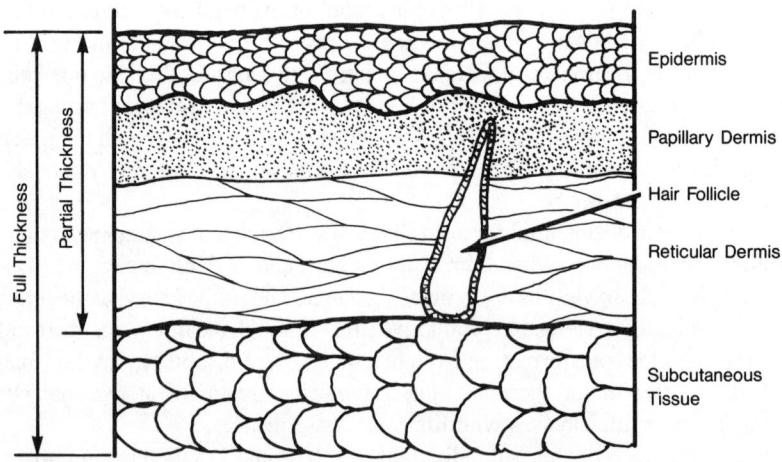

Figure 11-1 Normal Skin, Indicating Extent of Partial- and Full-Thickness Injuries

With significant skin loss, these homeostatic functions are impaired or lost, thereby rendering the victim susceptible to fluid loss, hypothermia, and infection. At the time of injury, the body begins to change physiologically (see Figure 11-2). There is loss of capillary integrity, with resultant sequestration of body fluids from the intravascular compartment to the interstitial and intracellular compartments, resulting in functional volume depletion. Initial fluid resuscitation must be calculated and then modified, based on physiological parameters, in order to maintain homeostasis. Patients with significant injuries become grossly edematous during initial fluid resuscitation. It is not unusual for an adult weighing 70 kg with a 50 percent body surface area injury to require 14,000 mL of fluid in the first 24 hours postinjury to maintain adequate renal perfusion.

Fluid resuscitation begins by using Ringer's lactate calculated from one of several formulas. The widely used Parkland formula is as follows: First 24 hours: 4 mL/kg/percent body surface area; administer one-half in the first 8 hours, one-half in the next 16 hours. After 24 hours, free water (5 percent dextrose) and colloid (5 percent albumin) are given, based on urine output, daily weight, and serum sodium concentration.

The mechanism of the injury may have prognostic implications. Burns may occur by flame, hot liquids, contact with hot objects, explosions, chemicals, electricity, or radiation. Seasonal variations exist. Summer brings Fourth-of-July celebrations and brushfires, while winter is darkened by Christmas-tree fires, by mishaps with heating devices or ovens, and by the homeless trying to keep warm with street fires.

Often there are extenuating social factors involved in burn injury, for example, child abuse and neglect, drug addiction, suicide, homicide, arson, and pyromania or other mental illness. Frequent admissions to large city burn centers include abused children with inflicted scald injuries, the homeless, substance abusers,

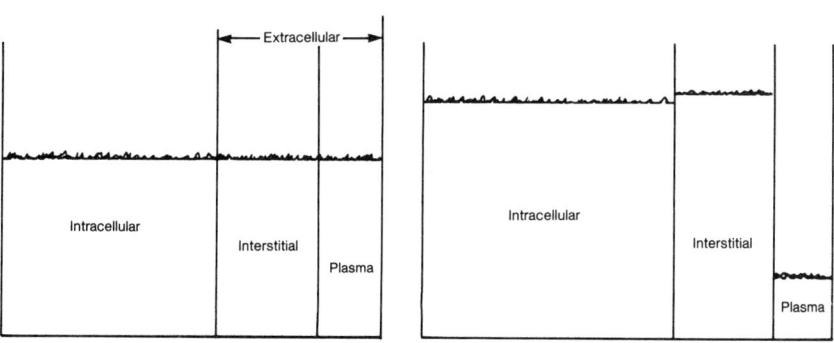

Figure 11-2 Shift of Body Fluids After Thermal Injury

children who play with matches, and the careless who smoke in bed. In addition, occupational dangers exist for firefighters, transit workers, factory workers, chemists, electricians, and those who work with volatile liquid and petroleum products. Children may gain access to corrosive household chemicals, while adults are commonly injured in household accidents.

The depth of injury may be immediately apparent; but, more often, burns require careful observation to determine whether or not surgery is needed, because the extent of the injury evolves over a period of days. The extent of injury may be roughly estimated using the "rule of nines," which indicates approximate body surface area (see Figure 11-3). In general, the extent and depth of the injury, along with the age of the individual, will determine the morbidity and mortality of the burn. The very young and old tolerate severe stress less well.

Wound Care and Potential Complications

There are many potential complications in burn injuries. Smoke inhalation may require prolonged endotracheal intubation and tracheostomy. Burn wounds may become infected. Pneumonia, intravenous line sepsis, urinary tract infections, and generalized sepsis constitute the majority of infectious complications.

A hypermetabolic response follows injury; thus, a high caloric diet is required if the patient is to survive the insult. This hypermetabolism and the resetting of the temperature-regulating mechanism of the hypothalamus explain the "fever" of burn patients. With the loss of large surface areas of skin, heat loss may be excessive. Ambient temperature should be maintained to keep the burn patient above 37 °C. This may require that the surgical team and burn center workers perform their tasks in extreme heat. Normal room temperature to the average person feels like the North Pole to burn victims.

General wound care consists of daily debridement and hydrotherapy and coverage of full- and partial-thickness burns with topical antibiotic creams. Depending on the institution, open or closed dressings are used. Systemic antibiotics are used only for documented infections and surgical prophylaxis. As tetanus prophylaxis is mandatory, this issue should be addressed upon admission.

The decision to operate is based on close inspection of the wounds. Obvious full-thickness injuries of large surface areas need grafting. Deep partial-thickness burns may require grafting to improve function or cosmesis. The timing of surgery may also be crucial. With severe injuries, operations to preserve life or limb may have to be performed under less than optimal circumstances. In recent years, early excision within one week of injury has become the standard.

The three most common topical chemotherapeutic agents are silver sulfadiazine (Silvadene), sodium mafenide (Sulfamylon), and silver nitrate, one-half percent.

Burn Surgery 139

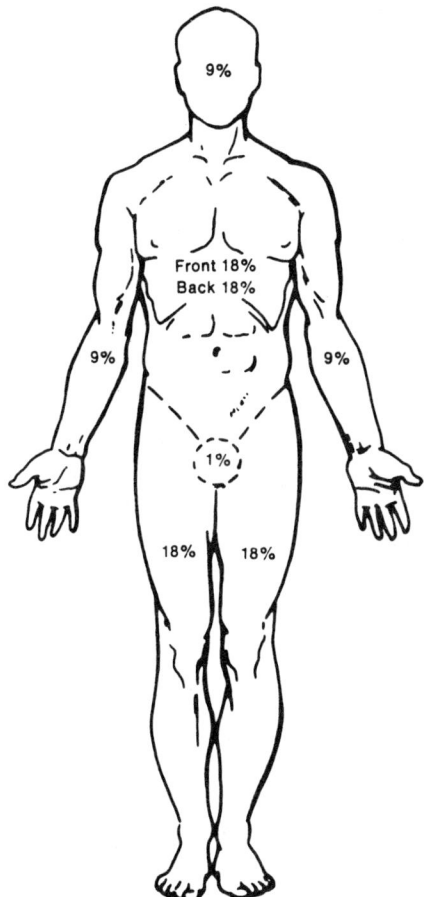

Note: The rule of nines is used to measure the percentage of body burned. Adding together the percent burned will give the nurse an estimate of the extent of body surface burned.

Figure 11-3 Rule of Nines for Burn Patients. *Source:* Reprinted from *Emergency Care in the Streets* by N.L. Caroline, P. 359, with permission of Little, Brown & Company, © 1983.

Silver sulfadiazine is opaque white, is painless upon application, and has moderate eschar penetration and a broad antibacterial spectrum. It is used preferentially for second- and third-degree burn wounds. Its disadvantages include transient neutropenia and formation of a pseudoeschar. Sodium mafenide is opaque white and has excellent eschar penetration and broad antibacterial spectrum; but it can be painful upon application, and it is a carbonic anhydrase inhibitor, which may cause metabolic acidosis. Silver nitrate has poorer penetration, less antibacterial activity, requires frequent dressing changes, and causes hyponatremia, hypochloremia, and discoloration of the skin. Nevertheless, it is an excellent agent for more superficial wounds (see Table 11-1).

Airway Management

The burn patient presents several unique challenges in airway management to the physician and nursing staff. Because of the possibility of smoke inhalation (lower airway injury), paralaryngeal swelling (upper airway injury), and anasarca associated with some burn injuries, obtaining an adequate airway may be difficult to almost impossible. A surgeon or anesthetist will frequently be called upon for assistance. In this regard, early assessment of the airway upon admission, by direct laryngoscopy or fiberoptic bronchoscopy, is mandatory. Endotracheal intubation should be performed early, with positive findings.

Bronchoscopy affords several advantages. First, the supraglottic, laryngeal, and tracheal anatomy may be closely examined. Supraglottic edema may be present and cause embarrassment of respiration without evidence of smoke inhalation. An injury involving superheated air or steam from an automobile radiator is an example. Evidence of smoke inhalation includes carbonaceous sputum and debris in the pharynx and tracheobronchial tree, erythema of the mucosa, or even ulceration and hemorrhage with sloughing of mucosa. Frequently, the serum carboxyhemoglobin will be elevated; although, with face-mask oxygen, carbon

Table 11-1 Topical Chemotherapeutic Agents

Agent	Advantages	Disadvantages
Silver sulfadiazine	Painless Moderate penetration of eschar Broad spectrum	Transient decrease WBC
Sodium mafenide	Excellent eschar penetration Broad spectrum	Painful Metabolic acidosis
Silver nitrate	Low cost Antibacterial activity best for superficial wounds	Bulky dressings Staining Electrolyte abnormalities

Burn Surgery 141

monoxide is washed out rapidly and may be normal upon admission. A severe respiratory injury greatly increases the morbidity and mortality of burn injuries. The respiratory tree is an additional large surface area that may be injured and prevent adequate gas exchange. Patients with such injuries usually must be stabilized for a longer period of time before operative intervention is safe. Bronchoscopy also may be used to intubate the patient, since the tube can be placed over the flexible instrument and "threaded" into the trachea. In a severely edematous patient, this may be the only way to secure an airway.

Thus, the burden of recognizing the potential of an airway injury is placed on the staff initially caring for the burn patient, and those responsible for airway management should be alerted early. Anticipation of airway compromise may avoid disaster. In particular, those caring for the airway should be cognizant of the fact that, if an endotracheal tube becomes dislodged, the patient may die or suffer permanent sequelae. Thus, rapid intubation or tracheostomy in such acutely injured patients is a unique and foreboding challenge.

Nasotracheal intubation is preferred to orotracheal intubation in the acute setting, for reasons of stability and patient comfort. Orotracheal tubes are particularly unstable in the pediatric population; thus, every effort to use nasotracheal tubes will prove beneficial. With uncuffed pediatric endotracheal tubes, just the slightest neck motion may cause extubation. In this regard, once the stable airway has been obtained, the ventilator-dependent patient must be restrained either chemically or physically from initiating self-extubation. Endotracheal tubes are secured with umbilical tape around the circumference of the head. Frequent adjustments must be made as edema increases and decreases. Care must be taken to prevent necrosis of the oral and nasal entrances, especially when these areas are burned.

A last resort in obtaining an airway when other methods have failed is emergent tracheostomy. As with other trauma victims, cricothyroidotomy is more expedient than a formal tracheostomy and is generally associated with less troublesome bleeding. This can be converted to a tracheostomy at a later time.

In sum, airway management is clearly of paramount importance.

Monitoring Criteria

The severely injured burn patient should be monitored carefully, with particular attention focused on acid-base balance, oxygenation, ventilation, hemodynamics, and wound care. Appropriate monitoring instruments should be used with a clear recognition of the risks, benefits, complications, and alternatives involved.

Criteria for intubation should include a compromised upper airway, as discussed above, and an inability to oxygenate or ventilate adequately. These factors may be associated with hemodynamic instability. Once the patient is ventilator-dependent, it is advantageous to maintain a normal to slightly acidic pH to facilitate oxygen transfer from hemoglobin to the tissues. Adequate serum phosphate, increased temperature, and acidic environment all encourage oxygen to rescue living tissue from anaerobic metabolism.

Intravenous access is the second priority after airway management. Peripheral veins should be used preferentially. However, in large burns, central access that is obtained early may prevent later futile and dangerous access attempts in the severely edematous state. All indwelling catheters should be placed, using sterile technique, and should be removed within 72 hours. In children, intravenous access is even more challenging. In such cases, access should be protected with sutures and splints, especially in severely injured children. Cutdowns are not recommended because of predictable bacterial infection due to the immunodeficiency state of severely burned patients and wound colonization. If needed, access may be obtained through burned areas.

Arterial lines are used for frequent monitoring of blood pressure and blood parameters, specifically arterial blood gases. Complications include distal embolization and thrombosis. Therefore, prior to insertion of a catheter in a radial artery, collateral flow to the palmar arch via the ulnar artery should be verified with an Allen's test. While compressing both the ulnar and radial arteries, the patient should be asked to open and close the hand. The ulnar should then be released and observations made for palmar blushing, which signifies adequate collateral flow.

Urine output is best measured in the ICU and intraoperatively with an indwelling urethral catheter. With healthy kidneys, urine output is an excellent measure of resuscitation. Normal urine output is 0.5 to 1.0 mL/kg/hr for adults and 1.0 mL/kg/hr for children.

Swan-Ganz catheters (flow directed, balloon tipped, pulmonary artery catheters) are used to obtain cardiac output measurements and to assess volume status, since the pulmonary capillary wedge pressure (PCWP) is an indirect determinant of left ventricular end-diastolic volume (LVEDV). Preexisting medical problems may justify its use pre-, intra-, and directly postoperatively (see Figure 11-4).

ECG leads should be placed on all ICU admissions and on patients in the operating suite, especially on patients with electrical injuries in which dysrhythmias are more common. With deep burns of the chest and upper extremities, needle-point leads should be used. In the operating room, alternate sites are selected out of the operating field.

A nasogastric tube is placed in patients with burns of greater than 15 percent body surface area in order to relieve gastric dilatation associated with the traumatic stress and to monitor gastric pH. Antacids are given every hour to keep the pH

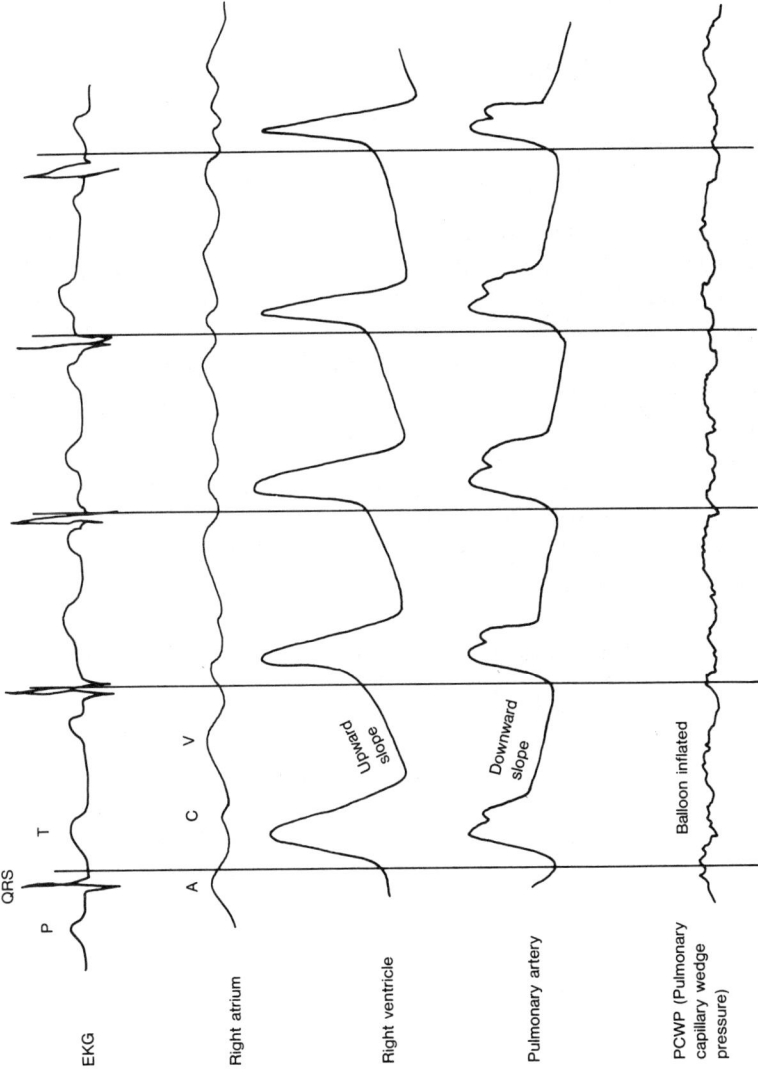

Figure 11-4 Pulmonary Artery Catheterization Wave Forms

greater than 5.0. This helps prevent Curling's stress ulcers of the stomach. Enteral feedings are begun when gastrointestinal function has returned.

SURGICAL PROCEDURES

In order to understand the needs of a patient in the immediate postoperative period, it is essential to consider what has previously occurred in the operating suite.

Just prior to surgery, the burn wounds are cleaned and placed in warm, normal saline-soaked, coarse mesh gauze dressings. Preanesthesia medications are given; and, upon arrival in the operating suite, the patient is made comfortable by courteous staff. The severely injured are transported with ventilatory assistance and monitoring equipment and are accompanied by physician and nurse. In many cases, physical therapists have made the appropriate splints prior to the operation; alternatively, these may be fashioned just after the procedure if splinting is deemed necessary.

As previously noted, monitoring equipment is introduced with clear awareness of the benefits, risks, and complications of each procedure. The placement of intravenous, intraarterial line, and pulmonary artery catheters and of endotracheal tubes is recorded and communicated to the postanesthesia staff prior to completing the procedure.

The majority of burn procedures involve excision of devitalized tissue, with placement of split-thickness skin grafts over a viable dermal, subcutaneous, or fascial bed. Early excision has the benefit of decreasing hospital stay, and it also frequently provides better functional results than does secondary healing. Graft "take" involves adherence and exchange of nutrients via capillary ingrowth. A healthy graft takes by one week postoperatively. The skin is harvested with a dermatome and will either be used as a sheet graft or be meshed to provide interstices for serum drainage and expansion to cover large surface areas. In the majority of cases, donor sites retain some dermis and will reepithelialize by one to two weeks.

The recipient bed is covered by the skin graft and fixed to the wound edges, using staples or sutures. Grafts may be approximated to one another, using sterile clips. A nonadherent dressing is applied to the fresh grafts. Next, the specific body section is immobilized to allow the graft to adhere to the underlying bed. Bulky dressings or splints should be used. Graft loss is usually due to inadequate immobilization, inadequate excision, or infection. Wounds should not be autografted if more then 10^5 organisms/g tissue are present by quantitative wound biopsy. In large burns with limited donor sites, graft failure may prove catastrophic, since weeks may be needed before recropping of previously used donor sites can be done.

Factors affecting the operation itself include the portion of the body to be grafted, the selection of donor sites, the size of the excision, and the hemodynamic stability of the patient.

Excision of 10 to 15 percent of body surface area is generally the maximum extent tolerated. Another guideline for maximal excision is blood loss of one circulating volume (about 5,000 mL in an adult). Donor sites are selected for skin quality, color matching, and sometimes for convenience, since repositioning a patient risks sheering grafts and contaminating donor sites. Each 10 percent of surface area grafted requires about five units of whole blood volume. Close cooperation is required between anesthesiologist, surgeons, and nursing staff to stay ahead of blood loss.

Nonadherent dressings are used to cover the grafted areas, while fine mesh gauze is generally applied to the donor sites. Dressings of flat trunk surfaces will maintain gentle pressure to discourage hematoma formation and to sustain the warm, moist environment ideal for epithelialization and healing. Splinting or otherwise dressed extremities should be handled with care. Every attempt should be made to keep the patient immobilized to prevent graft loss in the perioperative period, since capillary ingrowth cannot otherwise occur.

Other operations performed include simple debridement of wounds, application of homograft (cadaver skin), reconstructive surgery (not in the acute injury phase), tracheostomy, and other general surgery procedures required in the burn population.

In some burn centers, debridement is performed at the bedside or during hydrotherapy; otherwise, it is performed in the operating suite. Homograft is specially treated cadaver skin that is used as a temporary biologic dressing after excision. It is used when donor sites are not available and excision is necessary or when the quality of the excised bed is questionable. If homograft becomes adherent, autograft (from the patient) may be placed at a later date with more confidence.

Reconstructive surgery is performed for functional and cosmetic reasons. As mentioned earlier, burn wounds heal not only by epithelialization but also by contraction; thus, even months after the acute injury, contractures may form. Orbital burns may result in an ectropion, while web spaces between fingers may become hypertrophied even with grafting, necessitating reconstruction. Tracheostomies are performed when a patient becomes ventilator-dependent for more than one or two weeks. They are done to prevent tracheal stenosis and tracheoesophageal fistulae from occurring. Tracheostomies may be more difficult in the burn patient if the neck is edematous.

The burn population presents with at least the same surgically treated diseases as the general population. Acute cholecystitis, appendicitis, gastrointestinal bleeds from gastric and duodenal ulcers, diverticular disease, and tumors are all treated as in the unburned population. The stress of injury frequently induces spontaneous abortion in the severely injured pregnant patient. In addition, complications of the burn injury and iatrogenic complications may need surgical intervention. For example, septic thrombophlebitis of a peripheral vein from an indwelling catheter requires emergency surgical excision if pus is expressed from the puncture site. Escharotomies, incisions of eschar, are performed to release an extremity from its burned casing that is causing ischemia to the distal limb. To anticipate limb ischemia and prevent permanent damage to the farthest reaches of the extremity, ultrasonic Doppler flow velocity is monitored regularly and the extremity is kept elevated.

ANESTHETIC CONSIDERATIONS

The following are key elements in the anesthetic management of the burn patient:

- preoperative assessment
- airway management
- fluid management
- temperature control
- frequent transfusion of blood products

Optimal care of a patient scheduled for any surgical procedure begins with a thorough preoperative assessment. In particular, a complete history and physical exam, with review of the chart and laboratories, are starting points. The burn patient presents a greater challenge than most patients because of the larger constellation of physiological and anatomical changes.

The preoperative assessment should be based on a caring and supportive approach to the patient. This relationship with the patient builds confidence and lessens the anxiety far better than heavy sedation does. Preoperative medication should include a narcotic or benzodiazepine for sedation and an anticholinergic for antisialagogic properties (to decrease secretions). A patient recently burned and confined to a burn ICU will be anxious and in pain with increased autonomic system activity. An optimal preoperative medication should take these dynamics into consideration.

Burn Surgery 147

One must be totally aware of the patient's current clinical state. Close attention must be focused on evaluating the respiratory status of the individual, which includes assessment of radiographic findings. With critically ill patients who are intubated because of airway compromise, the condition of the patient and the status of the endotracheal tube should be noted. In our experience, we have found it helpful to check for airleaks around the cuff and to note how much pressure it takes to raise the patient's chest with acceptable ABGs. If the peak airway pressure exceeds 45 mm Hg, we prefer to have the ventilator delivered to the OR suite to ensure proper ventilation intraoperatively. ABGs are followed to assess any preoperative pneumonia or ARDS. This information sets the stage for optimal care perioperatively in that it minimizes the surprises that can occur when meticulous preoperative care is neglected in these very sick patients.

Special attention to the metabolic status of burn patients is a must. Depending on the percentage of body surface area involved and the depth of the wounds, these patients are very susceptible to hypothermia and hypovolemia. The volume status is best followed by monitoring urine output and through central pressure measurements. Temperature monitoring is a basic tool used before and during the operation.

A preoperative CBC, with platelets, electrolytes, and type and cross for blood, should be ordered. The historical risk of gastrointestinal bleeding dictates a watchful eye on the hemoglobin status. Availability of whole blood or packed cells and platelets is essential. The most common cause of perioperative bleeding is dilutional thrombocytopenia secondary to volume replacement with platelet-depleted packed cells.

Most burn patients are in a hypermetabolic state. It is therefore important to note preoperative tachycardia and sometimes mild temperature elevations that are consistent with a hypermetabolic state.

Anesthetic management of the burn patient requires alertness and precision that surpasses that normally required in the usual operative situation. To begin with, the burn patient is at a greater risk for perioperative morbidity and mortality than most patients, even in the hands of an experienced OR team that works with deliberateness and alacrity. Assessment of the airway should be the number one priority of the anesthesiologist. It must be kept in mind that laryngeal edema is a well-recognized source of morbidity and mortality.

The airway must be determined to be safe for either an intravenous induction or a more "controlled" awake nasal intubation. Once the endotracheal tube has been secured and placement confirmed by listening to both lung fields and watching for chest excursions on inhalation, intravenous induction can proceed.

In the patient with an uncomplicated airway and adequate volume status, thiopental (a rapidly acting barbiturate in the dose of 4–5 mg/kg) is given as a bolus, which induces unconsciousness within one or two minutes. Thiopental should probably not be used in any patient who has inadequate volume status. In the hypovolemic patient who is maintaining mean arterial pressure (MAP) by increased sympathetic tone, a thiopental bolus will be followed by profound hypotension or cardiac arrest. The cause of this precipitous fall in pressure is at least twofold. First, thiopental is a direct cardiac depressant with a potent negative inotropic effect on even healthy individuals. Second, it acts directly to depress the central neuraxis, thereby obliterating sympathetic tone. This may be the major cause of hypotension in the hypovolemic patient who is relying on increased sympathetic tone to maintain perfusion pressure of vital organs. In the case of profound hypotension after thiopental administration, a small dose of ephedrine (10 mg IV) with rapid infusion of a crystalloid solution (about 500 mL) should restore mean arterial pressure. Thiopental's central effect is transient because it is very rapidly redistributed by vessel-rich tissue groups (brain, heart, kidney, and liver) to vessel-poor tissue groups (muscle, fat).

Following administration of thiopental with unconsciousness and adequately controlled pressure, a dose of muscle relaxant should be given to facilitate laryngoscopy. Historically, the use of depolarizers (for example, succinylcholine) has been avoided because of the risk of hyperkalemia. Hyperkalemia results from the direct action of the depolarizer at the neuromuscular junction; if the rise is great enough, it may lead to widening of the QRS complex and progression to cardiac arrest. In particular, succinylcholine should be avoided in any patient with a burn from five days to six months postinjury.

The use of a nondepolarizer muscle relaxant that has a minimal effect on histamine release would place pancuronium (Pavulon) or vecuronium (Norcuron) as the agents of choice. To use an intubating dose, one would need to give Pavulon 0.1 mg/kg and ventilate by mask and wait for onset of the block. This technique has a disadvantage in that a nondepolarizer, when given in a dose large enough to facilitate intubation, becomes a long-acting muscle relaxant. This effect may require postsurgical controlled ventilation until the muscle relaxant has been metabolized.

It is interesting to note, however, that the burn patient does have a resistance to the nondepolarizing muscle relaxants. Possible explanatory factors derived from investigations include "components in the burn plasma" and proliferation of acetylcholine receptors in the postburn period.

Following induction of the patient, anesthesia can be maintained by several means. A pure narcotic-nitrous, oxide-oxygen technique may be employed, or a combination of narcotic-nitrous, oxide-halogenated hydrocarbon (such as Forane or Ethrane) may be used. Again, the preoperative state of the patient will determine which technique best suits the individual.

Of course, the issue of monitoring needs to be addressed. With all the improvements in monitoring devices and the incorporation of sophisticated monitors into the health care forum, the best monitor, and the only real responder to the clinical state of the patient, is the individual health care professional. It is not surprising that the American Board of Anesthesiologists has chosen the word *vigilance* as its motto and a lighthouse and beacon as its insignia. Minimal monitoring would include an ECG, a urinary catheter, a means to measure blood pressure accurately, and temperature monitoring.

In the case of a moderate tangential excision and split-thickness skin graft, where upwards of 8 units of blood may be lost, a constant visual display of the arterial pressure may be indicated. Swan-Ganz catheter placement and capnography are frequently used in the care of the critically ill patient, but they are no substitute for a well-planned and carefully conducted general anesthetic. Pulse oximetry and transcutaneous oximeters are simple to use and give a constant measure of O_2 saturation. In the hyperdynamic burn patient and especially in infants or neonates, they provide a better measure of oxygen carrying capacity and delivery than does the intermittent Pao_2 of an ABG.

The best measure of adequate volume replacement is urine output. This should be maintained at 1.0 to 1.5 mL/kg/hr. Volume replacement should be done with crystalloid solutions and should be roughly 6.0 to 8.0 mL/kg/hr, not including maintenance fluids. Replacement of blood should be prudent. It should be based on maintenance of the hematocrit of more than 30 percent and a platelet count of more than 50,000. Note that ten units of platelets will contain enough platelets to increase the count from 50,000 to 120,000.

With proper maintenance of blood volume by constant blood pressure and urine output measurement and with adequate oxygenation and ventilation, monitoring of the emergence of the patient from general anesthesia should require only close observation. The decision whether to ventilate postoperatively or to allow the patient to return to spontaneous ventilation will be addressed in the PACU.

All the agents used in the OR, with the exception of agents used to stimulate the CNS or cardiovascular system, have a respiratory depressant effect. All of the halogenated hydrocarbons and narcotics depress the central drive for ventilation.

POSTANESTHESIA CARE

Recovery from anesthesia is, for most patients, a smooth uneventful emergence from an uncomplicated anesthetic and operation. However, the postanesthesia nurse professionals should be specifically trained and skillful at the detection and treatment of all postoperative sequelae.

PACUs have been common only over the past 30 years, even though general anesthetics have been available since 1847, when ether was first publicly displayed at the Massachusetts General Hospital. However, as early as 1863 the following description of recovery rooms was noted by Florence Nightingale: "It is not uncommon, in small country hospitals, to have a recess or small room leading from the operating theater in which the patients remain until they have recovered, or at least recovered from the immediate effects of the operation."[1] Before the advent of postanesthesia care, patients succumbed "quietly" to common sequelae of general anesthesia. Today, good postanesthesia care is a must in any modern hospital setting.

For all patients entering the PACU, it is the anesthesiologist's role to ensure a smooth transition from the OR to the recovery room. The anesthesiologist does this by assisting the nurse who accepts the patient in the positioning of the patient and the recording of vital signs and by providing all information that is vital to the safety of the patient. In particular, the volume status of the patient, that is, the volume input and output from the time the patient was under the care of the anesthesiologist, should be clearly noted. The documentation should also include data on blood products, albumin, crystalloid, and urine output.

Along with the vital signs, a tidal volume should be recorded if the patient is still intubated; otherwise, the last tidal volume from the OR should be noted. Care should be taken to obtain a "core temperature" (esophageal or rectal) as soon as possible. Burn patients are very susceptible to hypothermia with the large areas of excised skin and fluid resuscitation that follows.

The following are the priorities of treatment, in order of importance:

1. Airway: O_2, tidal volume
2. Vital signs: BP, pulse, temperature, respiration
3. Monitoring: IV fluids, urine output
4. Patient comfort

All anesthetic gases depress the CNS, in particular the respiratory and cardiovascular center. Most patients are returned to the PACU with some residual gas still being respired because fat tissue acts as a depot that slowly releases to the venous pool. Therefore, hypoventilation and hypotension are commonly seen in the recovery room sometimes even after minor procedures. Where there is major blood loss and large doses of narcotics are given along with anesthetic gases, the incidence can be much higher unless close attention has been paid to the patient before leaving the OR suite.

The nurse should be aware of the total amount of narcotic and muscle relaxant given, when the last dose was given, and if the narcotic or muscle relaxant was reversed before the patient was able to return to a safe tidal volume.

In those patients who return from the OR with a core temperature of less than 35.0 °C, it is very important that the endotracheal tube be left in place until the patient has been warmed to greater than 36.5 °C. Hypothermia is frequently accompanied by hypoventilation and can slow the metabolism of muscle relaxants. In patients who have undergone major physiological trespass, it is simply wise to have one less vital sign to worry about. Whenever one is in doubt about the patient's ability to maintain a respiratory drive, it is best to err toward the side of ventilatory support. This ensures proper ventilation and allows time for both IV anesthetics and inhaled gases to be cleared by the liver, lungs, and kidneys.

Following arrival in the PACU and the recording of acceptable vital signs, all patients should receive O_2 by face mask, nasal cannula, or T-piece. Most patients will either be hypoventilating or will have increased shunt secondary to general anesthesia and position. It is not uncommon for burn patients to have a tachycardia for weeks after admission to the hospital. Such patients are in a hypermetabolic state with increased circulating catecholamines and steroids.

Regarding administration of narcotics for pain in the burn patient, it is not uncommon for this population to require "industrial dosing" of narcotics because of tolerance developed over several weeks of hospitalization, with the main symptom treated being pain. The mainstay for pain relief is morphine. It acts centrally in the periaqueductal gray area and thalamus to block pain transmission. Care must be taken to titrate to effect. Narcotics affect respiratory rate and not tidal volume; thus, a panting patient in pain can very quickly be made comfortable with a normal respiratory rate and tidal volume. However, in this case, though some may be good, more may not be better; and overzealous use of narcotics without proper time intervals to gauge effect may make a patient apneic.

Narcotic antagonists can be given intravenously to remedy this situation. Norcan in 0.1 mg doses should reverse a witnessed overdose. Until respiration spontaneously returns, the patient should either be ambued by face mask or intubated and ambued. The proper technique for ventilating a patient by mask is to extend the head and move the mandible anteriorly. This lifts the tongue away from the posterior pharynx and allows for ventilation of the lungs.

Drugs administered in the OR or recovery room are only one cause of hypoxemia. The differential in the postoperative patient includes the following:

- low inspired concentration of O_2
- hypoventilation
- areas of low V/Q relations
- an increased intrapulmonary right-to-left shunt.

The last named is the most common cause of postoperative hypoxemia. Basically, any process that upsets the normal balance of the lung-tissue–arterial-bed interface can cause shunting. Examples of this are atelectasis, bronchial obstruction from blood or secretions, pneumothorax, and pulmonary edema. When in doubt, help should be called for whenever it is suspected that a patient is hypoxic. All of the above diagnoses can be made by close inspection of the patient, auscultation with a stethoscope, and routine chest radiographs.

Another common postoperative complication is hypotension. In the burn patient, it is particularly important to assess accurately the volume status. Is the patient pale? Is the urine output low and color dark? Is the patient complaining of thirst? Or does the patient show signs of CNS depression, for example, hypoventilation, weak muscular tone, disorientation, or pinpoint pupils? Volume status and drug effects are the most common causes of postoperative hypotension, but cardiac and pulmonary disease should always be ruled out before one assumes a more benign etiology.

Hypertension is commonly seen in the recovery room. Usually, the cause is pain. Morphine IV is the most predictable and convenient means to alleviate pain. In the moderate-to-large size burns, subcutaneous injections are erratically absorbed, because blood is shunted away from the subcutaneous tissue while interstitial and intracellular edema is increased. Therefore, the IV route is customarily preferred. Other causes of hypertension are hypercarbia or drug effect, for example, clonidine withdrawal or vasopressor administration in the OR. Hypercarbia requires ABG confirmation and is likely to respond to aggressive respiratory therapy.

Postoperative bleeding in the burn patient is most likely due to dilutional thrombocytopenia. Routine CBC with platelet counts should be done; if oozing persists and the platelet count is less than 50,000–75,000, 10 units of platelets should be given. Other causes of postoperative oozing in the burn patient may be poor hemostasis, DIC, transfusion reaction, and previous bleeding disorder.

Difficult fluid management problems accompanying decreased urine output frequently require right-heart catheterization with a flow-directed, balloon-tipped pulmonary artery catheter. Distinctive waveforms of the right atrium, ventricle, pulmonary artery, and PCWP (pulmonary capillary wedge pressure) are illustrated in Figure 11-4.

Immobilization of grafted body sections is a primary concern, because any movement of graft over its fresh bed will affect eventual outcome and may stir up bleeding. Hematomas must be evacuated within the first three postoperative days or graft loss will occur in these areas. Both the cosmetic and functional results are affected by graft loss.

In sum, the following may be considered to be unique problem areas in burn patients that require continuing close postoperative attention:

- airway management
- hypothermia
- tachycardia

- tolerance to narcotics
- immobilization

Limbs are generally splinted or wrapped with bulky dressings. However, some body areas are more difficult to immobilize. These include the neck, axillae, perineum, and buttocks. An uncooperative patient can easily sheer grafts postoperatively. Extremities should be elevated, and distal vascular supply be checked frequently. Skin grafts of the back and buttocks may require that the patient be transported in a prone position from the OR until air-flotation or low-pressure beds are available in the ICU or burn unit.

Donor sites are, in essence, new partial-thickness injuries. In a physiological sense, one may view the postoperative patient as having just experienced another burn. Therefore, increased pain, insensible free water losses, and decreased temperature are the rule with large excisions. Donor sites are the source of most postoperative pain. Heat lamps are used for 15 minutes every hour to aid epithelialization, since this process is most efficient in a warm, moist environment. Topical antibiotics are used for ungrafted burns, as preoperatively.

NOTES

1. Florence Nightingale, *Notes on Hospitals*, 3d ed. (London: Longman, Green, Longman, Roberts, and Green, 1863), 89.

BIBLIOGRAPHY

Curreri, P. William, and Luterman, Arnold. "Burns." In *Principles of Surgery*. 4th ed., edited by S. Schwartz, G. Tom Shires, F. Spencer, and E. Storer, 269–288. New York: McGraw-Hill Book Co., 1984.

Feeley, Thomas W. "The Recovery Room." In *Anesthesia*, 2d ed., edited by Ronald D. Miller, 1921–1945, New York: Churchill Livingstone, 1986.

Goodwin, C.W. "Current Burn Treatment." In *Advances in Surgery*, edited by G.T. Shires, vol. 18, 145. Chicago: Yearbook Medical Publishers Inc, 1984.

Goodwin, C.W. "Major Burns." In *Principles of Trauma Care*, 3d ed., edited by G. Tom Shires, 163. New York: McGraw-Hill Book Co., 1985.

Morikawa, S., Safar, P., and DeCarlo, J. "Influence of Head-Jaw Position on Upper Airway Patency." *Anesthesiology*, 22 (1961):265.

Pruitt, B.A., and Goodwin, C.W. "Burns." In *Textbook of Surgery*, edited by D.C. Sabiston, 214–243. Philadelphia: W.B. Saunders, 1986.

Shuck, J.M., Pruitt, B.A., Jr., and Moncrief, J.A. "Homograft skin for wound coverage. A study in versatility." *Archives of Surgery* 98 (1969):472.

Tjeuw, Michael. "Burn." In *Anesthesiology: Problem-Oriented Patient Management*, edited by F. Yao and J.F. Artusio, Jr., 373. Philadelphia: J.B. Lippincott, 1983.

Chapter 12

Postanesthesia Care After Orthopedic Surgery

Ann Butler Maher, R.N., M.S.N.

GENERAL CONSIDERATIONS

The musculoskeletal system protects the body, gives it shape, and provides individuals with the ability to move.[1] In considering injury to the musculoskeletal system, whether planned as in surgery or unplanned as in an accident, a variety of components are involved. These include the bone, fascia, muscle, tendon, ligament, bursa, meniscus, and skin.

There are four categories of bone within the body; the classification is by shape.

1. *Long bones* are those whose length is greater than their width, such as the femur and humerus. Long bones have a shaft, the diaphysis, with two articular ends called the epiphyses. The flared portion of bone between the diaphysis and epiphysis is the metaphysis. Long bones are joined by joints.
2. *Short bones* are approximately equal in all three dimensions. Examples are the carpal bones of the hand and the tarsal bones of the foot.
3. *Flat bones* include the bones of the skull, scapula, and sternum. These bones serve a protective function.
4. *Irregular bones* are those that do not fit into any other category. They include the pelvic bones and the vertebrae and provide protection, support, and leverage.

Bone is formed by a dense, compact outer layer known as the cortex. Within the diaphysis of the long bones is a medullary cavity, which contains fat cells in loose fibrous tissue called the yellow marrow. At the ends of long bones and throughout short bones, the cortex surrounds a honeycomb-like organization of spongy cancellous bone composed of trabeculae. The trabeculae are arranged to respond to the stresses caused by weight transmission and muscle traction. Red marrow, composed mostly of immature red blood cells, is contained in cancellous bone. The periosteum is a fibrous tissue layer surrounding bone, except at the articular surface. Periosteum is osteogenic and plays an important role in fracture healing. The major blood supply to bone is delivered by the periosteal arteries and the nutrient (medullary) arteries.

Joints provide the connection between bones. They can be fibrous, cartilaginous, or synovial. *Fibrous (synarthrodial) joints* are connected by fibrous tissue and allow little or no movement. Examples are the sutures of the skull and the articulation between the radius and ulna. *Cartilaginous (amphiarthrodial) joints* are joined by cartilage, allow slight movement, and include the symphysis pubis. *Synovial (diarthrodial) joints,* which are freely movable, are characterized by a joint cavity between the bone ends. The two articulating surfaces are covered by hyaline membrane, which is smooth and resilient to pressure. The bone ends are surrounded and held in place by a capsule whose inner surface consists of synovial cells. These cells secrete a clear fluid into the joint cavity, which lubricates the opposing joint surfaces during motion and supplies nutrition to the relatively avascular cartilaginous surfaces. Some joints are completely or partially subdivided by fibrocartilaginous discs called menisci.

The capsules of fibrous and synovial joints are reinforced by tough, inelastic tissue bands or *ligaments* that stabilize the joint and limit excessive movement. Joint motion is produced by muscular forces. Muscles attach to bone indirectly through the connective tissue of the muscle. In some instances, the connective tissue fuses together to form a *tendon* composed of bundles of collagen fibers. Tendons are immensely strong and are often intertwined with capsular ligaments of the joints.[2]

Bursa, blind fluid-filled sacs, are normally found where tendons pass directly over the periosteum of the bone and thus are characteristically located around joints. They allow connective tissue surfaces to move smoothly over one another. Synovial tendon sheaths are specialized bursa into which tendons have ingrown. Bony surfaces demonstrate ridges and prominences for the origin and insertion of muscles; there are also grooves for the gliding of tendon over bone.

Sheets of connective tissue called *fascia* may surround one or more muscles, forming enclosures called compartments. Blood vessels and nerves are also enclosed in the extremity compartments.

Although growth of the skeletal system may appear to be completed at maturity, bone growth continues throughout life with the continual resorption of old bone and the laying down of new bone. With normal aging, there is a decrease in the flexibility of bone, predisposing the bone to breakage. In addition, conditions such as osteoporosis, osteomalacia, and hyperparathyroidism decrease the density of bone by increasing resorption, making the individual prone to fractures.[3]

SURGICAL CONSIDERATIONS

Surgical procedures for orthopedic problems can be classified in terms of their specific purposes:

- reporting of injury or damage to a part; this includes diagnostic evaluations using arthroscopy
- repair of a structure, such as a tendon or ligament; in the case of fractures, possibly involving the use of hardware
- realignment of structures, such as the spine in scoliosis or a long bone by osteotomy to shift weight bearing
- reconstruction of a part that has been damaged by trauma, a procedure that generally requires internal fixation or grafting of bone and/or tissue
- removal of a nonfunctional or dysfunctional structure that causes pain or impedes movement, such as the head of the radius in rheumatoid arthritis
- replacement of a part that has been destroyed by disease or trauma, such as the head of the femur, replaced with an Austin Moore prosthesis or total hip replacement

The major complications that may occur with any of the above are excessive bleeding and neurovascular impairment. Bleeding is a major consideration in surgery involving the hip and the spine because of the significant vascularity. Neurovascular impairment can occur secondary to operative positioning, prolonged tourniquet time, and delayed arterial repair. Total joint replacements that use methylmethacrylate may precipitate hypotension. The treatment is to administer extra fluids; this treatment is continued in the PACU.

ANESTHETIC CONSIDERATIONS

Anesthesia options in orthopedic surgery are more diverse than in some other specialties. Procedures on extremities may be done using local or regional blocks, as well as general anesthesia. When blocks of the brachial plexus are used, the patient needs to have the extremity protected because sensation may not return for hours after the surgery is completed. Anesthesia time may be extensive in patients undergoing spinal or major reconstructive surgery, such as replantation. This increases the potential for side effects, such as nausea and vomiting and prolonged respiratory depression.

Many orthopedic procedures are done on an outpatient basis, and this has implications for the choice of anesthesia. When general anesthesia is chosen, consideration is given to using anesthetic agents that are rapidly metabolized and excreted.[4] Nausea and vomiting are more common with general anesthesia.[5] Antiemetics may therefore be given preoperatively to reduce this problem. Alternatively, preoperative medications may be omitted entirely in some cases. In general, if preoperative medication is given, it is best to avoid use of tranquilizers, narcotics, or sedatives that have long durations of action.[6]

Maintenance of neurovascular function, reduction of pain, proper positioning and alignment, minimization of bleeding, and prevention of infection (maintenance of closed drainage systems) and edema are all common concerns following orthopedic surgery that the PACU nurse will encounter. Additionally, the PACU nurse must watch for such complications as compartment syndrome, fat embolism, and deep-vein thrombosis that can occur early in the postoperative period.

SPECIFIC PROBLEMS AND TECHNIQUES

Assessing Neurovascular Integrity

The primary consideration following orthopedic surgery is the maintenance of neurovascular integrity. All of the equipment and techniques employed in the postoperative period are utilized with this goal in mind.

Pulses, skin color, skin temperature, capillary refill, sensation, motion, and edema should all be monitored closely in the affected extremity, compared with the opposite extremity. Vascular parameters should be evaluated for changes in arterial versus venous flow (see Table 12-1). This is especially important following microvascular free flaps or replantation, since thrombosis is the major complication. Nerve function can be evaluated for both sensation and movement. Table 12-2 delineates the guidelines for normal nerve function in the major nerves of the upper and lower extremities.

Maintaining Alignment

Proper positioning and alignment are essential, not only to ensure adequate neurovascular functioning, but also to help prevent dependent edema, which exacerbates the edema secondary to injury and operative manipulation. A variety

Orthopedic Surgery 159

Table 12-1 Clinical Signs of Circulation

Parameter	Normal	Arterial Occlusion	Venous Occlusion
Color	pink	pale	cyanotic
Capillary refill	1 to 2 seconds	decreased, slow	increased, fast
Tissue turgor	full	hollow, "prunelike"	tense, distended
Temperature	warm	cool	

Source: Adapted from *Orthopaedic Nursing*, Vol. 3, No. 2, p. 12, with permission of National Association of Orthopaedic Nurses, © 1984.

---

of modalities are employed to assist care givers. These include casts, traction, external fixators, and immobilizers.

Casts

Casts may be constructed of plaster or synthetic fibers. If the patient has a plaster cast or plaster covered by ace bandages, the plaster will require hours to days to dry. When positioning the extremity, one should use the palms of the hands, not the fingers, to move the cast. This prevents indentations on the cast that can cause pressure on the underlying soft tissues. The casted extremity should be placed on a

---

Table 12-2 Evaluating Nerve Function

Nerve	Sensation	Motion
Peroneal nerve (major branch of sciatic)	Prick web space between great toe and second toe	Have patient dorsiflex ankle and extend toes at metatarsal phalangeal (MP) joints
Tibial nerve	Prick the medial lateral surface of the sole of the foot	Have patient plantar ankle and flex toes
Radial nerve	Prick the web space between thumb and index finger	Have patient hyperextend thumb, then wrist, and hyperextend the four fingers at MCP joint
Ulnar nerve	Prick the distal end of the small fingers	Ask patient to abduct all fingers with fingers flexed
Median nerve	Prick the distal surface of the index finger	Have patient oppose thumb and little finger, flex wrist

soft surface, such as pillows, making sure to use materials that breathe. Rubber or vinyl materials will increase the heat within the cast and prolong the drying time.

Bleeding is anticipated following many surgical procedures; and, since the plaster is porous, the cast will become stained with blood. Circling blood or drainage on the cast does not provide definitive information regarding the amount of bleeding, because staining varies with cast porosity. This practice also upsets many patients. In such cases, the physician should be queried regarding the amount of bleeding anticipated, and this should be used to guide the assessment. Excessive, continuous bleeding should be reported to the physician immediately. Synthetic casts dry within 15 to 30 minutes and are very rough. Care should be taken to protect the skin near the edges of the cast with tape and to cover the opposite leg or the patient's torso to prevent skin irritation or laceration.

Ice is usually applied to the cast over the operative site to minimize edema. Elevation further enhances venous return. When positioning a casted extremity, one should be careful to prevent the edges of the cast from causing compression of underlying soft tissues, which could result in neurovascular compromise. Elevation of the arm following hand surgery or replantation requires that the hand be placed with palm out, fingers slightly flexed, and the elbow at a 90° angle.

Following application of a spica, the patient's respiratory status must be closely observed. Although there may be a feeling of being confined the patient should not experience difficulty in breathing normally. If the patient has a shoulder or body spica, a cast cutter should be available in case cardiopulmonary resuscitation (CPR) is necessary. Also, in case CPR is necessary, one must know how to remove a body jacket following spinal surgery.

Traction

General guidelines for all types of traction include the following: The weights should be allowed to hang free, while maintaining alignment of the pulleys and end plates (such as the foot plate on Buck's traction) should not be allowed to rest against the foot of the bed or the pulley.

Skin traction can be applied with ace bandages over adhesive strips, or more commonly with commercial binders. The neurovascular status of the limb should always be checked distal to the traction apparatus. If there is a boot on the foot for Buck's traction, the toes should be checked (see Figure 12-1). The traction should be maintained in place unless otherwise ordered by the physician. Although a patient may have intermittent traction ordered, it is unlikely that it would be interrupted in the PACU.

Skeletal traction involves the application of weights directly to bone by insertion of Kirschner wires or Steinman pins into the proximal or distal end of a long bone but distal to the fracture (for example, a fracture of the midshaft of the femur

Orthopedic Surgery 161

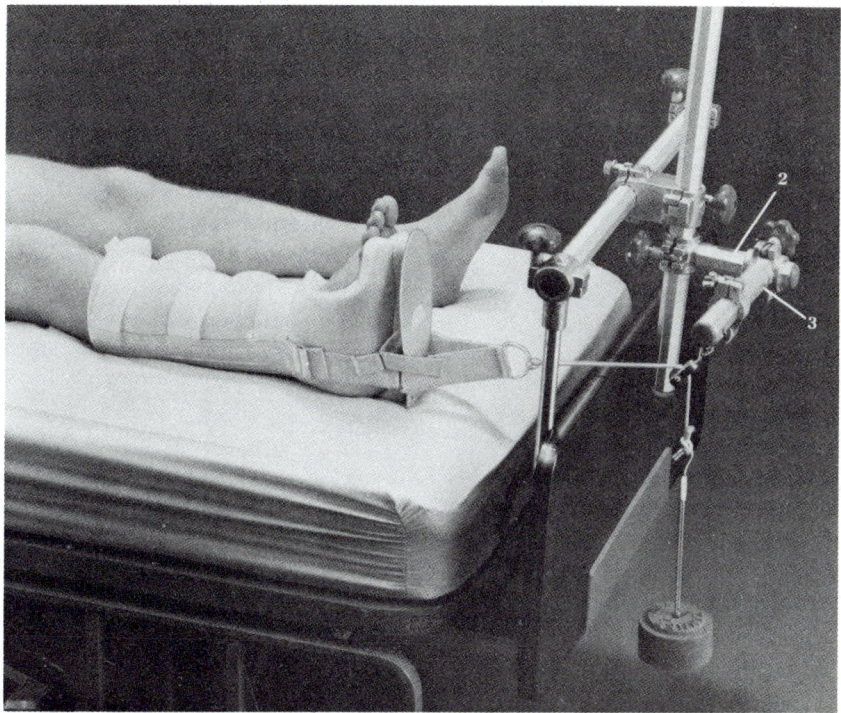

Figure 12-1 Buck's Unilateral Traction. *Source:* Reprinted from *The Traction Handbook*, p. 33, with permission of Patient Care Systems, Division of Zimmer, Charlotte, North Carolina, © 1980.

will have the pin inserted into the distal femur or proximal tibia). This type of traction is often "balanced," meaning that movement of the limb is compensated for by countertraction when the patient moves. This countertraction, provided by counterweights and the patient's own body weight, maintains the fracture site in alignment (see Figure 12-2). The neurovascular status of the limb should be checked distal to the fracture site, always in comparison with the uninjured extremity. Also, the insertion site of the wire should be checked for bleeding, which should be minimal or absent. Dressings should be applied or maintained at the pin sites, per hospital policy.

There are many approaches to pin site care, all of which, including benign neglect, appear to yield similar results in prevention of infection. The primary goals of pin site care are to promote the free drainage of fluid and minimize local tissue damage.[7] One should be sure, therefore, that traction attachments do not pull on or rub against the skin around the pins. If attachments, such as a Thomas splint with Pearson attachment for femur fractures, are part of the traction set-up,

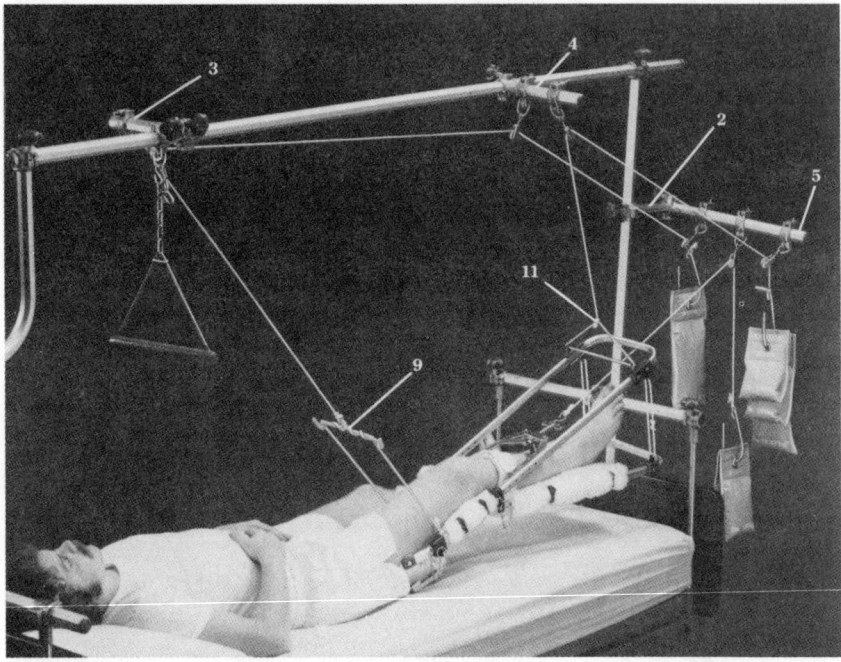

Figure 12-2 Balanced Traction and Thomas Leg Splint, Utilizing Skeletal Traction. *Source:* Reprinted from *The Traction Handbook*, p. 41, with permission of Patient Care Systems, Division of Zimmer, Charlotte, North Carolina, © 1980.

one must ensure that sufficient padding has been added where the limb rests against the apparatus to prevent skin breakdown or neurovascular compromise.

External Fixators

An external fixator is indicated when there is significant soft tissue damage or a fracture is too complicated to allow fixation with hardware or casting. Percutaneous pins are placed with a hand drill proximal and distal to the fracture site through stab wounds (see Figure 12-3). The pins may be through-and-through pins or half pins. The pins provide stabilization of the fracture fragments while allowing access to soft tissue for treatment or for placement of muscle and/or skin grafts. Pin care should follow the hospital's policy for skeletal traction. The pin insertion sites should be watched for tension on the skin. If the skin is tented, the stab wounds need to be extended. If this is not done, the site will probably develop a pin tract infection. In such cases, the extremity should be moved by using the longitudinal bars of the frame. In no case should the limb be handled near the

Orthopedic Surgery 163

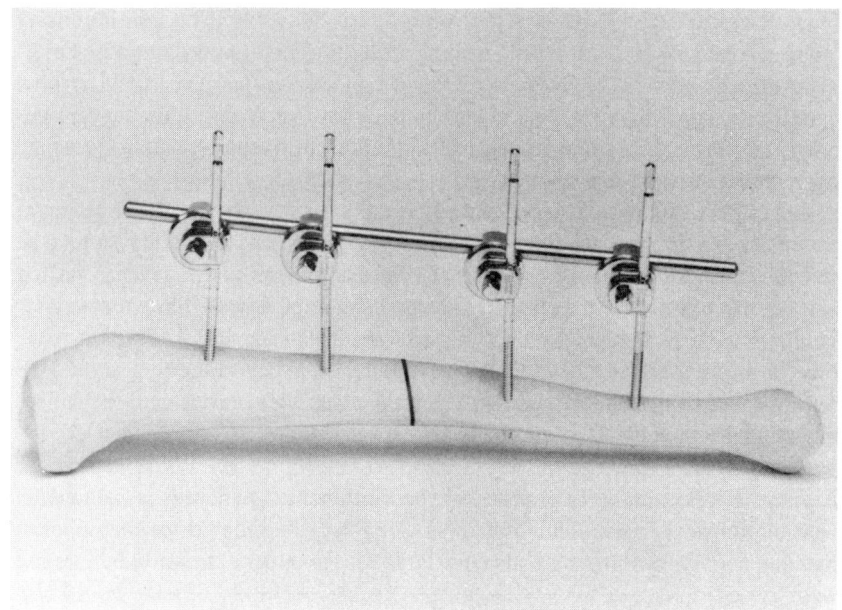

Figure 12-3 Unilateral Independent Pin Placement Frame. *Source:* Courtesy of Howmedica, Rutherford, New Jersey.

fixator; touching the extremity will be very painful for the patient and the fracture alignment may be disrupted. The limb should be assessed for neurovascular status below the fixator, and the injured tissue should be evaluated for signs of ischemia.

Immobilizers

Commercial immobilization devices are often applied instead of a cast. These devices are held in place by velcro bindings and maintain the joint in extension and flexion. Also commonly used following total hip replacement is the abductor pillow, which keeps the hips abducted. Maintaining abduction is essential to prevent the prosthesis from dislocating posteriorly. In such cases, one should examine the placement of the immobilizer or pillow to ensure that it is placed and secured properly following transfer from the operating table. Also, the neurovascular status distal to the device should be assessed.

Continuous Passive Motion

Continuous passive motion (CPM) is a technique for applying continuous range of motion to a joint, using a stationary, electronically controlled machine.[8]

Passive motion of weight-bearing joints, particularly if used continuously, reduces adhesions and stimulates healing, resulting in stronger fixation.[9] Originally utilized mainly following total knee replacement surgery, CPM is now employed postoperatively for a range of conditions, including total hip replacement, hip fractures, supracondylar and tibial plateau fractures, anterior cruciate ligament repair, and synovectomies.

The CPM machine is usually placed on the patient in the PACU. Maximum extension and flexion are ordered by the physician. The extremity should be observed to ensure that the limb is in correct alignment and that areas resting against the machine are padded. The affected joint should be evaluated for swelling, redness, tenderness, and pain. In some instances, the CPM will increase bleeding and therefore drainage; continuous, excessive bleeding should be reported to the physician. Because the knee can only flex and extend, the patient must remain on the back while the CPM is in place. Unless contraindicated, the patient may have the head of the bed raised for comfort and ease of respiration. Because of the immobility imposed by the machine, the patient is prone to deep vein thrombosis, and an antiembolic stocking may be ordered for the opposite extremity. CPM machines are also available for the upper extremity, but are not widely used.

COMPLICATIONS

Compartment Syndrome

Compartment syndrome occurs when there is an increase in the pressure within the muscle compartment caused by internal or external forces. Because the fascia that surrounds the compartment is inelastic, increased pressure can cause impaired arterial blood flow, leading to muscle ischemia, necrosis, and tissue death within several hours.[10] Although there are a variety of problems that may cause compartment syndrome, the three most common are fractures, soft tissue injury (crushing injury), and prolonged limb compression or postischemic injury (seen following arterial repair).[11] External causes are casts or compression dressings that are too tight. To prevent the syndrome from developing, some surgeons choose to perform prophylactic fasciotomy distal to arterial repairs.

Diagnosis is made primarily on the basis of clinical findings. Early recognition is important because irreversible damage may have already occurred by the time the patient develops conclusive clinical signs.[12] The signs of compartment syndrome include pain on passive motion of the fingers or toes, progressive pain that is unrelieved by narcotics, progressive loss of sensation and motion, and vascular compromise. The sensory deficit is more reliable in the early stages because every major compartment of the arm and leg has a major nerve running through it.[13] Normal pulses in the extremity do not rule out the presence of compartment syndrome, since smaller vessels are occluded long before larger arteries are compromised.

Compartment syndrome and arterial thrombosis have several common symptoms, but the two conditions can be distinguished. Arterial occlusion is characterized immediately by pale, cool skin with a very weak or absent pulse. In compartment syndrome, the skin is pink and the pulses intact until late in the clinical course.[14]

The diagnosis can be confirmed by measuring the pressure in the compartment using the needle technique, as described by Whitesides.[15] Continuous monitoring using the catheter technique is also possible, but unlikely in the PACU setting. Pressures over 30 mm Hg in a normotensive person are considered to be significantly elevated. However, there is disagreement about the specific pressure that requires surgical intervention, although 60 mm Hg is the upper limit. The patient fluid status is important in relation to the compartment pressure because vascular compromise will occur at lower compartment pressures in individuals who are hypotensive. Most patients with compartment syndrome can be diagnosed clinically, and the documentation of elevated pressure may be only confirmatory.[16] If the symptoms are in a casted extremity, immediate treatment is to bivalve the cast. If the symptoms do not improve within one hour, the patient is returned to the operating room for fasciotomy.

Postfasciotomy, the extremity may be placed in a dry, sterile, bulky dressing or be left open and covered with sterile, saline dressings. The dry dressing is more common following fasciotomy in orthopedic cases. The limb is elevated; and, following lower extremity fasciotomy, care must be taken to prevent plantar flexion of the foot.

Fat Embolism

Fat embolism syndrome (FES) occurs when fat molecules occlude the vasculature of the lung—producing respiratory distress. The primary etiological factors are long-bone fracture, and multiple trauma, although fat embolism following total hip and knee replacement has been documented.[17]

Diagnosis is made on a cluster of symptoms that are present in 60 percent of the patients within 24 hours following injury.[18] Initial signs and symptoms include air hunger with an increased pulse, increased respirations, and increased temperature. Changes in mentation are common but are difficult to evaluate if the patient has had general anesthesia or sedation. A Po_2 of less than 60 mm Hg, in the presence of the changes in vital signs and level of consciousness as noted above, is considered the diagnostic criterion of FES.[19] The petechial rash typically associated with FES does not appear until the second or third day and occurs in only 50 to 60 percent of cases.[20] Chest roentgenograms may reveal the presence of fluffy exudates within the lung fields. The changes are characteristic but not specific.

Treatment is administration of oxygen by mask or cannula. FES, unlike adult respiratory distress syndrome (ARDS), responds well to oxygen therapy. Steroids are also commonly given; they are believed to decrease the inflammatory response in the lungs.[21] FES can be a subclinical problem by itself, or it may be an etiological factor in the development of ARDS. In the latter case, management will be directed toward the ARDS.

Special Considerations

Patients with orthopedic trauma and those who have had surgery with a tourniquet in place are at high risk for development of thrombophlebitis. Application of antiembolic stockings in the PACU is a primary preventive measure.

Elderly patients who have undergone lengthy procedures, such as total joint replacements, may be hypothermic from the exposure time. These patients should be adequately covered and their temperature should be closely monitored while they are in the PACU.

Shoulder arthroscopy can generate copious amounts of drainage. Disposable diapers provide excellent absorbent pads that can easily be wrapped around the shoulder.

In sum, orthopedics is a diverse specialty and attention to these concerns will ensure a smooth postanesthesia course.

NOTES

1. Delores C. Schoen, *The Nursing Process in Orthopaedics* (Norwalk, Conn.: Appleton-Century-Crofts, 1986), 5.

2. James R. Hay and J. Gavin Reid, *The Anatomical and Mechanical Bases of Human Motion* (Englewood Cliffs, N.J.: Prentice-Hall, 1982), 26–28.

3. H. Courtland Stearns and Clare M. Stearns, "Orthopaedic Radiology," *Orthopaedic Nursing* 5 (1986):26–31.

4. Mary Dutka, "Elbow and Wrist Arthroscopy: Perioperative Nursing Care," *Orthopaedic Nursing* 5 (1986):29–34.

5. Nancy Bruton-Maree, "Outpatient Anesthesia for Orthopaedic Procedures," *Orthopaedic Nursing* 6, no. 2 (1987):30–37.

6. Patricia G. Cichlar, "Inpatient versus Outpatient Arthroscopy," in *Arthroscopy of the Knee*, ed. Nancy E. Hilt (Pitman, N.J.: National Association of Orthopaedic Nurses, 1983), 46–50.

7. Nancy J. Hoyt, "Infections Following Orthopaedic Injury," *Orthopaedic Nursing* 5 (1986): 15–24.

8. National Association of Orthopaedic Nurses, *Core Curriculum for Orthopaedic Nursing* (Pitman, N.J.: NAON, 1986), 99–100.

9. R. Salter, et al., "The Biochemical Effect of Continuous Passive Motion on the Healing of Full Thickness Defects in Articular Cartilage," *Journal of Bone and Joint Surgery* 62A (1980):1232–1251.

10. Jane Callahan, "Compartment Syndrome," *Orthopaedic Nursing* 4 (1985):11–18.

11. Scott M. Mubarak, "Recognition and Treatment of Compartment Syndromes," in *The Multiply Injured Patient with Complex Fractures*, ed. Marvin H. Meyers (Philadelphia: Lea and Febiger, 1984), 71–89.

12. C.H. Rorabek and I. Macnab, "Anterior Tibial Compartment Syndrome Complicating Fractures of the Shaft of the Femur, *Journal of Bone and Joint Surgery* 58A (1976):549–550.

13. Mubarak, "Recognition and Treatment," p. 76.

14. Ann Butler Maher, "Early Assessment and Management of Musculoskeletal Injuries, *Nursing Clinics of North America* 21, no. 4 (1986):717–727.

15. T.E. Whitesides et al., "Tissue Pressure Measurements as a Determinant for the Need of Fasciotomy," *Clinical Orthopaedics and Related Research* 113 (1975):43–51.

16. Mubarak, "Recognition and Treatment," p. 80.

17. P.F. Lanchiewicz and C.S. Ranawat, "Fat Embolism Syndrome Following Bilateral Total Knee Replacement with Condylar Prosthesis: A Report of Two Cases," *Clinical Orthopaedics and Related Research* 160 (1981):106.

18. C. McCollister Evarts, "The Fat Embolism Syndrome," in *The Multiply Injured Patient with Complex Fractures*, ed. Marvin H. Meyers (Philadelphia: Lea and Febiger, 1984), 67–70.

19. Judy Johnson, "Respiratory Complications of Orthopaedic Injuries," *Orthopaedic Nursing* 5 (1986):24–28.

20. W. Oh and M. Mohinder, "Fat Embolism: Current Concepts of Pathogenesis, Diagnosis, and Treatment," *Orthopedic Clinics of North America* 9 (1978):769–779.

21. Evarts, "Fat Embolism Syndrome," p. 68.

BIBLIOGRAPHY

Farrell, Jane. *Illustrated Guide to Orthopaedic Nursing*. Philadelphia: J.B. Lippincott, 1986.

Spiegel, Phillip G., ed. *Topics in Orthopaedic Trauma*. Baltimore: University Park Press, 1984.

Stearns, Clare, and Brunner, Nancy, eds. *OpCare—Orthopaedic Patient Care: A Nursing Guide*. Rutherford, N.J.: Howmedica, In press.

Trunkey, Donald R., and Lewis, Frank R. *Current Therapy of Trauma*—2. Toronto, B.C, Canada: Decker, 1986.

Chapter 13

Postanesthesia Care After Urological and Renal Surgery

Karen D. Spadaccia, R.N., B.S.N., C.C.R.N., C.E.N.

INTRODUCTION

The renal system involves many different functions and influences the activity of several other organ systems in the body. The system was once described to the author as "a small black box with water and waste products entering from one side and urine leaving from the other. When it works, great. When it doesn't, panic!" The individual who provided this description had a valid point, in that the kidney and its contiguous structures are necessary for life, and they must be repaired when not functioning appropriately. Six major functions of the renal system are listed in Exhibit 13-1. This chapter seeks to describe some of the complexities of the renal system and to address the management of patients undergoing urologic and renal surgery.

Exhibit 13-1 Function of the Renal System

1. regulation of the osmotic pressure of extracellular fluids by maintaining relative amounts of water and sodium
2. regulation of the electrolyte pattern of extracellular fluid
3. excretion of metabolic wastes
4. regulation of acid-base ratio
5. aid in the regulation of the volume of extracellular fluid
6. initiation of the renin-angiotensin cycle

First, some key terms should be defined:

- *Diffusion*: the movement of solutes across a semipermeable membrane; solutes are dissolvable substances, solvents are liquids capable of dissolving solutes, solutions are solutes dissolved in solvent.
- *Osmosis*: movement of a solvent through a membrane area of lower concentration to higher concentration of solutes.
- *Osmotic pressure*: determined by the number of particles of solute dissolved in a solution; increased particles lead to an increased pull for water.
- *Hydrostatic pressure*: force exerted by a liquid against a membrane wall.
- *Ultrafiltration*: filtration of fluids and dissolved substances across a semipermeable membrane at a very rapid rate due to high pressures within the system.
- *Milliequivalents*: number of electrical charges per unit of volume.
- *Active transport*: movement of dissolved substances against a concentration and/or electrical gradient.

ANATOMY OF THE RENAL AND UROLOGICAL SYSTEMS

The kidneys are bilateral retroperitoneal organs lying on either side of the vertebral column. They are approximately 5–7 cm wide and 11–15 cm long. The upper borders of the kidneys lie at the level of the T_{12} vertebrae, and the lower borders are at L_3. The left kidney is somewhat higher than the right, due to the presence of the liver on the right.

The functional anatomy of the systems comprises the following:

- *Renal cortex*: the outer portion of the kidney that is metabolically active. This is where aerobic metabolism occurs and ammonia and glucose are formed. It is the site of the renal capsules, proximal and distal convoluted tubules, and blood vessels.
- *Renal medulla*: the inner portion where glycolytic metabolism occurs, supplying energy needed for active transport. It consists of 8 to 18 radially situated cones or pyramids that converge into projections received by the sinuses of the renal pelvis.
- *Nephron*: the functioning unit of the kidney, comprising the glomerulus, tubules, and blood supply. Nephrons may be described as capillary loops that do not anastomose and are completely encapsulated by the tubules. There are approximately one million nephrons in the cortex of each kidney.

Urological and Renal Surgery 171

- *Vasculature*: Kidneys receive 20 to 25 percent of cardiac output or approximately 1,200 mL/minute via the renal arteries. The oxygen extraction is very high, and renal blood flow can be affected by several exogenous sources. These causes of variation must be kept in mind, since blood flow affects the amount of filtration and subsequent urine production. The renal veins exit the kidneys and empty into the inferior vena cava. Normal influences on renal blood flow are listed in Exhibit 13-2.
- *Ureters*: Transports urine to the bladder.
- *Bladder*: Holds urine flowing from the kidneys. When about 400 mL have collected, the desire to urinate causes contraction of the bladder muscle, thereby emptying the urine through the urethra.
- *Prostate gland*: Composed of 100 or more paraurethral glands (outer layer) and 100 or more periurethral glands (inner layer), surrounded by a capsule called Denonvillier's fascia. In males, the prostate gland surrounds the urethra.

PHYSIOLOGY OF THE RENAL AND UROLOGICAL SYSTEMS

Glomerular filtration occurs via the process of ultrafiltration, by which fluid and its accompanying constituents are forced out of the capillaries into Bowman's capsule. The average rate of filtration is 120 mL/minute (170–180 liters/24 hours). Despite the normal fluctuations in systemic blood pressure, the kidney has an autoregulation mechanism to ensure a constant rate. This mechanism involves the constriction and dilatation of afferent and efferent capillaries, thereby increasing and decreasing systemic capillary pressures in the kidneys. The effect is much the same as if one were to attach a smaller-diameter garden hose to a wider one;

Exhibit 13-2 Normal Influences on Renal Blood Flow

Renal blood flow is:
- higher in males than females
- increased during first and third trimester of pregnancy
- increased with age until maturity, then decreased in the elderly
- decreased with exercise
- increased in supine position
- increased in the afternoon
- decreased at night

the smaller hose would result in a higher pressure in the larger hose. The filtration remains relatively unaffected by pressures ranging from 70 mm Hg to 200 mm Hg.

As the filtrate that is produced passes through the tubules of the nephron, it is changed in volume and composition by the reabsorption of 168–169 liters of water and certain accompanying constituents. This reabsorption of solutes is relative to the osmotic pressure gradient created by the body's needs (see Table 13-1).

Thirst is a natural response to fluid loss.

Antidiuretic Hormone (ADH), which is manufactured by the hypothalmus and released by the pituitary gland, controls extracellular osmolality or fluid volume. The release of ADH is controlled by monitoring of the tonicity of extracellular fluid. For example, should the body become hypovolemic, thereby increasing solute concentrations, ADH is released. ADH has an affinity for the distal convoluted tubules of the nephron and will cause increased fluid reabsorption. This results in an increased extracellular volume and decreased urinary output.

It is important to note that several factors in addition to increased serum osmolality can cause an increased secretion of ADH. These factors are:

- pain
- stress
- unpleasant emotions
- morphine sulfate
- preparation of oxytoxin (Pitocin)
- chlorpropamide (Diabinese)
- several anesthetic agents
- IPPB or PEEP

Table 13-1 Approximation of Substances Filtered, Excreted, and Reabsorbed by the Tubules During a 24-Hour Period

Constituent	Amount Filtered	Amount Found in Urine	% Reabsorbed
Sodium	600 g	6.0 g	99
Potassium	35 g	2.0 g	94
Calcium	5 g	0.2 g	98
Glucose	200 g	0.0	100
Urea	60 g	35.0 g	35
Water	180 L	1.5 L	99
Amino acids	10 g	300.0 mg	97

Aldosterone, a hormone secreted by the cortex of the adrenal gland, acts directly on the tubules of the nephron to promote reabsorption of sodium. The effects of extracellular fluid volume are secondary to this, but no less important. The kidneys are responsible for maintaining the bicarbonate level in the carbonic acid-bicarbonate buffer system.

As extracellular fluid volume decreases and sodium levels increase, specialized cells in the kidney, called Polkiessen cells, are stimulated to release the enzyme renin into the cells. The cycle thus begun results in the release of aldosterone, which brings fluid volume and sodium levels back to normal (see Figure 13-1).

HISTORY AND PHYSICAL FINDINGS

Diseases affecting the urological system can be either masked by or confused with difficulties in other organ systems. Also, many patients hesitate in seeking assistance because of fear or embarrassment. Because of the close interrelationship with other systems and patient discomfort, history and physical findings must be closely scrutinized. When this is done, the disturbance can usually be placed in one of three categories: prerenal, intrarenal, or postrenal (see Table 13-2).

In obtaining a history, questions should elicit information concerning the following:

1. trauma to the urological system
2. changes in urine

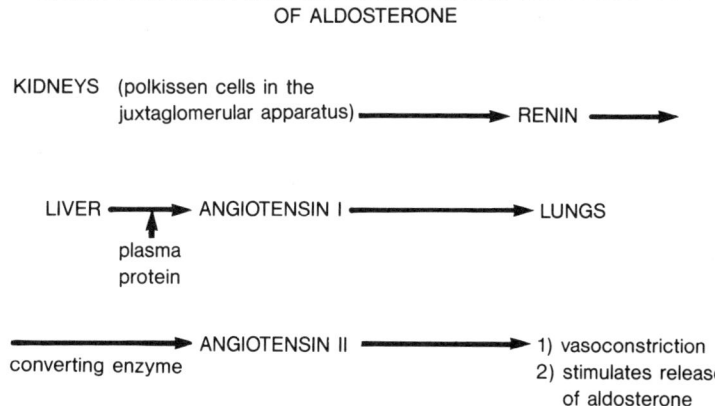

Figure 13-1 Renin-Angiotensin Mechanism Resulting in the Stimulation of Aldosterone

Table 13-2 Types of Renal Involvement and Possible Causative Factors

Site of Involvement	Possible Causative Agents
Prerenal—hemodynamic or cardiac in origin —decreased blood flow to the kidney	vascular disorders congestive heart failure shock embolus
Intrarenal—direct kidney involvement	glomerulonephritis acute renal failure chronic renal failure drugs diabetes
Postrenal—obstruction of flow of urine out of the kidney	urethral strictures prostatic hypertrophy carcinoma benign tumors infection calculi

- hematuria
- pyuria

3. problems in voiding

- incontinence
- frequency
- dysuria
- oliguria
- polyuria
- dribbling after normal voiding
- small streams
- difficulty

4. swelling in urogenital area

- scrotum
- vulva
- groin, abdomen, or flank

5. pain or tenderness in genitourinary tract
6. azotemia
7. dehydration
8. chills or fever
9. weight loss
10. possibility of metastases
11. sexual dysfunction
12. drug usage

The physical examination is directed by the responses in the history and is based on general appearances.

Laboratory studies include a urinalysis (see Table 13-3) and a study of serum electrolytes (see Table 13-4). They also include the following radiologic procedures:

- *KUB*: flat plate of abdomen looking at the kidneys, ureters, and bladder
- *IVP*: intravenous pyelogram injection of radiopaque dye and radiographic examination of ureters and bladder
- *cystography*: injection of radiopaque dye through a catheter into the bladder, thereby outlining the size and shape of the bladder, diverticular trabeculation, and ureteral reflux

Table 13-3 Normal Urinalysis Findings

Osmolality	>800 mOsm/kg
Bilirubin	negative
Calcium	Men: <275 mg/24 hours Women: <250 mg/24 hours
Creatinine	Men: 0.1–1.0 g/24 hours Women: 0.8–1.7 g/24 hours
Glucose	negative
Ketones	negative
Proteins	<150 mg/24 hours
Na	30–280 mEq/24 hours
Urea	64–99 mL/min
Specific gravity	1.025–1.032

Table 13-4 Normal Serum Values

pH	7.35–4.45
Na	135–145 mEq/L
K	3.8–5.5 mEq/L
Cl	100–108 mEq/L
Ca+	8.9–10.1 mg/dL or 4.5–5.5 mEq/L
Creatinine	Men: 0.2–0.6 mg/dL
	Women: 0.6–1.0 mg/dL
Glucose	80–100 mg/dL
Hct	Men: 42%–54%
	Women: 38%–46%
Hgb	Men: 14–18 g/dL
	Women: 12–16 g/dL

- *micturation cystogram*: x-rays taken of the bladder after the patient voids (prior to voiding, a radiopaque substance is instilled in the bladder to show the location of residual urine)
- *air cystogram*: used to identify filling defects caused by tumors, stones, or foreign objects
- *retrograde urethrography*: used to identify structures, trauma, or contractures of the urethral and bladder neck
- *tomography*
- *CAT scan*

In addition to the above, a cystoscopy (direct visualization of urethra and bladder), biopsy, and renal angiography (visualization of renal artery lesions and renal tumors) should be obtained.

SPECIFIC DISORDERS OF THE UROLOGICAL SYSTEM

Following is a detailed listing of 15 common disorders of the urological system:

1. Hydrocele

- Description: An accumulation of fluid within the serous sac of the scrotum. Classified as idiopathic or congenital.
- Presenting symptoms: Testicular mass.
- Diagnostic findings: Transillumination of the scrotum. Palpation reveals no palpable testes or indication that the testes is felt in the hydrocele sac.

- Surgical intervention: Hydrocele can be aspirated. Excision of the sac with inversion of tissue about the testis.
- Intraoperative complications: Bleeding, infertility.
- Postoperative management: Scrotal support, analgesics, carefully monitoring for signs and symptoms of infection.

2. Spermatocele

- Description: Retention cysts of the epididymus. Contain spermatazoa. Usually associated with scarring because of an inflammatory process or trauma.
- Presenting symptoms: Gradually enlarging sciotal mass with mild discomfort.
- Diagnostic findings: Palpation of mass distinct from the testis. Transillumination shows a cyst with fluid contents that are gray-white and contain inactive spermatozoa.
- Surgical intervention: Usually does not require treatment. If large enough, may require aspiration or excition.
- Intraoperative complications: Bleeding, infertility.
- Postoperative management: Scrotal support, analgesics, monitoring for signs and symptoms of infection.

3. Varicocele

- Description: Varicosities of the pampiniform venous plexus. More commonly associated with the left spermatic vein than the right. Usually seen between ages 15 and 30.
- Presenting symptoms: Dragging sensation or neuralgia of the testis.
- Diagnostic findings: Involved testis hangs lower, and a bruit may be palpable or audible near the spermatic cord.
- Surgical intervention: Treatment optional, since many tend to disappear spontaneously. If infertility is associated with the varicocele, ligation of spermatic vein may be warranted.
- Intraoperative complications: Bleeding, infertility.
- Postoperative management: Scrotal support, analgesics, wound management.

4. Torsion of testicle

   - Description: Sudden twisting of the spermatic cord, causing a partial or total obstruction of the blood supply to the testis.
   - Presenting symptoms: Sudden pain, followed by tenderness and swelling.
   - Surgical intervention: Serious emergency, requiring orchiopexy and, if gangerous, excision of the testis.
   - Intraoperative complications: Tendency for torsion is often bilateral, therefore orchiopexy of other testis should be done.
   - Postoperative management: Scrotal support, analgesics, antibiotics, wound management.

5. Urethral hypospadias

   - Description: Urethra opens on the ventral surface at the penis, and the distal urethra has not formed. Also there is marked curvature of the penis.
   - Presenting symptoms: Congenital abnormality noted on physical exam.
   - Surgical intervention: Corrective surgery involves straightening of the penis by removing the fibrous band causing the curvature. Then a tube is fashioned of skin leading from the intact urethra to the tip of the penis.
   - Intraoperative complications: Bleeding, sterility.
   - Postoperative monitoring: Monitoring for renal insufficiency, possibly due to the hydronephrosis caused by back pressure.

6. Epispadias

   - Description: Urethra opens dorsally on the penis.
   - Presenting symptoms: Congenital abnormality noted in physical exam.
   - Surgical intervention: Involves plastic repair of the opening and creation of an urethra.
   - Intraoperative complications: Bleeding, sterility.
   - Postoperative monitoring: Wound management, including catheter care. Strict asepsis to avoid infection.

7. Stricture

   - Description: Caused by scarring from old inflammation.
   - Presenting symptoms: Difficulty urinating; small stream.

- Diagnostic findings: Stricture is noted on x-ray or cystourethroscopy.
- Surgical intervention: May respond to dilatation or following two-step intervention: (1) direct visual urethrotomy, allowing excision of the stricture via an endoscopic procedure, and (2) Patch-graft urethroplasty of stricture, with graft of preputial or penile skin used to recreate the urethral section.
- Intraoperative complications: Bleeding, sterility.

8. (a) Benign prostatic hypertrophy, (b) prostatic cancer

- Description: (a) Seventy-five percent of males over 60 years of age have benign prostatic hypertrophy; of these, 50 percent will develop complete obstruction of the outflow tract. The disorder is caused by a hyperplasia of the inner glands of the prostate. This results in a distortion of the urethra and an obstruction of urine flow. (b) Prostatic cancer is the most common malignant growth in males, occurring in 20 percent of all males over the age of 50. Unlike benign prostatic hypertrophy, it involves the outer glands of the prostate.
- Presenting symptoms: (a) Urinary retention, nocturia, hematuria, hesitency, infrequency. Can progress to fever, chills, back pain, and renal colic. History of slowing of stream. (b) Prostatic cancer may produce no symptoms until it spreads to the urethra and/or bone, causing pain.
- Diagnostic findings: (a) Rectal exam reveals enlarged prostate; residual urine on catheterization; uroflometry; cystoscopy. (b) Rectal exam may be the only way to detect prostatic cancer.
- Surgical intervention: Four surgical approaches: (1) Transurethral (TURP)—resectoscope is introduced into the urethra and, under direct vision, the adenomatous tissue is resected, using a high frequency current; (2) suprapubic prostatectomy—the bladder is opened extraperitoneally, and the adenoma is resected; (3) perineal prostatectomy—approach is through the perineum, the prostate is detached from the rectum by cutting the rectourethralis muscle and the adenoma is removed; (4) retropubic prostatectomy—an incision is made just above the symphysis, the prostate is exposed, and the adenoma is removed.
- Intraoperative complications: With Surgical Approach 1—trauma to urethra, hemolytic reactions, water intoxication; with Surgical Approach 2—bleeding, damage to bladder, stimulation of sympathetic nervous system, resulting in severe bradycardias, hypotension, junctional rhythms; with Surgical Approach 3—damage to the rectum and

external sphincter; with Surgical Approach 4—bleeding because of involvement of prostatic venous plexus.
- Postoperative management: With Surgical Approach 1—monitor output (clot formation, bleeding), continuous bladder irrigations required, monitor fluid and electrolyte status; with Surgical Approach 2—monitor input and output, wound management, observe for development of urinary fistula; with Surgical Approaches 3 and 4—monitor input and output, wound management.

9. Bladder carcinoma

- Description: Majority of bladder cancers occur near the ureteral and urethral orifices. This suggests the possibility of a carcinogenic agent working on the mucosal membranes of the bladder. The cure and survival rates are directly related to the degree of invasion of the lesion.
- Presenting symptoms: Painless hematuria, any changes in frequency or urine.
- Diagnostic findings: Diagnosis is based on cystoscopy and biopsy, IVP, and air cystogram.
- Surgical intervention: Mandated by the extent of the tumor: Approach 1—destruction of tumor by means of electrocoagulation, either by transurethral resection or by open cystotomy; Approach 2—partial or total cystectomy, with diversion of urinary flow, ileal conduit or ureterorbal cutaneous anastomosis.
- Intraoperative complications: Approach 1—hemorrhage, bladder perforation, water intoxication; Approach 2—hemorrhage.
- Postoperative management: Monitor input and output, postoperative bleeding, fluid and electrolyte status.

10. Foreign bodies

- Description: A great variety of foreign bodies is found in the bladders of children and adults, for example, hairpins, matches, worms, balloons, candles.
- Presenting symptoms: Frequency, dysuria, foul-smelling urine, fever, hematuria.
- Diagnostic findings: X-ray and cystoscopic studies.
- Surgical intervention: Removal of object is done either transurethrally or through a suprapubic cystotomy.

- Intraoperative complications: Rupture of the bladder if transurethral.
- Postoperative management: Antibiotic management.

11. Injuries

    - Description: Bladder tears with leakage of urine into retroperitoneal or abdominal cavities; usually accompanies fractures or damage to other organs.
    - Presenting symptoms: History of trauma, either penetrating or blunt; tenderness.
    - Diagnostic finding: Cystography shows extravasation.
    - Surgical intervention: Prompt surgical closure of tear, placement of suprapubic catheter.
    - Intraoperative complications: Other organ system involvement.
    - Postoperative management: Monitor for infection, massive doses of antibiotics; monitor input and output.

12. Ureters, ureterocele

    - Description: Cystic dilatation of the bladder end of the ureter; caused by a congenital narrowing of the ureter, which can lead to back pressure, causing hydronephrosis, infection, or stone formation.
    - Presenting symptoms: Usually asymptomatic until problems from back pressure develop.
    - Diagnostic findings: Urograms and cystoscopy reveal a cyst body.
    - Surgical intervention: Removal of ureterocele is performed, and the ureter is reimplanted in the bladder.
    - Intraoperative complications: Bleeding, improper reimplantation and necrosis of ureter.
    - Postoperative management: Monitor output.

13. Ureteral stones

    - Description: Renal stones that have passed down; rarely do stones form in the ureters.
    - Presenting symptoms: Pain, hematuria.
    - Diagnostic findings: Show up as a filling deficit on IVP.

14. Kidney stones (urolithiasis)

- Description: Predisposing factors for stone formation: (1) foreign body, (2) vitamin-A deficiency, (3) urinary tract infection, (4) urine stasis, (5) metabolic disturbances.
- Presenting symptoms: Pain, hematuria.
- Diagnostic findings: IVP, KUB.
- Surgical intervention: Size and location of calculi determine surgical intervention; may be possible to resect the stone, or the entire kidney may have to be resected.
- Intraoperative complications: Bleeding.
- Postoperative management: Monitor input and output, fluid and electrolyte status.

15. End-stage renal disease

- Description: Many congenital anomalies and renal neoplasms require total resection of one or both kidneys, due to irreversible renal failure; also the kidneys can be destroyed by existing disease processes (see Exhibit 13-3).
- Presenting symptoms: Signs and symptoms of renal failure.
- Diagnostic findings: When a transplant is to be done, four tests are performed to ensure compatibility: (1) ABO Blood Typing—ABO antigens are present in red blood cells and most tissues; it is essential that the

---

Exhibit 13-3 Causes of Acute/Chronic Renal Failure

1. Polycystic disease
2. Neoplasms: Wilm's tumor, hypernephromas (all kidney tumors are considered malignant)
3. Vascular anomalies
4. Diabetes: development of vascular changes called diabetic neuropathy or Kimmelstiehl-Wilson disease
5. Gout: uric acid collects, causing stones and interstitial deposits
6. Sickle cell disease: nephropathy develops secondary to small multiple hemorrhagic and ischemic infarcts
7. B-hemolytic streptococci flu: acute glomerulonephritis causes an antigen/antibody activity
8. Renal calculi
9. Frequent cystitis
10. Congenital anomalies

Urological and Renal Surgery 183

donor and recipient be compatible. (2) White cell crossmatching—identifies the presence of circulating cytotoxic antibodies in the recipient. (3) HLA typing (human leukocyte antigen), major histocompatibility system—easily detected on leukocytes, but is also present on cell membranes of most body tissue. A genetic region of the sixth chromosome controls histocompatibility antigens. Four antigens have been isolated on the genetic region of each person. However, there are 30 different known antigens in the general population. Each offspring acquires one HLA region from each parent; therefore, there are four different types of possibilities, resulting in a one-in-four chance of offspring having the same HLA type. An identical HLA match has the best chance for survival. (4) Mixed lymphocytes culture (MLC)—determines the degree of incompatibility between donor and recipient by monitoring lymphocyte development.

- Surgical intervention: Renal transplantation.
- Intraoperative complications: Rejection (see Exhibit 13-4). Two types of lymphocytes are involved in rejection: (1) B-lymphocytes form antibodies; this response activates the kallikrein system, which deposits platelets and fibrin at the site of reaction. (2) T-lymphocytes produce cell-mediated immunity and become sensitized by contact with antigens; they release chemical factors called lymphokines, which destroy cells carrying specific antigens.
- Postoperative management: Monitor for rejection: oliguria, anuria, fever, hypertension secondary to fluid retention, weight gain, soft tender swollen kidney, malaise, changes in blood urea nitrogen (BUN), creatinine, clearance, electrolytes, changes in components of urine. Strict asepsis, wound management.

Exhibit 13-4 Forms of Rejection of Renal Transplants

1. Hyperacute	B-lymphocytes cause a reaction between antigens in the transplanted kidney and the recipients; occurs within minutes.
2. Accelerated	B-lymphocytes cause the same reaction, but it is delayed for 24–36 hours because the level of antibodies is not high enough at transplant.
3. Acute	Cellular immune response caused to t-lymphocytes; necrosis of kidney occurs one week to several months after transplant.
4. Chronic	Rejection occurs several months to years later and is a combination of b-lymphocytes and t-lymphocytes.

ANESTHETIC MANAGEMENT OF THE PATIENT WITH RENAL DISEASE

The choice of anesthetic agents and technique for the patient with renal disease, is aimed at providing an optimum perioperative course while minimizing the risk factors. The ability of the patient to tolerate adverse effects of anesthesia depends upon:

- normality of respiratory function
- normality of circulatory function
- homeostatic function of the liver, kidneys, endocrine, and CNS.

The selection of the anesthetic agent is based on:

- patient age, prior anesthetics, complicating disease
- nature of the operation
- habits and skills of the surgeon
- position required for the procedure
- emotional considerations

During preanesthetic evaluation, a numerical classification is assigned to each patient (see Table 13-5). Patients with underlying renal disease are automatically moved up one or two classes, depending upon the degree of involvement. In addition to assigning a classification, the anesthetist must take into account the renal system's response to various drugs. This information is also vital for the PACU nurse in evaluating postanesthetic responses.

Application of Agents

The uptake and elimination of inhalation drugs is predominantly accomplished by the respiratory system. However, certain agents have partial metabolism and excretion by the hepatic/renal systems; therefore, their effects may be prolonged. In addition, general anesthesia has been shown to cause decreased urine output and an increased urine osmolality. This can be attributed to the fact that there is a stimulation release of ADH and a reduction in glomerular filtration rate, perhaps due to hormonal factors, that is, increased renin stimulating the renin-angiotensin cycle.

The depolarizing muscle relaxants have no renal or liver metabolism. The nondepolarizing relaxants, with the exception of atracurium (Tracrium), are

Table 13-5 Physical Status Modifiers are Represented by the Initial Letter P Followed by a Single Digit from 1 to 6 Defined Below:

	Unit Values
P1—A normal healthy patient	0
P2—A patient with mild systemic disease	0
P3—A patient with severe systemic disease	1
P4—A patient with severe systemic disease that is a constant threat to life	2
P5—A moribund patient who is not expected to survive for 24 hours with or without the operation	3
P6—A declared brain-dead patient whose organs are being removed for donor purposes	0

The above six levels are consistent with the American Society of Anesthesiologists (ASA) ranking of patient physical status. Physical status is included in CPT-4 to distinguish between various levels of complexity of the anesthesia service provided.

Source: Reprinted from *Relative Value Guide—1985*, p. v, with permission of American Society of Anesthesiologists, © 1985.

---

metabolized via the hepatic/renal systems. Therefore, prolongation of block will occur when these agents are used. In such cases, reversal agents may be required to counteract the neuromuscular blocking.

Metabolism and excretion of intravenous agents are via the hepatic and renal systems. Therefore, the duration of action will be prolonged, and smaller doses must be given.

All local, anesthetic agents are metabolized in the liver and excreted in the urine. Therefore, blocks may be slightly prolonged in the presence of renal disease.

Adjunctive Treatment Modalities

As the incidence of renal failure increases, the frequency of the PACU staff being involved with treatment for renal failure will increase. Currently, three different types of alternative treatment modalities are available: peritoneal dialysis, hemodialysis, and continuous arteriovenous hemofiltration (CAVH).

Usually, peritoneal dialysis and hemodialysis are discontinued during the perioperative phase. Thus, the PACU nurse's role is limited to care of the

186 HANDBOOK OF POSTANESTHESIA NURSING

Exhibit 13-5 Indications for the Use of Continuous Arteriovenous Hemofiltration (CAVH)

General:	Hypervolemia resistant to diuretic therapy Hyperkalemia Azotemia Total parenteral nutrition (TPN) administration to patients requiring volume restriction
Special:	Cardiogenic pulmonary edema Refractory hypernatremia Hyperkalemia secondary to massive tissue destruction Cardiogenic shock Acute tubular necrosis Hepatic failure with profound acites Massive fluid retention

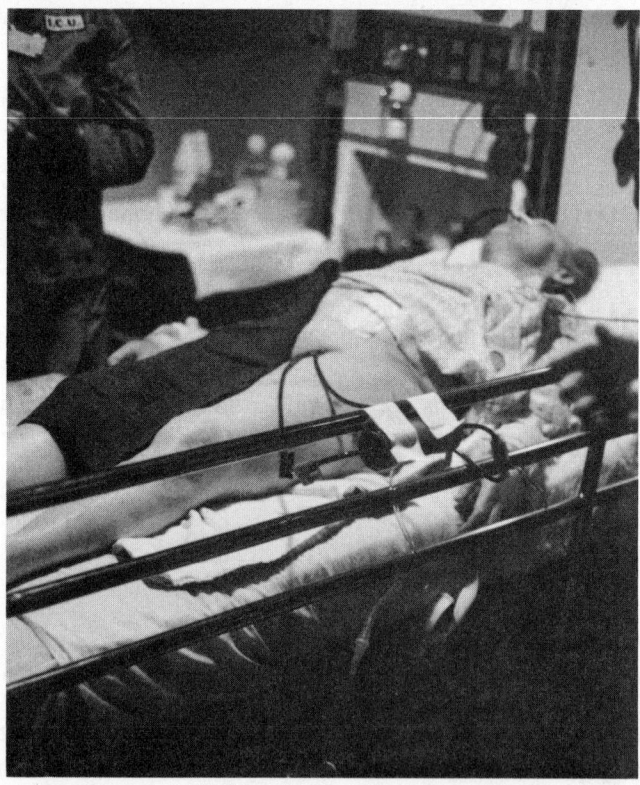

Figure 13-2 CAVH System in Operation in the PACU. *Source:* Courtesy of Amicon.

peritoneal Tenchkoff catheter or monitoring the patency of a Scribner shunt or AV fistula.

Since 1981, the new modality, CAVH, has gained popularity in the treatment of renal failure (see Exhibit 13-5 and Figure 13-2). In this procedure, a small filter containing multiple small transverse filaments is placed in a circuit formed from an artery and returning to a vein. Utilizing the principles of ultrafiltration and hydrostatic pressure, water, electrolytes, and low molecular weight substances pass through the filter and are collected in a standard urinary drainage bag (see Figure 13-3). Outputs average 600 mL/hr. The amount of filtrate produced is concurrently replaced by a comparable amount of intravenous solution. Thus, the system lowers the amount of toxins and fluids by appropriate electrolyte replacement and

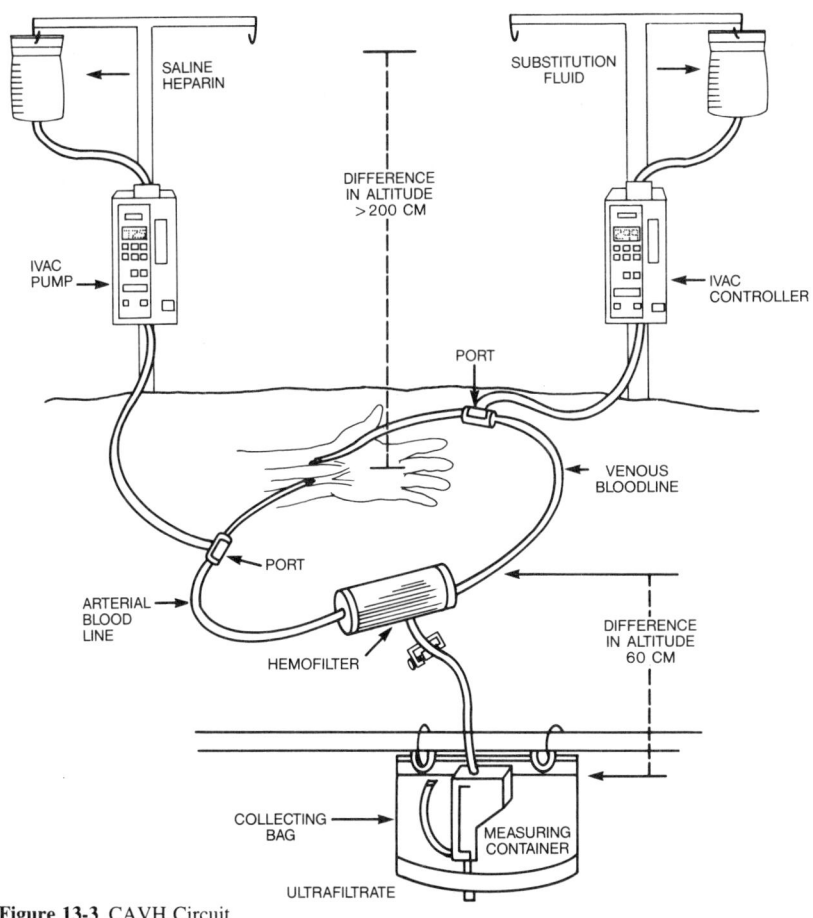

Figure 13-3 CAVH Circuit

slightly less volume. This is a continuous process (24 hours a day) that is controlled by the patient's own blood pressure. Therefore, it can be utilized on a hemodynamically compromised patient.

Patients with preexisting renal disease present a unique challenge to the PACU nurse. Monitoring should include the routine parameters of blood pressure, pulse, ECG, fluid intake and output, LOC, and temperature. In addition to these, the following parameters should be monitored:

- Urine: specific gravity, osmolality, creatinine clearance
- Serum: creatinine, BUN, NA+, K+, HCO_3
- CVP or pulmonary artery catheters to monitor fluid shifts.

BIBLIOGRAPHY

Brenner, B.M., and Rector, F.C. Jr., eds. *The Kidney*, 2d ed. Philadelphia: W.B. Saunders, 1981.

Eisenberg, Mickey S., and Copass, Michale K. *Emergency Medical Therapy*. Philadelphia: W.B. Saunders, 1982.

Fischbach, Frances. "Analyzing Urinalysis Results." *Dimensions of Critical Care Nursing* 2 (July/August 1983):225–232.

Fluid and Electrolytes. North Chicago, Ill.: Abbott Laboratories, 1970.

Frost, Elizabeth. *Recovery Room Practice*. Boston: Blackwell Scientific Publications, 1985.

Harrington, Joan D., and Brenner, Etta Rae, eds. *Patient Care in Renal Failure*. Philadelphia: W.B. Saunders, 1973.

Liechty, Richard D., and Soper, Robert T. *Synopsis of Surgery*, 4th ed. St. Louis, Mo.: C.V. Mosby, 1980.

Parrish, Alvin E. *Handbook of Nephrologic Emergencies*. New Hyde Park, N.Y.: Medical Examination Publishing Co., 1983.

Schruer, R., ed. *Manual of Nephrology*. Boston: Little, Brown & Co., 1981.

Part III

Addressing the Special Needs of Select Patient Groups

Chapter 14
Postanesthesia Care After Pediatric Surgery

John R. Charney, M.D.

Very frequently children, particularly infants, are erroneously considered to be "miniature adults." In fact, anatomic and physiological characteristics are constantly evolving from birth to adolescence. In order to provide appropriate care for the pediatric population, a basic knowledge of these particularities and their implications is essential.

ANATOMIC CONSIDERATIONS

Substantial differences exist in anatomic proportion between the neonate and adult. The surface-to-volume ratio is 70 times greater in the newborn than in the adult. At birth, the chest cavity is small relative to the size of the organs it contains. The abdominal contents are relatively large and tend to impinge upon the diaphragm. The ribs are more horizontal. The lower rib cage spreads because the cartilage is poorly developed.

There are significant differences in the structure and location of the upper airway. The infant larynx is situated at the C_2 vertebral level, while the adult larynx is located at the C_6 vertebral level. In the infant, the anterior attachment of the vocal cords to the larynx is inferior to the posterior attachment; in the adult, the two attachments are on an even plane. The epiglottis forms a more acute angle with the vocal cords in the infant than in the adult. The cricoid ring is in a semivertical position in the infant but in a nearly horizontal position in the adult. Moreover, the cricoid ring is the narrowest portion of the infant airway; the vocal cord opening is the narrowest portion of the adult upper airway.

The neonatal heart includes the foramen ovale and the ductus arteriosus, although these elements normally become dysfunctional within hours after birth. Anatomic closure does not occur for several months.

The newborn's organs are histologically immature; physiological functions are considerably altered.

The cardiopulmonary system is not fully developed at birth. The newborn lung contains only a small number of alveoli (about 8 percent of the number in the adult). The epithelium of the alveolar walls is cuboidal at birth but eventually becomes flat. Full alveolar maturation is not attained until ten years of age. A reduced amount of elastic tissue is present in the neonatal lung. Compared to the heart in the older child, the newborn heart contains fewer myocardial contractile elements. At birth, the diaphragm is deficient in fatigue-resistant muscle fibers.

The newborn liver is less developed. Endoplasmic reticulum, which is responsible for enzymatic function, is less abundant in the hepatocytes of the neonate. The Kupffer cells, which are responsible for endocytosis, appear to be functionally immature at this time.

The kidney is not fully developed at birth. In the neonate, the nephrons are heterogeneous and the proximal tubular volume is small in relation to the glomerular diameter. During the first few months of life, proximal tubular volume increases and the nephrons become homogeneous.

Neuromuscular maturation continues after birth. Myelination of the central nervous system is not complete in the newborn. The neonatal myocardial sympathetic innervation is incomplete, and the parasympathetic system predominates. The neonate has reduced muscle mass. During infancy, transformation of myotubules to mature muscle fibers and of slow-contracting to fast-contracting muscle takes place. Full ramification and segmentation of the myoneural junction, along with accelerating synaptic transmission, are achieved by two years of age.

Neonates have brown fat distributed in the nuchal region and behind the sternum. They lack subcutaneous fat.

Volume distribution differs according to age. In the neonate, 70 percent of body weight is water, compared with 60 percent in the adult. The extracellular compartment contains 60 percent of this water in the neonate and 30 percent in the adult.

There is increased red blood cell mass in the infant and young child. The blood volume is 90 mL/kg at birth, 80 mL/kg in young children, and 70 mL/kg in the adolescent.

PHYSIOLOGICAL CONSEQUENCES

The very high surface-to-volume ratio in the neonate necessitates a proportionate increase in metabolism, with subsequent adjustments in physiological function of the various organ systems. The metabolic rate in the infant is twice that in the adult; oxygen consumption is 6 cc/kg/min in the newborn, compared with 3 cc/kg/min in the adult. The anatomical differences between infant and adult organs also result in significant alterations in physiological function.

Cardiac Function

The cardiac output is 50 percent greater in the neonate than in the adult. Cardiac output depends on stroke volume and heart rate. Since the ventricles of the infant are less compliant, due to fewer myocardial contractile elements, stroke volume cannot be significantly increased. Therefore, the heart rate must be double that of the adult (130 to 150 beats/minute). The infant rate pressure product (systolic blood pressure × heart rate), however, remains comparable with that in the adult, since the normal systolic/diastolic pressure at term birth is 65/40. The heart rate decreases gradually until adolescence, while the blood pressure concomitantly increases.

Respiratory Function

The respiratory rate of the neonate (40 breaths/minute) is twice that of the adult, while the tidal volume (7 cc/kg) is comparable. At birth, gas exchange is less efficient because of the cuboid configuration of the epithelium lining the alveoli. During childhood, the epithelium flattens, which permits better gas exchange.

Because of the cartilagenous structure of the ribs, the newborn's chest wall is soft and thus very compliant. Lung compliance, however, is reduced, since little elastic tissue is present in the vicinity of the alveoli. If the infant's lungs become atelectactic, reexpansion will be difficult, since the chest wall is floppy and the lung relatively stiff. Without assisted or controlled ventilation, tidal volume and pressure cannot be increased sufficiently to overcome atelectasis. Crying helps open the small airways and the alveoli, while grunting during respiratory distress generates peak end expiratory pressure and thus counters to some extent collapse of the lung.

The ratio of dead space to tidal volume is 40 percent during the first month of life, then reduces to 30 percent.

The lung volume at which the small airways begin to close, or the closing capacity, is greatly increased in the newborn and infant. This is probably due to the small amount of elastic tissue in this age group.

After exhalation, a greater volume of air remains in the lungs of the infant than in those of the adult. Therefore, higher ratios of functional residual capacity to total lung capacity and residual volume to total lung capacity exist at birth.

Significant shunting of blood with a low Pao_2 (around 70 mm Hg) occurs at birth, since the ductus arteriosus and foramen ovale are still patent. The newborn's $Paco_2$ is around 33 mm Hg because of maternal hyperventilation toward the end of pregnancy. Plasma bicarbonate in the neonate is reduced at 20 mEq/liter (normal adult plasma level: 25 mEq/liter). These factors result in respiratory alkalosis balanced by metabolic acidosis, the pH being the same in both the neonate and the adult.

Thermoregulation

The high surface-to-volume ratio in newborns significantly affects thermoregulation. Heat is produced by a small volume of organs but is lost over a large surface area. In addition, the insulating subcutaneous adipose layer found in adults is deficient in infants. The infant produces heat by nonshivering, or chemical, thermogenesis (NST). The major source of this NST is the brown fat. Norepinephrine mediates NST.

Central and Peripheral Nervous System Function

During childhood, increasing myelination of the central nervous system, as well as maturation of the neuronal membranes resulting in more efficient neuronal discharge, lead to increased cerebral blood flow and metabolism. Between ages three and ten, cerebral blood flow is twice that of the adult.

The blood brain barrier in the newborn is permeable to macromolecules, but during infancy this barrier becomes impermeable to protein.

Synaptic transmission at the neuromuscular junction is slow at birth, but accelerates during the first two weeks of life.

Liver Function

Because of the reduced amount of endoplasmic reticulum, the infant liver presents with immature enzyme function. The activity of some of the conjugation enzymes (glucuronidase), cytochrome P-450 oxidative, and reductive enzymes is reduced at birth. Many drugs are therefore metabolized at a slower rate during the perinatal and early infancy period.

Kidney Function

Glomerular filtration rate is reduced in the newborn kidney. Tubular reabsorption, however, is even more limited, since the ratio of glomerular diameter to tubular volume is higher in the neonate. Bicarbonate is largely excreted in the urine, contributing to the lower plasma bicarbonate and metabolic acidosis in the newborn. Phosphate and amino acids are also highly excreted. Glucose and sodium are reabsorbed to the same extent in both the neonate and adult.

MONITORING

Appropriate monitoring is an absolute necessity in the postoperative care of the child emerging from an anesthetic. Heart rate, rhythm, and blood pressure monitoring is basic. Other parameters, such as temperature, ventilation, and oxygenation, must be watched closely, particularly in the very young population. In specific instances, such assessments as intracranial pressure measurements will also be indicated.

Decreases in heart rate, particularly in the infant, most likely indicate hypoxia, acidosis, and stress; vagal responses predominate in these situations in the young infant due to the immaturity of the sympathetic nervous system. In the face of significant changes in heart rate, one must immediately assess the adequacy of the child's oxygenation.

In postoperative patients with congenital heart disease, the care person must be particularly attentive to changes in cardiac rhythm. Conduction abnormalities are frequent in patients with these diseases, and they may become manifest in the postoperative period, whether or not the surgical procedure involved the heart itself.

The arterial blood pressure must be measured with a cuff of appropriate size. This cuff should encircle three-quarters of the arm. The cuff width varies according to age: 2.5 cm for the first year of life, 5 cm for age one to four, and 8 cm from age five to adolescence. A cuff that is too narrow or wide will give a spuriously high or low reading, respectively.

The body temperature should be checked with the use of a rectal thermometer. This thermometer must be carefully placed in the neonate, since abrupt insertion may result in perforation of the rectum. Hyperventilation and mouth breathing, which occur frequently in the postoperative period, may result in accelerated heat loss and cooling of the oral cavity, and therefore oral temperatures may give falsely low readings.

Respiratory movement and rate can be monitored by impedance pneumography, which translates chest wall motion into wave forms. However, this device cannot ensure that the patient is ventilating adequately, since chest or abdominal wall motion in the absence of air exchange will also translate into wave forms.

The pulse oximeter is an extremely useful monitor for early detection of hypoxia. It measures heart beat to beat oxygen saturation of hemoglobin. In addition to revealing hypoxia due to inadequate ventilation, this monitor may also uncover an impending disease process involving abnormal hemoglobin that is unable to carry oxygen, such as methemoglobinemia.

An apnea monitor is required postoperatively for preterm infants of less than six months postconceptual age. These infants are prone to apnea episodes for as long as 24 hours after surgery.

End tidal CO_2–O_2 monitoring is useful in intubated patients. Decreases in end tidal CO_2 (with concomitant increases in end tidal O_2) signal airway obstruction or pulmonary embolism; increasing end tidal CO_2 may indicate malignant hyperthermia.

Invasive monitoring for arterial blood pressure, central venous pressure, or pulmonary artery pressure is indicated in critical cases. Arterial catheterization is also helpful if extensive blood chemistry or blood gases are required. Pulmonary artery catheterization also permits cardiac output and mixed venous oxygen saturation measurements.

POSTANESTHESIA ASSESSMENT

The young postsurgical patient, particularly the neonate, very often presents in the recovery room with excessive drowsiness or even total unresponsiveness to stimulation. Failure to awaken in the postoperative period can result from residual anesthetics, drugs used intraoperatively for purposes other than anesthesia, electrolyte disturbances, intraoperative insult to the central nervous system, or physiological alterations.

The residual effects of anesthetics vary considerably in the neonate and infants, since their physiologic characteristics differ from that of the older child and adult. Prolonged muscle paralysis would be expected to result from those muscle relaxants whose elimination is dependent primarily on kidney function, such as d-tubocurare and vecuronium; but it appears that this prolongation is due more to the increased extracellular volume of distribution in the neonate than to the reduced glomerular filtration rate. Moreover, vecuronium has been shown to be eliminated faster in the older child than in the adult.

The effects of fentanyl in the neonate are quite variable. Cytochrome P-450, which is the enzyme system responsible for the metabolism of the narcotic in the liver, is immature in the neonate; and therefore fentanyl's metabolism is slowed. The expected result would be that more active narcotic is present in the neonate for a longer period of time. However, increased cardiac output with the resulting increased liver blood flow increases the rate at which fentanyl reaches the liver. This phenomenon may offset or actually override the effects of immature enzyme system and blood brain barrier, resulting in an accelerated awakening of the neonate.

The major problem with residual muscle relaxant or narcotic is respiratory depression. Residual muscle relaxant can be reversed with an anticholinesterase along with atropine (to block muscarinic cardiac effects), and residual narcotic can be reversed with naloxone. However, the duration of action of naloxone is shorter than that of morphine or large doses of fentanyl, and renarcotization may occur.

Inhalational agents are less soluable in infants than in adults. The infant's functional residual capacity is lower and the minute ventilation of infants is greater, since their respiratory rate is faster and their tidal volume per kilogram equivalent to that in the adult. Therefore, infants should recover relatively quickly from inhalational agents. Recovery from isoflurane is more rapid than from halothane because the solubility of isoflurane is less.

On occasion, drugs used intraoperatively for purposes other than anesthesia may be responsible for a continuing unconscious state postoperatively. For example, an obtunded child entering the recovery room with a lidocaine infusion started intraoperatively because of ventricular arrhythmias should be suspected of having toxic plasma levels of this drug, and the infusion should be stopped until a blood level is measured. Many antibiotics (for example, aminoglycosides) and calcium channel blockers prolong the effects of muscle relaxants.

Electrolyte disturbances, particularly hyponatremia, should be suspected in a child who is unresponsive after surgery if the child has some underlying predisposing disease. Infusion solutions lacking sodium that are used intraoperatively should also be suspect.

A child can be obtunded as a result of episodes of intraoperative hypoxia with neurological sequelae or intraoperative intracranial hemorrhage. Neurological evaluation and certain diagnostic procedures, such as a computerized axial tomography (CAT) scan, must be done immediately so that prompt, appropriate measures (for example, cerebral resuscitation) may be undertaken.

Various physiological alterations may also be implicated. Hypotension, acidosis, or hypothermia may delay awakening by themselves or by prolonging the effects of anesthetic or paralyzing agents used intraoperatively. Anemia is very often the cause of delayed arousal. Hypercarbia must also be suspected, particularly in the infant, as anesthetics substantially reduce effective ventilation.

In summary, delayed awakening and unresponsiveness can result from a variety of causes. The anesthetic record must be carefully evaluated, and all unusual events occurring during surgery and anesthesia must be reported. Appropriate clinical and laboratory examinations must then be done.

VENTILATORY MANAGEMENT

Very often, the postoperative unconscious or semiconscious state is associated with respiratory depression. It is therefore essential to evaluate and monitor carefully the ventilatory status of every child in the recovery room.

Extubation of any child should be done only after certain criteria have been met. The small infant should be vigorous with good muscle tone. In the older child, various parameters should be measured: the maximum inspiratory force should be greater than 25 cm H_2O and the forced vital capacity greater than 10 cc/kg. The older child should have an adequate hand grip and be capable of lifting the head.

The child must be carefully observed in the immediate postextubation period, since various problems may arise during this time. Any evidence of hypoxia, as indicated by the color of the child or by oximeter, must be treated with oxygen and, if the situation appears critical, with positive pressure ventilation. Auscultation of the chest, arterial blood gas measurement, and a chest x-ray must be done immediately.

Obstruction of the Endotracheal Tube

The most common cause of respiratory distress in the intubated child is obstruction of the endotracheal tube. Mucous plugging, blood clot, and cuff herniation are major causes of obstruction. The cuff should be deflated and the tube vigorously suctioned, and then lavaged with normal saline if suctioning is unsuccessful in clearing the mucus or blood from the airway. However, a blood clot or a thick mucous plug may not be dislodged from the end of the endotracheal tube, even with vigorous suctioning and lavage; in such cases the tube must therefore be changed. An end tidal CO_2–O_2 monitor will reveal obstruction by indicating a rapid decrease in end tidal CO_2 due to the inability of CO_2 to exit in the airway, and a rise in end tidal O_2 because oxygen cannot get by the obstruction to the lung.

Laryngospasm may ensue after the endotracheal tube has been removed. If the child has partial laryngospasm, lifting of the mandible forward by grasping the angles of the lower jaw will generally be sufficient to break it. One should avoid the use of positive pressure by mask in cases of partial laryngospasm; a huge amount of pressure is required to break laryngospasm, and it may convert a partial laryngospasm into a total one. Total laryngospasm may require treatment with succinylcholine followed by reintubation.

Upper Airway Obstruction

Upper airway obstruction is also a potential problem in the postoperative period. Subglottic edema may result from prolonged intubation or the use of an inappropriately large endotracheal tube during the operation. Subglottic edema manifests itself clinically by inspiratory stridor, often associated with substernal and intercostal retractions and nasal flaring. Auscultation will confirm the inspiratory wheezing-type sounds. These sounds will be heard not only in the chest but also in the neck and cheek, thus confirming the upper airway origin of the respiratory distress.

Treatment of subglottic edema consists of the administration of intravenous dexamethasone, 1 mg/kg, and racemic epinephrine aerosol, .05 mL/kg/dose (maximum .5 mL). If severe, 2.25 percent racemic epinephrine should be administered diluted to 5 mL normal saline, every two hours.

Lower Airway Problems

Respiratory distress in the postoperative period can also be due to lower airway problems. The lungs must be carefully auscultated after extubation. Diminished breath sounds and dull percussion may indicate atelectasis, which can occur rapidly by mucous plugging of the lower airways. Vigorous chest percussion and coughing will prevent serious plugging. The chest x-ray will show a dense shadow in the affected area, with narrow intercostal spaces and a shifted mediastinum to the atelectactic lung. The pulse oximeter will indicate falling oxygen saturations. Reintubation with lavage, suction, and administration of positive pressure to inflate the collapsed lung is necessary. Rarely, bronchoscopic aspiration is required.

An asthmatic child is prone to postoperative bronchospasm. Expiratory wheezing is evident. A chest x-ray will show hyperexpansion of the lungs. An arterial blood gas measurement is important to determine the degree of respiratory failure; hypoxemia is invariably present. A $Paco_2$ of below 35 mm Hg is compatible with a well-compensated respiratory status, whereas a $Paco_2$ of 40 mm Hg or above is indicative of respiratory failure. Oxygen must be administered to all children presenting with wheezing. Aminophyllin IV, 5 to 7 mg/kg over 15 minutes, should be started and then maintained at 1 mg/kg/hr as a continuous infusion. Bronkosol 1 percent (.5 mL diluted 1:3 with saline in O_2 aerosol) or Alupent inhaler treatments should also be administered. If the asthma is severe, an isoproterenol infusion should be considered. Ketamine infusion has been used successfully.

Pulmonary Edema

Bilateral rales heard on auscultation indicate pulmonary edema. The chest x-ray will show cloudy densities extended outward from the hilar regions. Rose-colored sputum may be present.

There are several causes of pulmonary edema. Fluid overload is the most common. If the pulmonary edema is not too severe in the older child, administration of oxygen via face mask or nasal prongs and IV furosemide, 1 mg/kg may be sufficient treatment. If severe, reintubation and positive pressure ventilation with the addition of peak end expiratory pressure (PEEP) may be necessary.

Other, more dramatic causes of pulmonary edema exist. These include pulmonary edema due to neurogenic insult, to severe airway obstruction, or to the administration of certain drugs to an already hypoxic child. The probable underlying mechanism of these types of pulmonary edema is pulmonary vasoconstriction.

Neurogenic pulmonary edema may occur in the postoperative period following procedures associated with head trauma (for example, cranioplasty for basal skull fracture). This type of pulmonary edema is vasoactive-mediated, with cerebral vasoconstriction followed by generalized vasoconstriction and centralization of fluid toward the lung. It should be suspected in any postoperative neurosurgical patient with sudden onset of clinical signs of pulmonary edema and must be treated with a vasodilator, preferably an alpha blocker, such as phentolamine (1 mg IV), as well as with furosemide. A computerized axial tomography of the brain should be done to detect postoperative intracranial bleeding, which may have triggered the mechanisms leading to this type of edema.

Severe airway obstruction may cause pulmonary edema in the child who develops hypoxic pulmonary vasoconstriction. The work of breathing is greatly increased in the child with airway obstruction, and this will decrease pleural pressure and increase venous return to the heart, increasing preload leading to the pulmonary edema.

In children with prolonged hypoxic pulmonary vasoconstriction, the administration of succinylcholine for reintubation may cause florid pulmonary edema. Succinylcholine may cause histamine release, which will increase capillary permeability and edema, thus exacerbating the effects of increased pulmonary vascular resistance. In infants, pulmonary hemorrhage may even ensue. Reintubation with controlled ventilation with PEEP and the administration of phentolamine and lasix are generally required to treat this type of pulmonary edema.

Pneumothorax

Falling oxygen saturations with tachypnea, asymmetric chest expansion, and auscultatory signs of diminished breath sounds and hyperresonance to percussion are signs of pneumothorax, which is most often due to intraoperative hyperventilation. The chest x-ray shows a mediastinal shift away from the absence of lung markings on the affected side. Chest tube insertion is mandatory in this situation.

Respiratory distress with unilateral absent breath sounds on auscultation and dullness to percussion may indicate fluid accumulation in the pleural space due to placement of a central venous catheter into that space (dextrothorax). The chest x-ray will reveal obliteration of the diaphragmatic angle with the rib cage and upward concavity of the liquid level on the affected side. Surgical injury of the thoracic duct results in chylothorax.

Pulmonary Embolism

Pulmonary embolism is a rare cause of sudden postoperative respiratory distress, but it must be suspected in any child who was immobilized for any length of time prior to surgery (for example, prior to orthopedic surgery for lower limb fracture) or who has a predisposing disease process (antithrombin III deficiency). Tachypnea, tachycardia, and pain on inspiration are presenting symptoms. Hemoptysis is a late sign indicating pulmonary infarction. The pulse oximeter shows decreasing oxygen saturations. The chest x-ray will be negative unless atelectasis or pulmonary infarction are already present. Because of increased right heart pressures proximal to the embolic obstruction, the ECG will show evidence of right ventricular hypertrophy. Right bundle branch block, right QRS axis deviation, an S_1Q_3 or $S_1S_2S_3$ pattern, and ST changes are other ECG signs indicating pulmonary embolism. A sudden drop in end tidal CO_2 in an intubated, mechanically ventilated child may be the first indication of massive pulmonary embolism.

Treatment with heparin must be initiated immediately if pulmonary embolism is suspected. An angiogram must be done to confirm its presence.

Adult Respiratory Distress Syndrome

Adult respiratory distress syndrome may occur in the immediate postoperative period in massively septic or severely traumatized children. ARDS results from pulmonary capillary leak with both alveolar and interstitial edema and loss of lung compliance. The chest x-ray is normal initially, but the lungs gradually become hazy. Tachypnea and falling oxygen saturation are the initial symptoms. Arterial blood gases confirm the hypoxemia. The Pa_{CO_2} will be low initially because of the tachypnea. On auscultation, breath sounds are initially clear; but, as the interstitial edema compresses the airway, wheezing sounds become evident. Rales will be heard when the edema accumulates in the alveoli.

Treatment includes mechanically controlled ventilation. PEEP must be added in order to improve functional residual capacity and compliance.

Should reintubation be necessary, appropriately sized endotracheal tubes should be inserted. If internal diameter is used as a measurement for proper tube size, the formula is 4 + age in years/4. Alternatively, the French unit, which is an approximate measurement of external tube circumference in millimeters, may be used to determine adequate tube size; the formula for the French unit is 18 + age in years. Visualization of the vocal cords is more difficult in the infant, due to the differences in the anatomy of the upper airway. If the endotracheal tube does not pass through the narrow cricoid ring in the infant, intubation with a smaller tube should be attempted. An air leak around the tube at an airway pressure of 15 cm H_2O should be present in order to limit the possibility of subglottic edema. Uncuffed tubes should be inserted in infants.

The type of ventilator to be used for the child in the recovery room depends on the child's age and size. A time-cycled, pressure-limited, volume-variable ventilator is preferable for the newborn and infant, since their lungs are very small. Various parameters, such as inspiratory and expiratory duration and peak inspiratory pressure, can each be adjusted with the time-cycled ventilator. A volume-cycled respirator is desirable for the older child.

FLUID AND ELECTROLYTE MANAGEMENT

Maintenance and Replacement Fluids

The postanesthesia care person must ensure adequate fluid administration postoperatively. Such administration will depend primarily on fluid and blood losses and replacement that occurred during surgery.

Basically, all patients receive maintenance fluids. These fluids are based on the average water and electrolytes lost by the lungs, skin, stool, and urine relative to the metabolic rate. Thus, maintenance fluids are to be given as follows:

- 100 mL/kg/day for the first 10 kg of body weight
- 50 mL/kg/day for 10 to 20 kg + 1,000 mL
- 20 mL/kg/day for more than 20 kg + 1,500 mL

Calculation of maintenance fluid based on surface area is as follows: 2,000 mL/m^2/day (approximate surface areas being .20 m^2 for the newborn, .50 m^2 for a one-year-old, .75 m^2 for a five-year-old, 1.00 m^2 for a nine-year-old, 1.50 to

Pediatric Surgery 203

1.70 m² for the young adult). This method of fluid administration is particularly useful in the pediatric intensive care setting.

Adequate maintenance electrolyte requirements are 2 to 4 mEq/kg/day (50 mEq/m²/day) of sodium and 2 to 3 mEq/kg/day of potassium. This is provided by the addition of 30 mEq/liter of sodium and 20 mEq/liter of potassium to the solution (that is, dextrose 5.0 percent in .2 percent NaCl with 20 mEq/liter KCl).

Replacement fluid must also be administered postoperatively in cases of dehydration. One can quickly assess the state of hydration in a child by clinical examination. Dry mucosa, sunken fontanelle (in an infant), tachycardia, and tenting and mottling of the skin due to poor capillary filling are all signs of significant dehydration. Periorbital and peripheral edema are signs of overhydration.

Dehydration must be treated vigorously to avoid a state of shock. Hematocrit, electrolytes, and arterial blood gases must be evaluated in order to detect and treat any additional disturbances, such as anemia, hypo- or hypernatremia, or hyperchloremic or lactic acidosis.

Anemia and coagulation abnormalities resulting from surgery must be corrected in the immediate postoperative period. The normal hematocrit of the newborn is above 50 (with the majority of the hemoglobin still being fetal, HbF); that of the one-month-old is 40, with a physiological drop to the low 30 range at four months of age; thereafter, it is between 35 to 40.

Generally, when 10 percent of the blood volume is lost, the deficit should be replaced completely with packed red blood cells. The quantity of packed red blood cells needed to restore the hematocrit to a desired value can be estimated by the following formula:

$$\frac{(\text{blood volume} \times \text{desired hematocrit}) - (\text{blood volume} \times \text{present hematocrit})}{\text{hematocrit of packed red blood cells}}$$

The hematocrit of packed red blood cells is generally 65.

Various factors may influence the hematocrit. A low hematocrit may be due to a dilutional effect secondary to hyperhydration, while an elevated hematocrit may be due to a concentration effect secondary to dehydration.

Continuous postoperative bleeding may be secondary to defective hemostasis due to dilution of platelets and/or clotting factors occurring during surgery. In this situation, platelets should be given if the count (normal: 200,000 to 400,000) is less than 100,000; one unit of platelets will increase the count by 12,000. If the partial thromboplastin time (normal: 45 to 65 seconds in the newborn, 37 to 50 seconds in the child) is prolonged, indicating a deficit in factor VIII, fresh frozen plasma should be given. Severe dehydration will inevitably lead to a state of shock.

Fluid therapy for shock is divided into three stages:

- First stage: Expand extracellular volume by infusing 20 mL/kg of Ringer's lactate or 10 mL/kg of 5 percent albumin over one hour. Perfusion to the various organs should thereby improve.
- Second stage: One-half the amount of the calculated total replacement fluid should be given over eight hours, in addition to the calculated maintenance fluid.
- Third stage: The remaining one-half of the replacement fluid should be infused over the next 16 hours, in addition to the maintenance fluid. Intracellular fluid losses should thereby be replaced. Urinary output should attain 1 to 2 mL/kg/hour.

The total amount of replacement fluid can be estimated as follows: Body weight in kilograms × percent dehydration/100 = deficit in liters.

Electrolyte Disturbances

Often significant dehydration is accompanied by electrolyte disturbances, particularly sodium. Serum sodium levels of less than 120 mEq/liter should be corrected according to the following formula:

$$(\text{desired sodium concentration} - \text{actual sodium concentration mEq/liter}) \times \text{normal body weight (kg)} \times \left(\frac{\% \text{ body weight that is total body water}}{100}\right)$$

The sodium deficit must not be corrected too rapidly, since sodium overload must be avoided. Sodium overload can result in cerebral edema or hemorrhage in young infants. Rapid correction can also result in osmotic demyelination in all patients. Serum sodium should not be increased by more than 10 mEq/liter/day.

Hypernatremia associated with dehydration very rarely occurs intraoperatively. In this case, water shifts from the intracellular to the extracellular compartment. Clinically, the symptoms differ somewhat from those of other types of dehydration. The child presents with lethargy and fever. The skin is thick and doughy. The child may have a shrill cry. Hypernatremic dehydration must be corrected slowly, since a rapid decrease in serum sodium will result in intracellular flooding, leading to cerebral edema. The serum sodium must not be dropped by more than 10 mEq/liter/day.

Often, lactic acidosis—or, in the case of hypertonic dehydration, hyperchloremic acidosis—is associated with dehydration. Correction of water deficit and the electrolyte disturbances are generally sufficient, and bicarbonate therapy is usually not necessary.

Other important electrolyte disturbances include hypo- or hyperkalemia. Hypokalemia in the postoperative period can parallel dehydration particularly associated with the use of diuretics or resulting from the administration of a large quantity of fluids devoid of potassium. ECG changes, such as a prolonged QT interval and flat T waves, may be detected. Judicious treatment with supplemental potassium, in addition to that given for maintenance, is necessary.

Hyperkalemia can be a postoperative complication in children with preexisting renal disease. Infants recovering from open-heart procedures may also present with residual hyperkalemia, due to those cardioplegia solutions containing high concentrations of potassium. ECG changes may show peak T waves and widened QRS complexes. If serum potassium levels are above 6 mEq/L or if ECG changes are present, immediate treatment is mandatory. Treatment consists of dextrose 10 percent solution infusion, .1 unit/kg insulin IV, and sodium bicarbonate, 1 mEq/kg. These will shift potassium from the extracellular to the intracellular compartment. Calcium chloride, 30 mg/kg, should be administered to protect the heart from the toxic effects of the hyperkalemia. Peritoneal dialysis might be considered in extreme cases. When the hyperkalemia is moderate and asymptomatic, kayexalate, a potassium exchange resin, can be given as an enema.

Osmotic Diuresis

Continuing dehydration in the postoperative period may result from osmotic diuresis. Osmotic diuresis in the postoperative period is common in diabetic children. Infants recovering from open-heart procedures during which the priming solution used to initiate cardiopulmonary bypass contained dextrose may also present with osmotic diuresis. Blood and urine sugar levels are substantially elevated. Large amounts of fluid may be required over several hours to compensate for the excessive urinary output. Insulin therapy is indicated for both the diabetic and the nondiabetic child.

PAIN CONTROL

Postoperative pain relief in children can be accomplished safely with proper dosage and titration of analgesics. Some examples:

- Codeine: .5 mg/kg/dose every four hours, subcutaneously
- Meperidine: .5 mg/kg/dose every four hours, intravenously
- Morphine: .1 mg/kg/dose intravenously every four hours

The care person must be certain that postoperative pain is not related to an underlying complication (for example, pulmonary embolism, sickle cell crisis, acute intermittent porphyria) that may need immediate therapy.

UNUSUAL PROBLEMS

Some unusual disease processes may become manifest during the postoperative period. A few deserve mention since immediate appropriate care is mandatory.

Malignant Hyperthermia

A disease that requires prompt, aggressive treatment is malignant hyperthermia. This disease entity is characterized by a substantial, sustained depletion of calcium from the sarcoplasm reticulum, resulting in increased skeletal muscle metabolism with muscle contracture and an enormous production of heat. The hypermetabolic state necessarily alters physiological function, with marked increases in oxygen consumption with carbon dioxide and lactic acid production. Venous Po_2 and pH thereby decrease. These metabolic changes translate clinically by extreme fever (body temperature often exceeds 42 °C), profuse sweating, tachypnea, tachycardia, cyanosis, skin mottling, respiratory and metabolic acidosis, and rhabdomyolysis with increased serum myoglobin and myoglobinuria leading to eventual renal failure. Other consequences include hyperkalemia and an activated sympathetic system, contributing to immediate cardiac complications, such as arrhythmias and congestive heart failure. Disseminated intravascular coagulation is another potential complication.

Malignant hyperthermia is often triggered by the administration of succinylcholine or halothane or by postoperative pain or stress. Children with a family history of the disease or with musculoskeletal disorders, such as strabismus, kyphoscoliosis, hernias, or large muscle bulk, are susceptible to malignant hyperthermia. Supplemental monitoring postoperatively, such as end tidal CO_2 if the patient is still intubated, should be considered in any child at risk.

Treatment of malignant hyperthermia includes the following:

- immediate surface cooling with ice and cold blankets, and visceral cooling via cold intravenous infusions
- administration of dantrolene (a direct acting skeletal muscle relaxant that probably acts by slowing calcium release from the sarcoplasm reticulum), 1 to 2 mg/kg over two minutes intravenously, which may be repeated every five to ten minutes, up to a total dose of 10 mg/kg
- hyperventilation to correct the respiratory acidosis
- sodium bicarbonate (2 mEq/kg) to correct the metabolic acidosis and hyperkalemia
- insulin and glucose (.5 units/kg insulin and .5 g/kg of glucose) to correct hyperkalemia
- procainamide, 15 mg/kg, to treat ventricular arrhythmias
- diuretics to maintain urinary output in order to prevent renal damage from myoglobinuria

Sickle Cell Anemia

A child with sickle cell anemia must be carefully monitored in the postoperative period. Factors that induce sickling of red blood cells include cold stress, hypoxia, dehydration, acidosis, and hypotension. Postoperative pain may be due to sickling rather than the surgery.

Sickling can result in a number of clinical entities, such as organ infarction by vascular occlusion or enlargement by red blood cell sequestration, hemolysis, or bone marrow suppression. The two main therapeutic objectives are:

1. Prevention of reduction of hemoglobin (as it is the reduced form that sickles) by keeping oxygen bound to it; this is accomplished by maintaining adequate ventilation and oxygenation to avoid rightward shift of the oxygen dissociation curve (a shift to the right will increase unloading of oxygen from the hemoglobin).
2. Prevention of hyperviscosity; adequate amounts of crystalloid should be administered to maintain relative hemodilution.

Acute Intermittent Porphyria

Severe abdominal pain mimicking an acute abdomen may be associated with acute intermittent porphyria (AIP), a genetic disorder involving the biosynthesis of heme. This disease rarely occurs before puberty.

Liver cytochrome P-450 enzyme-inducing drugs, particularly the barbiturates and dilantin, will provoke the clinical symptomatology. Demyelination of the nervous system is the underlying pathological disturbance. Central, cranial, and autonomic nervous system symptoms, such as paraplegia, facial palsy, and tachycardia, are frequently associated with the abdominal pain (which is probably due to autonomic-mediated gastrointestinal spasm).

The urine, which is initially colorless, turns dark on standing. The Watson-Schwartz test will detect the presence of porphyria, and ion-exchange chromatography will quantify porphyrin precursor.

Treatment of an AIP crisis consists initially of the administration of 10 to 20 grams/hour of glucose or of Hemin, an iron containing metallo-porphyrin, 4 mg/kg over 20 to 30 minutes. Glucose and hemin block an enzyme in the biosynthetic pathway, which is overactivated during acute episodes of the disease.

Congenital Heart Disease

Congenital heart disease usually includes atrial or ventricular septal defects that allow shunting from one side of the heart to the other.

Right-to-left shunting is a serious problem in the postoperative period, particularly in the infant. Crying, stress, hypoxia, acidosis, and hypercarbia all increase pulmonary vascular resistance and therefore create pressure gradients, forcing the unoxygenated blood from the right side of the heart to the left and into the systemic circulation. Desaturation of the arterial blood occurs with resulting cyanosis. In such cases, air must not be allowed to enter the venous circulation, since it will pass from the venous into the systemic circulation and air embolus in various organs, particularly the brain, may result.

The child must therefore be kept adequately oxygenated and ventilated. Pain medication should be administered as needed. Morphine should be used cautiously, since it increases pulmonary artery pressure. Systemic hypotension must be avoided to prevent a high pulmonary to systemic pressure gradient.

Particular attention must be paid to the infant who may be very agitated following surgery. Droperidol, .1 mg/kg IM, may be administered in this instance. Droperidol is not only a major tranquilizer of the butyrophenone group, it is also a powerful alpha blocker. Alpha blockers dilate the pulmonary vasculature (and, to a lesser extent, the systemic vasculature), thereby limiting or reversing right-to-left shunting.

A child with congenital heart disease who has postoperative respiratory depression due to intraoperative heavy narcotization should be mechanically ventilated rather than reversed with naloxone. Naloxone is a pure antagonist that will reverse not only the respiratory depression but the cardiovascular depression and analgesia as well, causing hypertension, tachycardia, pain, and agitation. Right-to-left shunting or congestive heart failure may ensue. Naloxone, therefore, must be carefully titrated, if used at all.

Tetralogy of Fallot is a congenital heart disease that deserves particular mention. This disease entity includes obstruction to the right ventricular outflow tract (infundibular stenosis), as well as a ventricular septal defect, right ventricular hypertrophy, and a rightward deviated aortic arch. Tachycardia must be avoided, since a fast heart rate will severely limit the time blood has to flow through the already obstructed outflow tract. Tachycardia can eventually lead to infundibular spasm, completely shutting down the outflow tract. A beta blocker (for example, propranolol, .01 mg/kg) may be used to reduce the heart rate. Phenylephrine, an alpha agonist, 2 µg/kg, which increases systemic vascular resistance (and, to a lesser extent, pulmonary vascular resistance) and also reduces heart rate by a baroceptor reflex, may be administered in cases of tachycardia with systemic hypotension.

Generally, the heart rate should be slower and the systemic blood pressure higher in cases of valvular stenosis. However, in cases of valvular regurgitation, a faster heart rate and a lower systemic blood pressure (and therefore a reduced afterload) are required to limit backflow of blood and to force more forward flow.

Methemoglobinemia

Cyanosis may be due to methemoglobinemia. Methemoglobinemia may be precipitated in certain individuals by drugs containing amide groups (lidocaine, benzocaine, or prilocaine—used topically or parenterally) or nitro groups (nitroglycerin, used frequently during pediatric open heart procedures). It is caused by the accumulation of methemoglobin, an oxidation product of hemoglobin.

Methemoglobin is not capable of reversibly binding to oxygen. Therefore, the oxygen-carrying capacity of blood is reduced. In addition, the remaining normal hemoglobin has a greater affinity for oxygen. The oxygen dissociation curve shifts to the left, diminishing the unloading of oxygen to the tissues. Cyanosis is the first clinical sign; then, as methemoglobinemia becomes more important, tachycardia, dyspnea, headache, and lethargy ensue. Methemoglobinemia can be a particularly serious complication in an anemic child.

The blood appears chocolate brown due to abnormal pigment. Since it directly measures oxygen saturation, the pulse oximeter shows a decrease in oxygen saturation commensurate with the degree of methemoglobinemia. An arterial blood gas, however, shows a normal Pa_{O_2}, since oxygen tension is not affected.

The methemoglobinemia can be identified by spectrophotometry. Treatment consists of methylene blue, 2 mg/kg IV, which reduces methemoglobin to hemoglobin.

CARDIOPULMONARY LIFE SUPPORT

Basic Cardiac Support

Basic CPR techniques vary somewhat between the infant and the older child because of anatomical and physiological differences.

Artificial ventilation is provided by the following techniques: In the infant, the head should be placed in a sniffing position in order to align the oropharynx and the airway. The rescuer's mouth is placed over the nose and mouth of the infant to create a seal. The breaths delivered must adequately expand the chest to maximize effective ventilation, but excessive pressure must be avoided to prevent pneumothorax.

In the older child, the head is tilted backward to hyperextend the neck. The rescuer's mouth should be placed over the victim's mouth with a tight seal, and the nose should be pinched. Again, chest expansion must be adequate and not excessive upon delivery of each breath.

There are two techniques for chest compression for infants. One is the two-finger technique, in which two fingers are placed over the sternum at the upper third of the chest where the infant ventricles are located. The other technique involves encircling the chest with both hands and with the thumbs over the sternum. The sternum is to be compressed one-half inch.

The technique for older children is much the same as for adults: the heel of one hand should be placed on the sternum at the lower half of the chest (the ventricles lie lower in the chest in the older child and adult than in the infant). Compressions are then accomplished by downward pressure by one or two hands, depending on the size of the child. The arms should be fully extended. The sternum is to be compressed one and one-half inches.

The rate of compressions for infants is 100 per minute and for children 80 per minute, with one insufflation interposed for every five compressions.

Other resuscitative techniques have been described. Abdominal binding and spontaneous compression-ventilation apparently improve cerebral perfusion pressure and cerebral blood flow.

The following three-stage technique should be used for intubation of the infant:

1. Hold the laryngoscope handle with the left hand and place the laryngoscope blade carefully in the mouth. Sweep the tongue leftward.

2. Position the tip of the blade in the vallecula.
3. Elevate the tongue and attached epiglottis to expose the glottic opening. Do not tilt the blade. If the glottic opening is not visible, lift the epiglottis after placing the tip of the blade under it.

If pharmacological therapy is required, the following guidelines should be followed:

- Ventilate the child with 100 percent oxygen; no subsequent drug will work on an anoxic heart. The chest must rise symmetrically upon ventilation (if there is no underlying lung disease) and breath sounds on both sides must be heard equally to auscultation. No sounds must be heard in the abdomen.
- Administration of atropine, .01–.03 mg/kg, will increase the heart rate, which, particularly in the infant, will raise the cardiac output.
- Sodium bicarbonate will reverse metabolic acidosis if the patient is being adequately ventilated. Ideally, an arterial blood gas should be drawn so that the dose of bicarbonate needed can be calculated by the formula: Base deficit × bodyweight × (% of body weight that is extracellular fluid/100). Since bicarbonate remains in the extracellular compartment, one-half of this calculated dose is given. If an arterial blood gas is not immediately available, 1 to 2 mEq/kg of sodium bicarbonate should be administered. If the infant weighs less than five kilograms, the sodium bicarbonate must be diluted 1:1 in sterile water, since the full-strength solution may cause intracranial hemorrhage due to the hyperosmolar effect of sodium and the increased cerebral blood flow due to increased CO_2 in the blood.
- Administration of epinephrine, .01 mg/kg IV; as an infusion, the initial dose is 1 µg/min. Epinephrine is an alpha and beta agonist drug. It therefore increases heart rate and myocardial contractility as well as systemic vascular resistance. Mechanical activity becomes more responsive to electrical activity after administration. Epinephrine converts the irregular, low amplitude and low frequency ventricular fibrillation, which is unresponsive to defibrillation electric shock, to the more regular, higher amplitude and higher frequency ventricular fibrillation that is responsive to electric shock. Epinephrine may also improve cerebral perfusion pressure and cerebral blood flow during cardiopulmonary resuscitation. It has no effect on the severely acidotic heart. It is inactivated if given simultaneously with sodium bicarbonate.
- Administration of calcium chloride, 20 to 30 mg/kg. Calcium chloride may be administered if epinephrine is ineffective in restoring adequate cardiac function, since calcium also increases myocardial contractility. The positive

inotropic action depends on the presence of activated ionized calcium. Calcium chloride contains the ionized form of calcium and is therefore the best solution to use. Calcium will precipitate bicarbonate if both are given simultaneously. Calcium potentiates the cardiac effects of digitalis and therefore must be administered with extreme caution in a digitalized child.

Prognosis

Recent evidence indicates that mixed venous blood gases may be of great prognostic value. A low mixed venous pH and a rapidly rising mixed venous P_{CO_2} during resuscitation may reflect severe irreversible myocardial failure and a poor prognosis.

Advanced Cardiac Support Drugs

Isoproterenol is a pure beta agonist that increases heart rate and myocardial contractility. It also reduces peripheral vascular resistance. The drug is given as an infusion, and the initial dose is .1 μg/kg/min, increasing by .1 μg/kg/min to a maximum of 1.0 μg/kg/min.

Dopamine, a weak catecholamine precursor of norepinephrine, is administered as an infusion. It has three levels of activity, depending on the dosage:

1. dopamine activity (at 1 to 2 μg/kg/min), which increases mesenteric and renal blood flow and urinary output (is useful in cases of oliguria)
2. beta agonist activity at 3 to 10 μg/kg/min
3. alpha agonist activity at doses greater than 10 μg/kg/min

Higher doses of dopamine are required for cardiac effect in infants because of the reduced amount of contractile elements in their myocardium.

Dobutamine is a powerful inotropic drug. It exists as a racemic mixture, such that alpha activity counterbalances beta activity. Thus, there is less increase in heart rate or blood pressure than with dopamine. Dobutamine is particularly useful in low cardiac output states, tending to redistribute blood volume from the right to the left side of the heart. Dosages range from 2 to 10 μg/kg/min.

Levophed, a norepinephrine solution, has predominantly an alpha adrenergic, but it also has some beta adrenergic action. It is usually given during resuscitation only as a last resort when all other measures have failed. It increases blood pressure primarily by peripheral vasoconstriction. It is administered by infusion, .1 to 1.0 μg/kg/min.

Treatment of Tachyarrthymias

Ventricular Fibrillation

Ventricular fibrillation is treated by electric shock. The initial energy dose used should be 2 joules/kg, increasing to 4 joules/kg if the lower dose is ineffective. Oxygenation must be optimized and acidosis treated before defibrillation can be effective.

The energy dose must be reduced in the digitalized child, since the effects of digitalis on the myocardium are potentiated by electric shock. Otherwise, irreversible cardiac arrest may ensue.

Ventricular Tachycardia

In cases of ventricular tachycardia, lidocaine is the initial treatment of choice. Lidocaine is a Type I-B antiarrhythmic agent that reduces both the action potential (AP), and the effective refractory period (EFP)—the AP more than the EFP. The IV dose is 1 mg/kg/dose. It may be administered as an infusion, 20 to 50 μg/kg/min.

Procainamide is a Type I-A antiarrhythmic agent that increases EFP and AP (increasing EFP more than AP). This drug may be used in ventricular tachycardia refractory to lidocaine. Dosage is 2 mg/kg/dose intravenously given over 5 minutes, then repeated every 15 minutes. The child must be monitored with an ECG and a continuous blood pressure measurement, since widening QRS, lengthening of the QT interval, or hypotension indicate toxicity.

A torsade de pointe rhythm—which is essentially an atypically bidirectional ventricular tachycardia where the QRS polarity alternates above and below the isoelectric line—may result from the prolonged QT interval. The treatment of choice for a torsade de pointe rhythm is isoproterenol, which shortens the QT interval. Type I-B antiarrhythmics, such as lidocaine, may be effective in that they also shorten the QT interval. Other Type I-A antiarrhythmics, such as quinidine, must not be used in the presence of a torsade de pointe rhythm, since they all lengthen the QT interval.

Cardiac arrest may occur rapidly following the administration of procainamide.

Bretyllium is useful in the treatment of refractory ventricular tachycardia and fibrillation. It appears to have a biphasic action, first stimulating and then inhibiting catecholamine release. Dosage is 5 mg/kg IV given rapidly for ventricular fibrillation, and 5 mg/kg IV given over ten minutes for ventricular tachycardia.

Supraventricular Tachyarrhythmias

Paroxysmal supraventricular tachycardia is most effectively treated by verapamil, a calcium channel blocker. The doses are .1 to .3 mg/kg (maximum: 5.0 mg) intravenously. Propanolol, .01 mg/kg, is also effective.

Atrial fibrillation may be treated with digoxin. The dose is 10 μg/kg. Vomiting, diarrhea, nausea, visual disturbances, and arrhythmias—particularly ventricular premature contractions and atrial tachycardia with block—are signs of toxicity. Phenytoin is useful in treating atrial tachycardia with block. Serum potassium level should be within normal limits.

Verapamil may also be used, provided that the atrial fibrillation is not associated with preexcitation syndrome due to ectopic conduction pathways (as in Wolff-Parkinson-White syndrome), since the normal pathways, but not the ectopic conduction, will be blocked. In this situation, ventricular fibrillation may result.

BIBLIOGRAPHY

Andres, J.M., Mathis, R.K., and Waler, W.A. "Liver Disease in Infants." *Pediatrics* 90(1977):686.

Avroy, F., and Martin, R. *Berman's Neonatal-Perinatal Medicine*, 3d. ed. 785–786. St. Louis, Mo.: C.V. Mosby, 1983.

Biller, J., and Yeager, A. *The Harriet Lane Handbook*, 9th ed., 22. Chicago: Yearbook Medical Publishers, 1980.

Chandra, N., Rudikoff, M., and Weisfeldt, M.L. "Simultaneous Chest Compression and Ventilation at High Airway Pressure during Cardiopulmonary Resuscitation." *Lancet* 1(1980):175–178.

Colucci, W., Wright, R.F., and Brunwald, E. "New Positive Inotropic Agents in the Treatment of Congestive Heart Failure: Mechanisms of Action and Recent Clinical Developments." *New England Journal of Medicine* 314(1986):290–299.

Cook, D.R. "Muscle Relaxants in Infants and Children." *Anesthesia Analgesia* 60(1981):335.

Dripps, R.D., Eckenhoff, J.E., and Vadam, L.D. *Introduction to Anesthesia*, 5th ed., 364–387. Philadelphia: W.B. Saunders, 1977.

Fisher, D., Castagnoli, K., and Miller, R.D. "Vecuronium Kinetics and Dynamics in Anesthetized Infants and Children." *Clinical Pharmacology and Therapeutics* 37(1985):402–406.

Fisher, D., et al. "Pharmacokinetics and Pharmacodynamics of d-Tubocurarine in Infants, Children, and Adults." *Anesthesiology* 57:(1982):203–208.

Goldsmith, S., and From, A. "Arsenic-Induced Atypical Ventricular Tachycardia." *New England Journal of Medicine* 303(1981):1096.

Graef, J., and Cone, T. *Manuel of Pediatric Therapeutics*, 2d., ed. 197–204. Boston: Little, Brown & Co., 1980.

Greenbaum, D., and Marschall, K. "Adult Respiratory Distress Syndrome." *New York Medical Quarterly*, 2(1980):27–30.

Gregory, G. *Pediatric Anesthesia*, 323–326. New York: Churchill Livingstone, 1986.

Hinkle, A. "Fluid and Blood Replacement in Pediatrics." *Thirty-Fifth Annual Refresher ASA Course Lectures* 131(1984):1–6.

Isselbacher, K.J., et al. *Harrison's Principles of Internal Medicine*, 9th ed., 494–500, 1551–1552. New York: McGraw-Hill, 1980.

Johnson, K.L., Erickson, J.P., Holley, F.O., and Scott, J.C. "Fentanyl Pharmacokinetics in the Pediatric Population." *Anesthesiology* 61(1984):A–441. (abstract)

Krishna, G., Haselby, K.A., and Rao, C.C. "Current Concepts in Pediatric Anesthesia with Emphasis on the Newborn Infant." *Surgical Clinics of North America* 61(October 1981):997–1012.

Life Support, sec. VII, VIII, X, XVI, XVII. Dallas, Tx.: American Heart Association, 1981.

Luczun, M.E. *Post Anesthesia Nursing: A Comprehensive Guide,* 169–189. Rockville, Md.: Aspen Publishers, 1984.

Miller, R.D. *Anesthesia,* 2d. ed., 1755–1766, 1971–1988. New York: Churchill Livingstone, 1986.

Neimann, J.T., et al., "Hemodynamic Effects of Continuous Abdominal Binding During Cardiac Arrest and Resuscitation." *American Journal of Cardiology* 53(1984):269–274.

Robotham, J.L. "Effects of Positive and Negative Pressure Ventilation on Cardiac Performance." *Clinics in Chest Medicine* 4(1983):161–187.

Silverman, W., and Sinclair, J. "Temperature Regulation in the Newborn Infant." *New England Journal of Medicine* 274(1966):92.

Sterns, R.H., Riggs, J.E., and Schochet, S.S., Jr. "Osmotic Demyelination Syndrome Following Correction of Hyponatremia." *New England Journal of Medicine* 314(1986):1535–1542.

Strube, P.J., and Hallam, P.L. "Ketamine by Continuous Infusion in Status Asthmaticus." *Anaesthesia* 41(1986):1017–1019.

Swaiman, K., and Wright, F. *The Practice of Pediatric Neurology,* 2d. ed., 765–769. St. Louis, Mo.: C.V. Mosby, 1982.

Tandberg, D., and Sklar, D. "Effect of Tachypnea on the Estimation of Body Temperature by an Oral Thermometer." *New England Journal of Medicine* 308(1983):945.

Theodore, J., and Robin, E.D. "Speculations on Neurogenic Pulmonary Edema." *American Review of Respiratory Disease* 113(1976):405–410.

Weil, M.H., et al. "Difference in Acid-Base State Between Venous and Arterial Blood During Cardiopulmonary Resuscitation. *New England Journal of Medicine* 315(1986):153–156.

Yao, F., and Artusio, J. *Anesthesiology: Problem Oriented Patient Management,* 331–337. Philadelphia: J.B. Lippincott, 1983.

Yen, R., Tran, B., and Charney, J. *Intraoperative Methemoglobinemia Due to Lidocaine Jelly.* Forthcoming.

Chapter 15

Postanesthesia Care After Obstetrical Surgery

Farida Gadalla, M.D.

GENERAL CONSIDERATIONS

The pregnant patient, as well as the patient in the immediate postpartum period, must be considered apart from the nonpregnant female, due to the anatomical and physiological changes of pregnancy. Exhibit 15-1 and Table 15-1 provide an overview of anatomical and physiological changes in pregnancy.

SURGICAL PROCEDURES

Obstetrical surgical procedures can be categorized as follows:

- Surgical procedures performed during pregnancy. These may or may not be pregnancy-related. The most common pregnancy-related surgical procedure is a cerclage operation performed to tighten an incompetent cervix. An appendectomy is the most common nonobstetrical surgical procedure, constituting about 65 percent of nonobstetrical surgical procedures.
- Surgical procedures performed for delivery, for example, caesarean section.
- Surgical procedures performed postpartum, such as bilateral tubal ligation.
- Emergency procedures, such as total abdominal hysterectomy following either vaginal and caesarean deliveries.

Exhibit 15-1 Various Systemic Changes in Pregnancy

1. Cardiovascular System

    - ↑ ↑ ↑ Blood volume (plasma > RBC volume)
    - ↑ ↑ ↑ ↑ Cardiac output (↑ stroke volume and ↑ heart rate)
    - ↓ ↓ Total peripheral resistance
    - ↓ Mean arterial BP
    - ± CVP
    - Vena caval and aortic compression in supine position

2. Gastrointestinal System

    - ↓ Gastrointestinal motility and gastric-emptying time
    - ↓ Volume of gastrointestinal secretions
    - ↑ Gastric acidity
    - ↓ Lower esophageal tone (progesterone)
    - Therefore, pregnant patients after the first trimester should always be considered as having a "full stomach" and must be considered at risk for regurgitation and aspiration.

3. Central Nervous System

    - MAC decreased
    - Sensitivity to local anesthetics changed
    - Engorgement of epidural veins
    - Decrease in size of epidural space

4. Skin and Mucous Membranes

    - Mucous membranes are more friable during pregnancy, and the mucosal capillaries are engorged. Therefore insertion of nasal airways and nasotracheal and nasogastric tubes are to be avoided.

5. Metabolic

    - O_2 consumption is increased by 20 percent, requiring modification in technique by both surgeon and anesthesiologist and necessitating special care in the PACU.

ANESTHETIC CONSIDERATIONS

The anesthetic considerations for the pregnant patient are dictated by the anatomical and physiological changes of pregnancy. The actual drugs used to maintain an anesthesia are of little significance to mother and fetus. It is, however, essential to maintain oxygenation and placental blood flow in order to ensure fetal well-being. The following formula applies:

Table 15-1 Changes in the Respiratory System During Pregnancy

Variable	Direction of Change	Average Change
Minute ventilation	↑	50%
Alveolar ventilation	↑	70%
Tidal volume	↑	40%
Respiratory rate	↑	15%
Dead space	No change	
Airway resistance	↓	36%
Total pulmonary resistance	↓	50%
Total compliance	↓	30%
Lung compliance (alone)	No change	
Chest wall compliance (alone)	↓	45%
Arterial P_{CO_2}	↓	10 mm Hg
Serum bicarbonate	↓	5 mEq/L
Arterial pH	No change	
Arterial P_{O_2}	↑	10 mm Hg
Total lung capacity	↓	0–5%
Functional residual capacity	↓	20%
Expiratory reserve volume	↓	20%
Residual volume	↓	20%
Vital capacity	No change	
Closing volume	No change or ↑	
Oxygen consumption	↑	20%

Source: Adapted from *Anesthesia for Obstetrics* by S.M. Shnider and G. Levinson, p. 4, with permission of Williams & Wilkins Company, Baltimore, © 1987.

$$PBF = \frac{UABP - IUP - UVBP}{Ripl + Re}$$

where:
PBF = placental blood flow
UABP = uterine artery pressure
IUP = intrauterine pressure
UVBP = uterine venous pressure
Ripl = intrinsic vascular resistance of placental vessels
Re = extrinsic resistance imparted by tone of myometrium

To maintain placental blood flow, it is essential to maintain the left-lateral tilt position, and a fluid load must be given immediately before anesthesia. This is especially important prior to regional anesthesia, which causes sympathetic blockade and interferes with the patient's ability to compensate for circulatory insufficiency.

Due to the decrease in anesthetic requirements during pregnancy, relatively small doses of both local and general anesthetics are needed. Similarly, when an epidural technique is used, smaller volumes are needed to fill the epidural space, which is more vascular in the nonpregnant state.

Ketamine (Retalar) causes increased uterine tone, thus decreasing placental blood flow, and should be used only in small doses and when the benefits in supporting the blood pressure outweigh the potential disadvantage.

Diazepam (Valium) may be given in small doses during labor and caesarean section. In larger doses, it may cause respiratory depression, decreased muscle tone to the baby, and an increase in the incidence of neonatal jaundice.

The overall aim of the anesthesiologist is to maintain the mother's physiological status while administering drugs that are relatively safe for the baby and making sure that the baby is well-oxygenated. While performing general anesthesia, the patient must be oxygenated prior to induction. All inductions are carried out using a rapid sequence technique, and all patients are intubated with a cuffed endotracheal tube to protect against aspiration following regurgitation. It is best to avoid nasal airways and nasogastric tubes, since the nasal mucosa is friable and tends to bleed secondarily to the capillary engorgement. During general anesthesia in the second and third trimesters, the patient is always intubated orally, using a smaller-than-average endotracheal tube (for example, a 7 mm tube) because of engorgement of all mucous membranes. The patient must remain intubated until she is awake and alert enough to protect her airway, since aspiration can occur on emergence as well as induction.

The most commonly used premedicant drug during pregnancy is 0.3N sodium citrate, which is a nonparticulate antacid that raises the gastric pH and protects against acid pneumonitis. The general anesthetics most often used are those tried by the test of time, such as thiopental (Pentothal), morphine, meperidine hydrochloride (Demerol), inhalational agents, and muscle relaxants. The newer synthetic narcotics are not approved for use during pregnancy.

Inhalational agents are used in surgical procedures in which the baby is not to be delivered because they cause uterine muscle relaxation, improve uterine blood flow if the blood pressure is maintained, and are presumed to protect against premature labor. In both low and high concentration, they protect against maternal recall that could otherwise occur when N_2O/O_2 are being used in a 50/50 concentration.

POSTANESTHESIA CARE

The following surgical, medical, and anesthetic considerations are pertinent to specific obstetrical procedures.

Obstetrical Surgery 221

Elective Abortion

If done during the first trimester, elective abortion is usually a short procedure carried out by mask. There are no special precautions other than watching for excessive bleeding and noting the use of oxytocin (Pitocin) with its side effects, such as hypotension, or the use of ergonovine maleate (Ergotrate), which may cause hypertension, tachycardia, nausea, and vomiting.

If the abortion is in the second trimester, prostaglandins may have been used. These have numerous unpleasant side effects, such as nausea, vomiting, tachycardia, arrhythmias, and changes in blood pressure. As noted earlier, during second-trimester procedures, the endotracheal tube must remain in place until the patient is alert and able to protect her airway. If dilatation and curettage are used to complete an abortion or miscarriage, the same considerations as noted above for elective abortion apply.

Vaginal Delivery

Patients may be brought into the PACU following a complicated vaginal delivery, especially if they have received a general anesthetic. If they have received a general anesthetic, it is essential not to extubate until the patient is responsive. One must also ensure that the uterus is contracting down adequately, as the inhalational agents cause uterine relaxation. Obviously one must also watch for postpartum hemorrhage.

Surgery During Pregnancy

In surgery for problems during pregnancy—for example, cerclage, appendicitis, and ovarian cysts—apart from the routine postoperative care, the aims of PACU personnel are to:

- maintain maternal homeostasis and hence fetal well-being
- monitor the fetus to detect and remedy any abnormality
- monitor for uterine contractions
- prevent premature labor

On arrival in the PACU, it is essential that the patient not be extubated until she is awake. She is maintained on supplemental oxygen, and a wedge is placed under her right hip to prevent aorto-caval compression and subsequent decrease in uteroplacental blood flow. The patient must be well-hydrated to help maintain uteroplacental blood flow and to decrease the chances of onset of premature labor.

The most common occurrence following surgery, especially under regional anesthesia, is a drop in blood pressure. This must be treated immediately by increasing intravenous fluids and administering ephedrine (Ephedrine sulphate) IV in 5–10 mg doses. Ephedrine is the drug of choice because it increases the blood pressure primarily by central adrenergic stimulation and has minimal effects on uterine blood flow; whereas drugs like phenylephrine (Neo-Synephrine) and norepinephrine (Levophed) have mainly adrenergic effects, causing a decrease in uterine blood flow.

The fetus is monitored using an external doppler ultrasound device that picks up the fetal heart rate. The normal rate is 120–160 beats per minute, and there should be a baseline variability of about 6 beats per minute. However, some drugs, such as narcotics, sedatives, and inhalational anesthetics, decrease the beat-to-beat variability. It is important to correlate the fetal heart changes with the uterine contraction to determine the presence of late deceleration, which is a sign of fetal distress (see Figures 15-1, 15-2, and 15-3). Fetal tachycardia is an early sign of fetal distress.

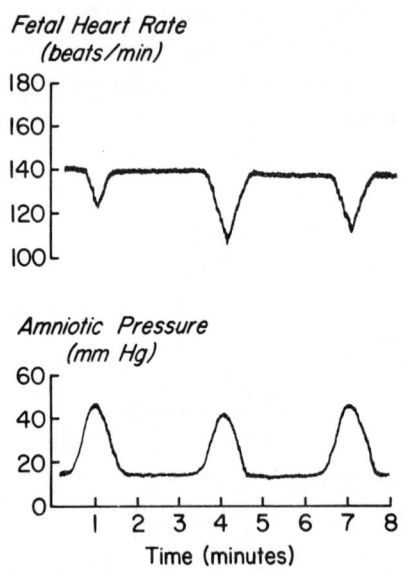

Figure 15-1 Early Deceleration. *Source:* Reprinted by permission of Elsevier Science Publishing Co., Inc. from R.H. Schwarz, *Handbook of Obstetric Emergencies* p. 77. Copyright 1984 by Medical Examination Publishing Company, Inc.

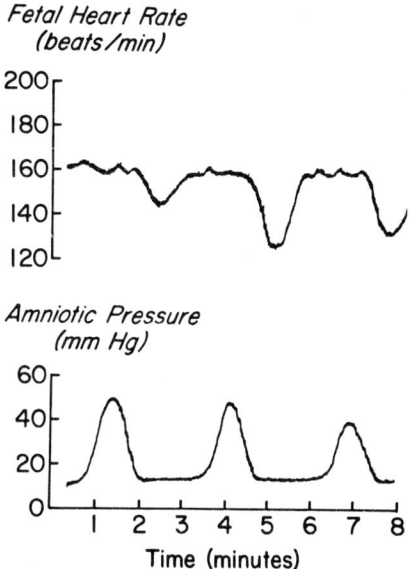

Figure 15-2 Late Deceleration. *Source:* Reprinted by permission of Elsevier Science Publishing Co., Inc. from R.H. Schwarz, *Handbook of Obstetric Emergencies* p. 79. Copyright 1984 by Medical Examination Publishing Company, Inc.

In many institutions, tocolytics are used routinely after this surgery during pregnancy to prevent premature labor. The tocolytes most commonly in use are magnesium sulfate and b agonists, such as ritodrine (Yutopar) and terbutaline (Brethine). These are used as continuous infusion, and the uterus is monitored for presence of contraction.

Ectopic Pregnancy

Ectopic pregnancy is pregnancy that has implanted outside the endometrial cavity. Ninety-five percent of these occur in the fallopian tube, and rupture may occur. A ruptured ectopic is an acute surgical emergency. The patient is frequently in shock due to intraabdominal hemorrhage. She is also in severe pain, and is, as usual, considered to have a full stomach. Postoperative care should include maintenance of hydration, transfusion if necessary, close monitoring of vital signs and urine output, and observation for bleeding disorders.

Disseminated intravascular coagulation (DIC) is a medical condition that may complicate such obstetrical procedures as ectopic pregnancy, abruptio placenta, amniotic fluid embolus, and procedures with extensive blood loss. In this condi-

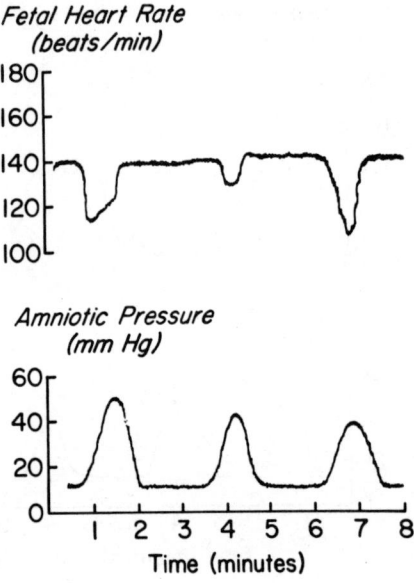

Figure 15-3 Variable Deceleration. *Source:* Reprinted by permission of Elsevier Science Publishing Co., Inc. from R.H. Schwarz, *Handbook of Obstetric Emergencies* p. 80. Copyright 1984 by Medical Examination Publishing Company, Inc.

tion, the clotting mechanism is accelerated, fibrin is deposited, and subsequently the fibrinolytic system is activated, leading to clinical bleeding diatheses (see Table 15-2).

Therapy consists of:

- monitoring
- maintaining hemostasis
- administering oxygen
- administering clotting factors (fresh frozen plasma)
- heparinization, to inhibit the clotting mechanism until factors have been restored (last resort)

Caesarean Section

The most common surgical procedure in the field of obstetrics is obviously the caesarean section, involving 25 to 30 percent of deliveries in the larger medical centers of the United States. The choice of anesthetic for an elective caesarean section is an epidural anesthetic. The drugs commonly used are (1) lidocaine

Table 15-2 Blood Coagulation Studies: Normal, Pregnant, and DIC Values

Normal Values	Pregnancy	DIC
Platelet count 150,000–400,000/min^3	Same	Lowered
Quick prothrombin time 75–125%	Shortened	Lengthened
Partial thromboplastin time 30–45 sec.	Shortened	Lengthened
Thrombin time 10–15 sec	Shortened	Lengthened
Fibrinogen assay (or titer) 200–400 mg%	300–600 mg%	Decreased
Fibrin split products	Negative	Measurable
Factor V assay 75–125%	Same	Decreased
Factor VII assay 50–200%	May be increased	Decreased

Source: Reprinted by permission of Elsevier Science Publishing Co., Inc. from R.H. Schwarz, *Handbook of Obstetric Emergencies* p. 48. Copyright 1984 by Medical Examination Publishing Company, Inc.

(Xylocaine), with intermediate onset and intermediate duration; (2) chloroprocaine (Nesacaine), with fast onset and short duration; and (3) bupivacaine hydrochloride (Marcaine), with slow onset and long duration.

Today, it is common practice to inject epidural narcotics to give postoperative analgesia. Preservative free morphine (Duramorph) is in use and gives prolonged analgesia (24–35 hours). However, it has a number of side effects, such as itching, respiratory depression, urinary retention, nausea, and vomiting. Pruritis, which occurs in 65 percent of patients, can be counteracted by naloxone hydrochloride (Narcan) IV; the patient must be monitored closely postoperatively for approximately 24 hours.

A suggested monitoring schedule and order form for use after application of epidural morphine is shown in Exhibit 15-2.

Epidural fentanyl citrate (Sublimaze) has been used with success and fewer side effects in doses of 50–100 mg; however, the pain relief is of a much shorter duration, approximately three to four hours. With this narcotic, respiratory depression has not been found to be a problem.

Whether the patient has had regional or general anesthesia, the postoperative care consists of checking the uterus to make sure it is contracting down, checking for postoperative bleeding and, as noted earlier, counteracting the side effects of such drugs as ergonovine maleate (Ergotrate) and prostaglandins that may have been used.

Exhibit 15-2 Suggested Monitoring Schedule and Order Form for Use After Administration of Epidural Morphine

---

1. The patient has received the following:

    Morphine _____ mg
    Route: Epidural _____ Intrathecal _____
    Date _____
    Time _____

2. No p.o., IM, IV, or s.c. narcotics are to be given for 20 hours, except by order of an anesthesiologist: telephone # _____, beeper # _____
3. Check and record respiratory rate every 30 minutes for 12 hours, then every hour until 24 hours following epidural or intrathecal narcotic administration.
4. Narcan (naloxone) ampule (1 mL, 0.4 mg) must be readily available at the nursing station for immediate administration.
5. Oxygen flow meter with nipple adapter and self-inflating bag with mask must be immediately accessible, either at nursing station or on emergency cart.
6. Call house officer or anesthesiologist (telephone # _____, beeper # _____) if the patient has evidence of airway obstruction, change in respiratory pattern, decreased respiratory effort, or respiratory rate below 11.
7. If respiratory depression is present, house officer or nurse may administer Narcan 0.1–0.2 mg IV, and repeat as necessary.
8. Call anesthesiologist (telephone # _____, beeper # _____) if patient complains of severe itching, urinary retention, excessive nausea, or vomiting or appears unexpectedly somnolent.

Source: Reprinted from *Anesthesia for Obstetrics* by S.M. Shnider and G. Levinson, p. 134, with permission of Williams & Wilkins Company, Baltimore, © 1987.

Preeclampsia and Eclampsia

Preeclampsia and eclampsia are very serious conditions that may accompany pregnancy. Preeclampsia is a condition that may occur after 20 weeks gestation; it is characterized by hypertension, generalized edema, and proteinuria. Eclampsia is accompanied by convulsions.

The disease affects multiple organ systems and is essentially a condition of vasoconstriction, possibly due to increased renin, angiotensin, aldosterone, and catecholamines. Intravascular volume and protein content are decreased; and, because of subsequent placental insufficiency, fetal well-being may be jeopardized by even small drops in blood pressure (see Figure 15-4).

The definitive treatment of this condition is delivery of the baby. However, in rare cases, the condition may persist or deteriorate following delivery. The aim of

Obstetrical Surgery 227

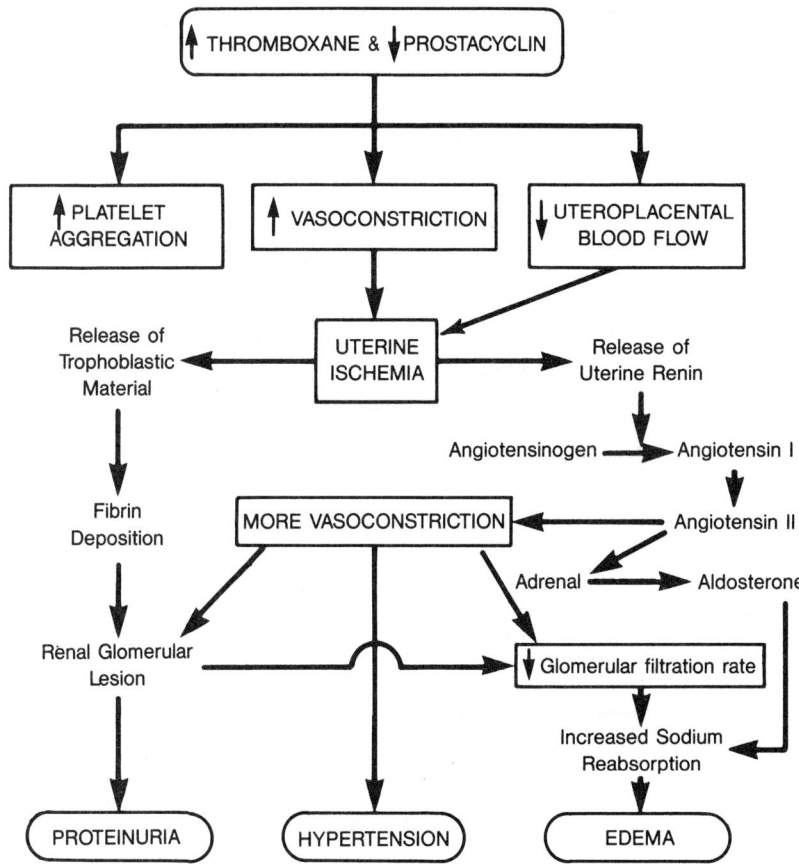

Figure 15-4 Proposed Scheme of Pathophysiological Changes in Toxemia of Pregnancy. *Source:* Reprinted from *Anesthesia for Obstetrics* by S.M. Shnider and G. Levinson, p. 227, with permission of Williams & Wilkins Company, Baltimore, © 1987.

therapy is to provide adequate hydration to improve circulation, minimize vasospasm, and decrease CNS hyperactivity.

Magnesium sulfate is the drug of choice in controlling preeclampsia and eclampsia. It reduces hyperreflexia and depresses uterine activity and acts as an anticonvulsant, a sedative, and a mild vasodilator. However, reg SO_4 levels must be monitored for side effects that recur with increasing levels (see Table 15-3). Also, it must be given with care when there is renal impairment, since magnesium is excreted by the kidneys.

Table 15-3 Effects of Increasing Plasma Magnesium Levels

Plasma mg (mEq/liter)	Effects
1.5–2.0	Normal plasma level
4.0–8.0	Therapeutic range
5.0–10	Electrocardiographic changes (P–Q interval prolonged, QRS complex widens)
10	Loss of deep tendon reflexes
15	Sinoatrial and atrioventricular block
15	Respiratory paralysis
25	Cardiac arrest

Source: Reprinted from *Handbook of Obstetric Emergencies* by S.M. Shnider and G. Levinson, p. 230, with permission of Williams & Wilkins Company, Baltimore, © 1987.

In the PACU, the patient must be watched carefully for the development of eclampsia, and convulsion precautions must be available at the bedside. In brief, the following monitoring procedures are maintained:

- CVP is monitored in moderate and severe cases.
- Urine output is monitored.
- Patient is watched for developing seizures.
- Patient is watched for developing pulmonary edema.
- Magnesium levels are maintained within the therapeutic range of 4–8 mg/liter.

BIBLIOGRAPHY

Baden, J.M., and Brodsky, J.B. *The Pregnant Surgical Patient.* Mt. Kisco, N.Y.: Futura Publishing, 1985.

Covino, B.G. and Scott, D.B. *Handbook of Epidural, Anaesthesia and Analgesia.* Orlando, Fla.: Grune & Stratton, 1985.

James, F.M. and Wheeler, A.S. *Obstetric Anesthesia: The Complicated Patient.* Philadelphia, Pa.: F.A. Davis Co., 1982.

Ostheimer, G. *Handbook of Obstetrical Anesthesia*. New York: Churchill Livingstone, 1984.

Schwarz, R.H. *Handbook of Obstetric Emergencies*. New Hyde Park, N.Y.: Medical Examination Publishing Co., 1984.

Shnider, S.M., and Levinson, G. *Anesthesia for Obstetrics*. Baltimore, Md.: Williams & Wilkins, 1987.

Chapter 16

Normal and Abnormal Hemostasis in the Surgical Patient

Barry J. Zadeh, M.D.

PHYSIOLOGY OF HEMOSTASIS

Blood Vessels

Hemostasis, the control of blood vessel integrity, is one of the central homeostatic functions in chordate organisms. The initiating step in this process is injury to the wall of a blood vessel. This is followed by a series of sequential events that are interrelated and interdependent.

The first effect of injury to a vessel is vasospasm involving the vessel in the area of the injury. The nature of this vasoconstriction varies with the type of injury, the nature of the blood vessel, and its location in the body. Injuries that transect a blood vessel are likely to produce marked vasospasm with rapid cessation of bleeding. Tangential injuries, on the other hand, cannot constrict circumferentially and are effectively splinted open by the vasospasm, resulting in prolonged blood loss. Vein injuries are less dependent on vasoconstriction as a primary hemostatic process than arteries. The smooth muscle in their walls is much less developed, and the pressure in the vessel is much lower. In general, bleeding from veins is therefore much less than from arteries, and active vasoconstriction is less important. The location of the blood vessel also is critical in the vasoconstrictive process. Tissues vary in the density of their support stroma. Vessels in cancellous bone are prevented from constricting by their rigid matrix, and bleeding from bone is relatively greater than from similar injuries in soft tissues.

The processes that mediate vasospasm are not completely understood, but they are certainly multifactorial. The blood vessel begins to contract within one-tenth of a second of injury, implying that a reflex mechanism is responsible for earliest vasospasm. The vessel remains contracted for prolonged periods of time, indicating that a secondary factor supervenes. A variety of tissue and platelet factors are released in the second phase of hemostasis; these are potent vasoconstrictors, and they probably produce this effect until a formed clot is in place. In addition, the increase in tissue tension resulting from extravasated blood and fluid and decreased pH in the area results in a decrease in blood flow to the area by shunting of blood through alternate vascular beds.

Platelets

Platelets circulate in the blood as semispherical structures or discocytes, which are 1–5 μm in diameter (see Figure 16-1). These are cellular fragments that are released from the cytoplasm of megacaryocytes in the marrow and, as such, are not true cells. They have no nucleus, but they do have a highly organized and complex cytoplasm. In the inactive state, the platelet has a smooth appearance and is covered by a glycocalyx 20–30 nm thick. The membrane itself is a highly ordered lipid bylayer that is rich in arachidonic acid and has a net positive charge on the external surface. The membrane is characterized by multiple apertures, .05–.20 μm in diameter, that connect the surface with an internal canalicular structure. Beneath and associated with the surface is a network of microtubule and microfilament systems that function as a cytoskeleton. These elements maintain the surface topography and connect the surface with an array of specialized organelles that are needed during the homeostatic process. In addition to mitochondria and a limited Golgi apparatus, the cytoplasm contains three specialized organelles: the dense bodies, alpha granules, and lysosome/peroxisomes. The main contents of each of these organelles are listed in Table 16-1. In addition to these membrane bound organelles, the cytoplasm also contains reserves of glycogen and a large pool of actin, myosin, and other contractile element precursors.

Following injury to a vessel wall, the second phase of hemostasis entails the formation of a plug of platelets to close the defect. The series of mechanisms by which platelets perform this function are categorized as adherence, activation, aggregation, and platelet release reaction. The normal circulatory system is a continuous structure lined by a specialized cell, the endothelia, whose membranes produce a micromilieu with which platelets do not normally adhere. The endothelia, like the platelets, express a net positive charge on their external surface, which serves to inhibit platelet contact. In addition, the endothelia produce

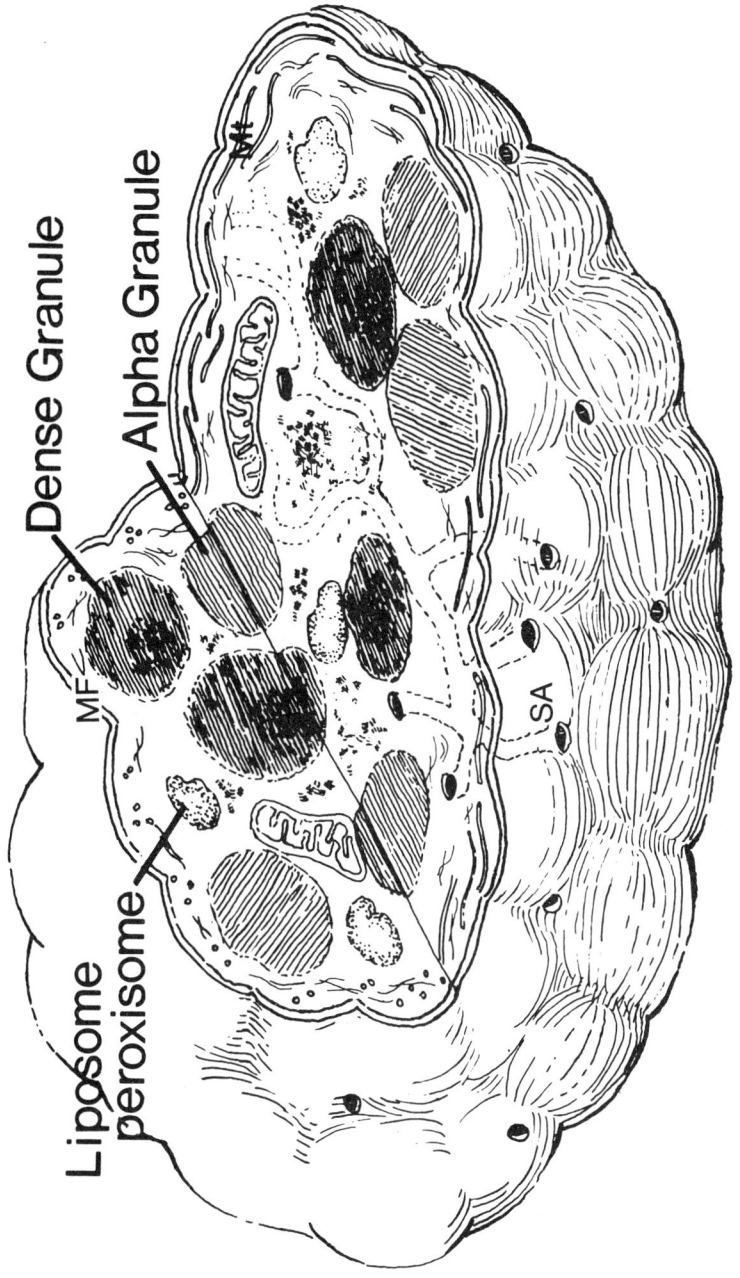

Figure 16-1 Platelet Morphology

Table 16-1 Content of Platelet Granules

Dense Bodies	Alpha Granules	Lysosomes/Peroxisomes
ADP	Albumin	Hydrolytic enzymes
Antiplasmin	Beta-Thromboglobulin	
ATP	Factor V	
Calcium ions	Factor VIII:vWF	
Epinephrine	Fibrinogen	
Norepinephrine	Fibronectin	
Pyrophosphate	PDGF	
Serotonin	Platelet Factor 4	
	Thrombospondin	

prostacylin, an arachidonic acid derivative, which is a potent inhibitor of platelet activation.

Injury to the vessel disrupts these protective mechanisms and also results in exposure of underlying structures containing collagen. The platelet surface contains binding sites for collagen that allow adherence at the site of injury. This binding reaction results in morphological changes in the platelet surface and internal structures. The first alteration is a change in the smooth surface architecture with the development of numerous spiny processes and pseudopods, termed echinocyte morphology. This change increases the surface area available for interaction with the surface, and the platelet spreads over the injured surface. Simultaneously, the activated platelets undergo a cell surface change called a "flip flop," and the net charge on the surface goes from positive to negative. At this point, the activated platelet begins to release the substances stored in the specialized organelles and cytoplasmic pools. Hydrolytic enzymes in the lysosomes and cellular cations provided by this reaction allow cellular cyclooxygenases and lypoxygenases to interact with membrane arachidonic acids, and a potent group of prostaglandin derivatives are produced.

The combined effect of these series of steps is to produce an environment in which platelet adhesion and continued activation is promoted. Circulating platelets are recruited and act further to accelerate the process. The entire area of vessel and endothelial injury participates in the reaction, and a primary plug of loosely associated platelets forms. The release of potent vasoconstrictors into the local environment ensures that vasospasm persists. At this point, a temporary cessation of bleeding occurs, a stagnant environment exists in which the clotting cascade can progress, and primary hemostasis is complete.

Clotting

In order for the temporary hemostasis resulting from platelet plug formation to result in prolonged or permanent repair, an additional series of reactions must occur. The most prominent of these is the development of a tight fibrin meshwork that binds to and ensnares the platelet plug. The process involved in clot formation is a cascading series of events involving circulating plasma proteins, cations, and lipoproteins derived from injured tissue or platelets. The final result of these reactions is conversion of soluble fibrinogen in the circulating blood to an insoluble polymer of fibrin interwoven into the platelet plug. The present numerical nomenclature of the factors involved is shown in Table 16-2. These reactions are not dependent on the presence of a primary platelet plug, but they are facilitated and accelerated by it.

The first step in the cascade is activation of one of two pathways by the products of vessel injury. The basis of the extrinsic pathway is the activation by and use of tissue thromboplastin in the clotting cascade. This factor is a lipoprotein, which serves to form a complex with Factor VII. In the presence of calcium ion, this complex is activated and acts on Factor X to produce Factor Xa, the active form of the factor. In the presence of Factor V and calcium ions, Factor Xa combines with the lipoprotein moiety of tissue thromboplastin to produce the extrinsic prothrombin activator complex. Tissue thromboplastin thus has a central role in both activation of the pathway and conversion of prothrombin to its active form.

The intrinsic pathway is independent of tissue lipoprotein and, in its place, uses a platelet lipoprotein, platelet Factor III, in a similar role. The intrinsic pathway is activated by the contact of Factor XII with collagen or other surface-related factors. In the presence of certain mediators, a short cascade occurs until Factor IXa is formed. This factor associates with Factor VIII and platelet Factor III to produce a complex in the presence of calcium ions that activates Factor X.

Table 16-2 Clotting Factors

Factor	Alternate Nomenclature
I	Fibrinogen
II	Prothrombin
III	Tissue thromboplastin
IV	Calcium
V	Proaccelerin
VII	Proconvertin
VIII	Antihemophiliac globulin
IX	Christmas factor
X	Stuart-Prower factor
XI	Plasma thromboplastin antecedent
XII	Hageman factor
XIII	Fibrin stabilizing factor
Platelet Factor III	Platelet phospholipid

At this point, the pathways unify, and either platelet Factor III or tissue thromboplastin can serve as the lipoprotein matrix of prothrombin activator. In the environment of vessel injury and a primary platelet clot, both pathways are induced and fibrinogen is rapidly converted into fibrin monomers. The final step in the reaction is the formation of cross-linked fibrin polymers by activated Factor XIIIa. The fibrin fibers then bind to and ensnare the platelets in a firm lattice. Figure 16-2 outlines the factors involved in these reactions.

With the development of a platelet-fibrin mesh, the stage is set for the completion of the permanent hemostatic plug. The processes involved in this step are a complete dissolution of the platelet cytoskeleton, release of remaining granule

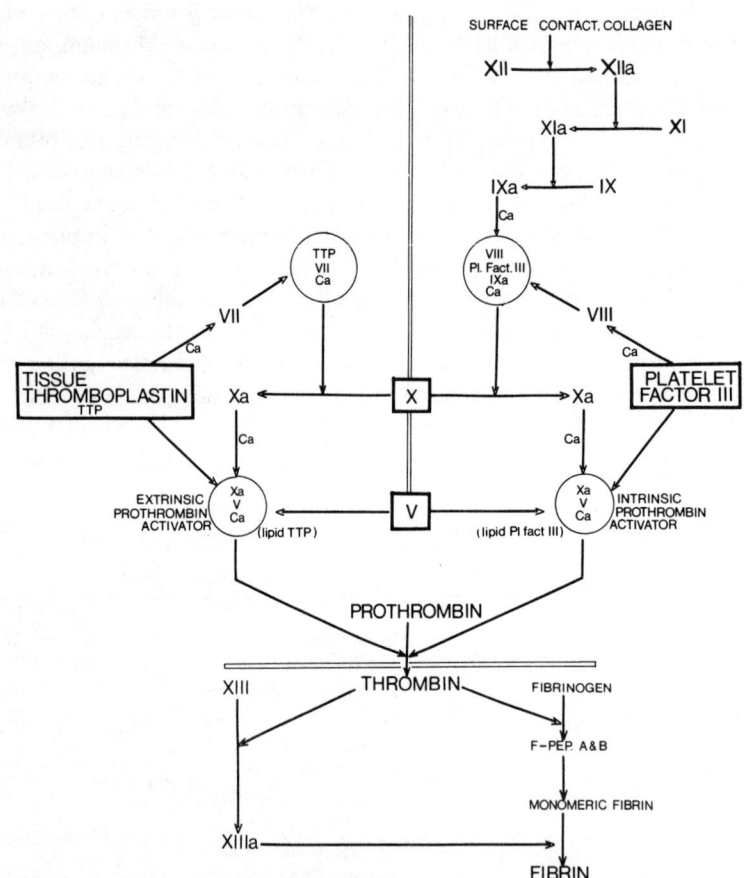

Figure 16-2 Clotting Cascade

Normal and Abnormal Hemostasis   237

stores, fusion of the plasma membranes, and polymerization of actinomyosin stores into a functioning contractile apparatus. The fully formed actinomyosin filaments then contract to exert tension on the clot. The combined platelet and fibrin skeleton with trapped RBCs and WBCs produces a secure structure that prevents further bleeding and allows a framework for repair of the vessel wall. Figure 16-3 presents a summary of the events in hemostasis.

SURGICAL TECHNIQUES

Most bleeding during surgery is not the result of abnormalities in hemostasis but rather the effect of creating a wound in which normal hemostatic mechanisms are

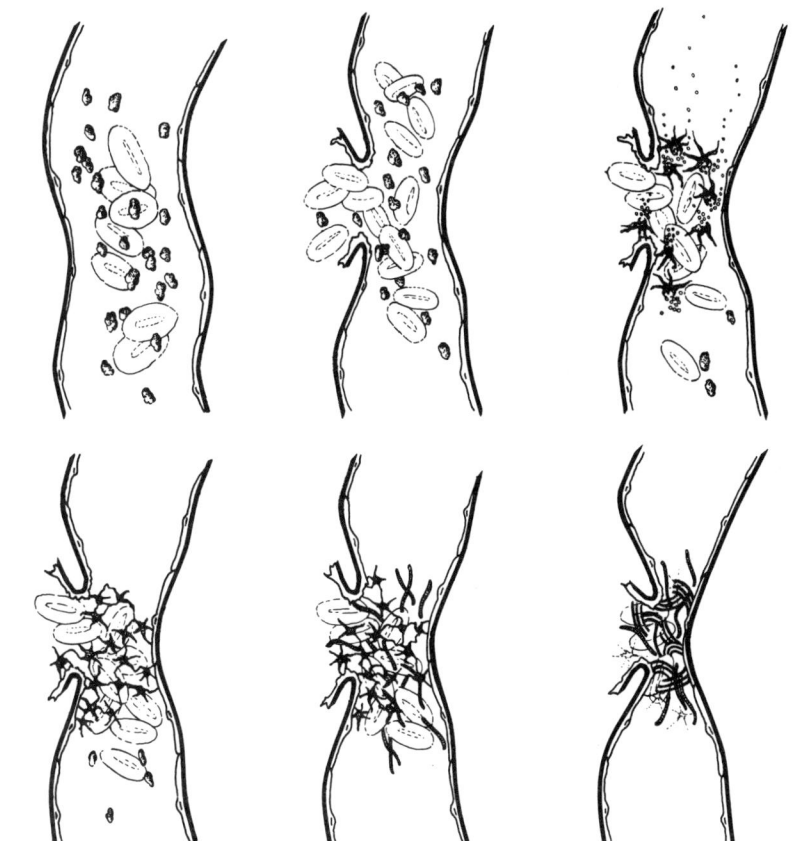

Figure 16-3 Summary of Hemostatic Mechanisms

hindered. To ensure adequate visualization of fine tissue structures, the wound is left widely opened and the compressive properties of tissue are not allowed to exist. Many anesthetic agents in widespread use are potent vasodilators that suppress reflex vasospasm of injury. In some cases, it is necessary for the surgeon to divide vessels too large for control by hemostatic mechanisms. Normal primary clot formation takes five to ten minutes to occur, and in this time significant blood loss can occur in a wound of any significant size. It is therefore not practical for the surgeon to rely on normal hemostatic mechanisms alone to provide for control of bleeding.

In the effort to provide an optimal environment for each operation, the surgeon tries to provide mechanical control of bleeding in as short a time as possible and to provide an environment that allows for maintaining normal clotting in the postoperative period. To accomplish these goals during diverse procedures and in all tissue locations, a wide variety of local mechanical techniques and adjunctive measures have been developed.

Mechanical Techniques

Suture control of bleeding vessels is the principle technique used in surgical hemostasis. First used in antiquity, the technique was lost during the Middle Ages until Ambrose Pare reintroduced it in 1552. While suture materials were initially crude, progress in materials manufacturing over the last century has resulted in the availability of a wide variety of suture materials in many sizes and textures. The two most important advances in suture control of bleeding were made in the earliest part of the 20th century. At that time, the improvements in suture and needle design allowed Alexis Carrel, in 1906, to develop vascular suture techniques. These techniques allowed the surgeon to add repair of large vessels to ligature as a means of accomplishing hemostasis while preventing tissue injury. Concurrently, William Halsted introduced the concept of fine suture ligature, involving only the vessel itself. This method ensures hemostasis while preventing injury to surrounding structures. Finally, in 1911, as a means to increase speed and facilitate application in delicate tissues, Harvey Cushing developed silver clips as an alternative to ligature. With improvements in clip appliers since that time, this technique has become a valuable adjunct to suture ligature in certain procedures.

Active compression is another technique used to aid in hemostasis. The open wound is an environment in which blood vessels are not subjected to the compressive forces that control bleeding in a closed hematoma. The use of direct pressure on a bleeding vessel causes stasis to occur and promotes clot formation. The simplest means of applying compression is to use the digit. To direct compression over larger areas, laparotomy pads or sponges are employed. When prolonged compression is necessary, surgical adjuvants like Surgicel may be used in conjunction with sutures. In this manner, prolonged compression with absorbable materials can be maintained into the postoperative period.

Cautery, using heat, electric current, or laser light, is a means of obtaining mechanical hemostasis by actively coagulating the proteins in the blood and cut ends of vessels to produce a hemostatic plug. Direct heat from brands was used since before recorded memory to stop bleeding but was abandoned by physicians after the Middle Ages because of the extensive injury it produces to surrounding structures. In 1928, electrocautery with a grounded current was introduced by Bovie and Cushing to facilitate hemostasis in neurosurgical procedures. The use of a controlled current was shown to be selective for blood vessels because of decreased electrical resistance in blood.

The advantages of rapid hemostasis with limited tissue injury, coupled with the advent of nonvolatile anesthetics, shortly thereafter led to the widespread use of cautery in many diverse situations. In the control of bleeding from vessels in the 100 μm to 2 mm range, cautery has replaced ligature and clip placement in the hands of most surgeons because of the extreme decrease in time involved in its use. The perceived drawback of cautery is that tissue necrosis not seen with fine ligature technique may result in poor wound healing. In practice, however, the time-saving advantage and lack of foreign body allow cautery to be used with no demonstrable increase in infection rates or wound dehiscence.

The use of laser light energy to produce cautery is the newest mechanical method to be developed. Its greatest utility to date has been in conjunction with endoscopy, where suture and electrocautery are not practical. Whether or not in the future an expanded role for laser cautery is likely remains unclear; much will depend on possible future advances in practical delivery systems.

Surgical Adjuvants

A wide spectrum of chemical agents has been used to aid in hemostasis in the surgical wound. Some chemical agents produce vasoconstriction, others augment platelet function or activate clotting factors, while still others function simply by providing a matrix for mechanical compression. In general, these agents are used in those situations in which multiple small vessels are injured and are not amenable to direct mechanical measures. In addition, they can be effectively used in situations in which mild defects in hemostatic mechanisms produce abnormal bleeding in the local wound without evidence of systemic bleeding.

When augmented vasoconstriction is needed, epinephrine is the topical vasoconstrictor used most frequently. It can be used on mucosal surfaces, like the bed of a tonsillectomy procedure, or superficially. It is commonly used after burn wound excision where dense edema and hyperplasia of the dermis prevent vasoconstriction in neovascular beds.

Cocaine is another agent widely used as a vasoconstrictor. However, due to potent side effects in the central nervous system and the potential for abuse, its application has unfortunately been limited. A clear indication for its use is surgery on the upper respiratory tract, where relatively small doses can produce marked constriction of mucosal vessels.

Collagen, as noted above, is a potent activator of both platelets and the intrinsic clotting pathways. For this reason, various forms of collagen have been used topically to promote local hemostasis. Early in the century, fresh tissue was used in the surgical wound with some success. However, issues of sterile technique and marketing resulted in the development of more refined substances containing collagen compounds. The first of these, Gelfoam, and other similar products were derived from denatured collagen. Although this substance was shown to be effective in promoting hemostasis, further investigation indicated that the mechanism of action was not the direct activation of the clotting pathways. The process of preparing and sterilizing collagen causes denaturation and results in the loss of direct hemostatic properties. Processed collagen sponges appear to act by providing a matrix for blood accumulation and compression of small vessels. To overcome this problem, a process to obtain intact collagen from tissues was developed, and the result is now available as microcrystalline collagen (Avitene). When applied to the wound, this product directly activates platelets and can augment clot formation.

As participants in the clotting cascade, thrombin and fibrin have also been used to aid in local hemostasis. They function to add substrate to the local environment and to circumvent the clotting cascade, and they may also stimulate platelet activation. They can be used topically in solution or incorporated into inert carriers. The greatest success of these agents has been achieved when they are used with cellulose sponges. These inert sponges, Oxycel or Surgicel, function as the carriers of thrombin or fibrin and prevent dilution by washout. While the chemical agents are promoting activation of clot formation, the sponges themselves are converted by hydrolyzing agent in the blood into a sticky gelatenous mass. The entire complex then forms a macroclot that exerts compressive force on the bleeding vessels to further promote hemostasis. An advantage of this system is that all components are absorbable and can be left in place if necessary.

ABNORMALITIES OF HEMOSTASIS

Defects in the hemostatic mechanism may be present in a patient prior to surgery, or they may develop during the operation. The defects that are present preoperatively are diverse in nature; they may be overtly manifested or subclinical, and they may be present from birth or acquired.

Congenital Defects

Congenital abnormalities in hemostasis are much less common than acquired ones. The most common congenital abnormalities are inherited autosomal recessive deficiency states in clotting factors caused by point mutations in the coding sequence of the gene.

Hemophilia

Hemophilia A, classic hemophilia, is the most common of all hereditary defects of hemostasis, affecting 10 to 12 of each 100,000 live births. It is a sex-linked recessive disorder characterized by a deficiency of circulating Factor VIII. The penetrance of the defect is highly variable and incomplete, with clinical severity almost totally dependent on the degree of deficiency in circulating factor. In most individuals, levels below 15 percent of normal produce spontaneous episodes of bleeding. When levels are from 15 to 40 percent, bleeding may occur only with trauma or surgery. At levels greater than 40 percent, bleeding is unusual. The spontaneous bleeding typically affects joints or results in prolonged epistaxis. Milder defects may bleed only after dental extractions or minor surgery. However, with severe deficiency states, spontaneous intracranial, retroperitoneal, or retropharyngeal bleeding can occur.

Since Factor VIII participates only in the intrinsic clotting pathway, tests for laboratory abnormalities are restricted to the partial thromboplastin time (PTT) test. Prothrombin time (PT), bleeding time, and thrombin time are all normal. However, during major surgery, bleeding may be massive due to the failure of stable clot formation. Therefore, if surgery is contemplated on a known or suspected hemophiliac, every attempt must be made to correct the deficiency of Factor VIII preoperatively.

After obtaining accurate baseline Factor-VIII levels, appropriate amounts of Factor VIII concentrate or cryoprecipitate are administered, beginning six to eight hours preoperatively, to achieve normal levels in the plasma. In severe deficiency states, this may approach 50 units per kilogram (fresh frozen plasma, FFP, contains .06 units/mL; Factor VIII concentrate and cryoprecipitate contain 9.0 to 10.0 units/mL). In principle, 0.4 to 0.6 units/kg should be replaced for each percentage point below normal. The level should be rechecked as close to the time of surgery as possible; it is maintained postoperatively for one to two weeks, depending on the extent of the procedure. The half-life of replacement Factor VIII is 8 to 12 hours; therefore, one-half of the loading dose should be repeated every 12 hours to maintain normal levels.

Hemophilia B (Factor IX), plasma thromboplastin antecedent (PTA) deficiency (Factor XI), and Hageman trait deficiency are other hereditary defects in the intrinsic pathway. These defects produce a pattern of laboratory abnormalities similar to hemophilia A, but they are much less common. Factors IX and XI deficiencies, although usually less severe than hemophilia A, may produce abnormal surgical bleeding. When a deficiency state exists for one of these factors, therapy parallels that for hemophilia A. Levels of each factor should be raised to near normal values and maintained for the early postoperative period. Factor IX is available as a concentrate from pooled plasma and has a half-life of 12 to 24 hours. Factor XI is not available in purified form but can be replaced with FFP. Factor XII deficiency is interesting in that it is associated with extremely prolonged PTT values but rarely produces abnormal bleeding after major surgery. The importance of this condition lies in its contrast with other disorders of the intrinsic pathway that are associated with abnormal bleeding.

Hereditary deficiencies in Factors VII, V, X, and XIII are very rare, but they produce characteristic laboratory abnormalities when they are present. Factor VII participates exclusively in extrinsic clotting and deficiencies result in an isolated prolongation of the PT. Factors V and X are contributors to both clotting systems, and deficiencies increase both PT and PTT. Factor XIII deficiency results in normal laboratory studies but can be diagnosed by quantitative factor levels when suspected.

Platelet Function Disorder

There are three hereditary disorders of platelet function, and all are exceedingly rare. In contrast to the deficiency disorders of clotting factors, these disorders are characterized by qualitative defects.

Thrombasthenia is a condition characterized by normal platelet number, a very prolonged bleeding time, and bleeding from minor trauma to mucous membranes. The defect is a failure of the platelets to aggregate appropriately in response to ADP. During surgery, bleeding is likely to be massive. Treatment relies on the use of large volumes of platelets until a normal bleeding time is obtained. Platelets are transfused as fresh, cold, stored platelet-rich plasms. If used within five days, the half-life of these platelets ranges from 24 to 72 hours. Platelet counts have no meaning, and postoperative replacement therapy must be governed by clinical judgment and bleeding times.

Another disorder, platelet release dysfunction, is characterized by a history of easy bruising and prolonged bleeding from mucous membranes. It is caused by an, as yet uncharacterized, defect in platelet membrane function. Platelet adherence functioning is unimpaired, but activation is incomplete and appropriate aggregation does not occur. Fortunately, the defect is usually mild and untoward bleeding is uncommon except during major surgery. When indicated, the defect can be corrected by administration of exogenous platelets.

Macrothrombocytic thrombopathia is the rarest of congenital platelet defects. It is characterized by the presence of large, irregular-shaped platelets. These platelets fail to release platelet Factor III, and clot formation is markedly impaired.

Von Willebrand's disease is an autosomal dominant trait that affects the production of von Willebrand's factor, a protein involved as an intermediate in both the intrinsic pathway and the platelet adhesion. The disorder is characterized by a Factor VIII deficiency with prolongation in PTT and a qualitative platelet defect in the surface activation process, which results in a prolonged bleeding time. Significant spontaneous bleeding is unusual, but prolonged bleeding after surgery is common. Replacement therapy before surgery entails use of cryoprecipitate, which not only increases Factor-VIII levels but also results in the production and release of von Willebrands factor. As with other hemostatic disorders, therapy should continue into the postoperative period. Parenthetically, the use of Desmopressin (DDAVP), while useful in chronic management of patients with von Willebrand's disease, has not yet been fully defined during surgery on patients with this disorder.

Acquired Defects

In contrast to congenital disorders, acquired defects in hemostasis are very common in surgical patients. They can precede surgery or develop during the operation itself. While often multifactorial, isolated platelet or clotting pathway defects also occur. Quantitative and qualitative platelet defects are the most common causes of abnormal hemostasis in the surgical patient.

Quantitative

Thrombocytopenia is defined as a quantitative deficiency in platelet numbers without any associated platelet function abnormalities. It is due to either a decrease in platelet production and release, or as a consequence of decreased time in the circulation as clinical manifestations of the quantitative deficiency syndromes. Normal platelet counts are 150,000–450,000/mL. A reduction in number to 75,000–150,000/mL is well-tolerated during surgery if all other hemostatic mechanisms are normal. Counts below 60,000–75,000/mL result in abnormal bleeding during surgery. Spontaneous bleeding into the subcutaneous tissues with minor trauma or prolonged bleeding from mucous membranes is seen with counts of 20,000–40,000/mL. Levels below 15,000/mL are extremely dangerous, with the potential to develop intracranial or gastrointestinal bleeding. Diffuse bleeding during and after surgery will almost invariably occur after major procedures if the platelet count cannot be maintained above 25,000/mL.

Abnormalities of production are most commonly seen in myeloproliferative disorders; they are also due to aplasia of the marrow. Acute and chronic leukemias result in thrombocytopenia by producing both a mass effect in the marrow and also by generating and releasing local and systemic factors that inhibit the maturation and release of platelets from the marrow. The improved survival of patients with these disorders recently and the more aggressive approaches taken today to deal with their intercurrent surgical conditions often necessitates operative procedures in this group.

The chronic nature of the condition and the very low platelet levels complicate preoperative therapy. Very often, prior platelet transfusions have been required, with resulting formation of platelet and sera-specific antibodies. The presence of these reactive antibodies produces two unfavorable reactions. First, platelet half-life in the circulation is reduced, necessitating increased platelet transfusion before, during, and after surgery. Second, an allergic-type hyperpyrexia and related platelet transfusion reactions occur. In the setting of a major operation, these reactions are both confusing and potentially dangerous. Serious consideration should be given to pretreating patients with this disorder with diphenhydramine (Benadryl) and steroids. Yet, despite these limitations, it is usually possible to perform major surgery safely in these very ill patients.

Aplasia of the marrow occurs as an expected side effect of chemotherapy or as an unusual complication during use of many commonly prescribed drugs. When this condition is produced as a side effect of chemotherapy a pancytopenia usually results. In this case, the hemostatic defect shares many properties with the thrombocytopenia of myeloproliferative disorders and is managed in much the same manner. Instances of aplasia secondary to idiosyncratic drug reactions are much more varied; they may include total and severe aplasia or involve only one precursor pool.

The diagnosis of this disorder rests on the presence of thrombocytopenia and a bone marrow biopsy that shows decreased megacaryocyte numbers. The condition is usually temporary and will resolve with a discontinuation of the offending agent. If continuation of the agent is mandatory or if the aplasia is permanent, surgery should be deferred until the platelet count can be raised to levels of at least 60,000/mL during major procedures and maintained at that level for at least one week.

Decreased survival time of circulating platelets is also a common cause of isolated thrombocytopenia. Idiosyncratic autoimmune reactions to a large number of pharmacological agents result in increased destruction in the spleen. Differentiation from aplasia is then based on the observation of an increased number of megacaryocytes in the marrow.

Idiopathic thrombocytopenic purpura (ITP) is a syndrome characterized by a similarly increased destruction of circulating platelets in the spleen, but here no specific underlying cause can be defined. While cessation of the cause usually corrects drug-induced thrombocytopenia, patients with ITP often require splenectomy. The preoperative management of the patient with ITP involves a course of treatment with steroids as a primary therapeutic agent. Only when steroid therapy fails is a splenectomy performed. During the preoperative period, every attempt is made to maintain platelet numbers over 60,000/mL with steroids, but platelet transfusions are not given except under extreme conditions. However, platelet packs are prepared and may be used after the spleen has been removed in the operating room and during the recovery period.

Qualitative

Qualitative defects in platelet function are at least as common as quantitative defects, but they are more difficult to identify and characterize. They may be due to extrinsic causes, or they may be secondary to intrinsic defects in the platelet, as seen in certain myeloproliferative disorders. Furthermore, platelet adhesiveness, aggregability, and release reactions may be affected individually or in combination. This category of hemostatic defects is especially interesting in that routine surgical screening tests do not identify the defects; they are, therefore, the cause of most cases of unexplained surgical bleeding.

In our society, the agent most likely to produce these abnormalities is the cyclooxygenase inhibitor aspirin. Even though the increase in bleeding time is prolonged, massive bleeding is unusual during surgery after aspirin ingestion. However, since the effect of aspirin on platelets is not reversible, it is prudent to discontinue the use of aspirin-containing agents for at least one week before any major surgery.

Uremia produces an abnormal bleeding time in the setting of normal platelet numbers. The defects in platelet function associated with uremia are complex and not clearly understood, but the result is an impaired ability of the platelet both to adhere to collagen and to aggregate in the presence of ADP. Patients undergoing hemodialysis have a less pronounced form of platelet dysfunction because this process in some way reverses the defect associated with uremia. When surgery is necessary in these patients, it is advisable to optimize metabolic function through dialysis in the immediate preoperative period. The treatment of bleeding that occurs should include the use of both fresh platelets and clotting factors when indicated.

The presence of acquired defects in clotting factors is also a common occurrence in surgical patients. Most often, the causes are primary liver disease, the use of anticoagulants, vitamin K deficiency, or diffuse intravascular coagulation (DIC).

The three prominent disorders of liver function that impair hemostasis are alcoholic cirrhosis, hepatitis, and obstructive jaundice. All are common and occur in the surgical patient. The disorder of clotting factors results from a deficiency in production and release by the liver cell and includes all clotting factors except Factor VIII. Due to the relative sensitivity of Factors VII and V to lowered plasma levels, the extrinsic pathway is more prominently affected with a marked elevation in the PT. In the cirrhotic patient, this defect may be compounded by the presence of thrombocytopenia of secondary hypersplenism. The treatment of factor deficiency from obstruction involves the use of vitamin K and relief of the obstruction. These measures will result in a fairly rapid return of clotting factor levels to normal. If emergency surgery is required, FFP should be administered until the PT is within normal range. The use of vitamin K is not efficacious in the treatment of cirrhotic disorders. In such cases, FFP should be used in the preoperative preparation of the patient, and fresh blood and platelets should be considered if continued bleeding occurs in the operative or postoperative period.

Anticoagulants are utilized on an acute or chronic basis in the management of numerous medical disorders, and their use may be ongoing in patients being considered for surgery. In addition, anticoagulants are used during surgery in low doses to prevent the formation of deep vein thrombosis and in high doses to produce systemic anticoagulation during certain vascular procedures.

Heparin is a relatively short-acting compound that combines with a plasma protein, heparin cofactor, to become a potent antithrombin complex. This agent has the advantages of a rapid onset of action and a short half-life in the plasma, and it has the additional property of having a specific antagonist, protamine sulfate. Heparin may therefore be used safely in the preoperative period; it should be discontinued three to five hours before surgery. When employed during surgery, reversal can be achieved within minutes and monitored by automated ACT in the operating room.

The major disadvantage of heparin as an anticoagulant is that it cannot be used orally. For this reason, Coumadin is the drug of choice in most instances where chronic anticoagulation is required. The mechanism of action of this drug is to cause a state of relative vitamin K deficiency by specifically blocking the action of this cofactor in the formation of prothrombin and Factors VII, IX, and X. This results in impaired clotting in the extrinsic pathway and a prolongation of the PT. To correct this deficiency, it is possible to simply stop the drug and wait three to five days, stop the drug and give Vitamin K for reversal over 24 to 48 hours, or to continue the agent and use FFP during the perioperative period to correct the factor deficiencies. The specific course of action will be based on the rationale for chronic anticoagulation and the nature of the operative procedure to be performed.

Diffuse intravascular clotting (DIC) is a group of disorders that have in common the nonspecific activation of the clotting factor pathways and, in some cases, platelets at sites remote from endothelial injury. The injury can be considered a final common end point of several conditions that share a set of mediators. These mediators include substances that have tissue thromboplastin-like activity, endotoxin, and antigen-antibody complexes.

The leading causes of DIC in surgical patients are gram-negative sepsis, major trauma, and complications of pregnancy. The specific defects in hemostasis that result include thrombocytopenia; deficiencies in Factors V, VIII, and XIII and in prothrombin and fibrinogen; and an accumulation of fibrin split products and fibrin monomer. These defects result in a prolongation of the PT, the PTT, and the bleeding time; the appearance of RBC fragments on the blood smear; and absolute hypofibrinogenemia and the appearance of fibrin split products. The correction of these changes is based on the removal of the inciting cause. If this cannot be done, the disorder is rapidly terminal. After resolution of the activating process, the replacement of platelets and clotting factors can be performed under the guidance of appropriate laboratory results. In the past, the use of heparin was advocated to lessen the severity of the consumptive coagulopathy, but such use has been found to be very dangerous and should now be used only in extreme situations.

ABNORMAL SURGICAL BLEEDING

Preoperative Screening

All patients undergoing surgery should be considered in terms of the risk of abnormal bleeding they may represent. To determine this risk is a complex process that includes patient-related factors in the history, physical examination, and laboratory examination and factors related to the nature and extent of the operation itself. Preoperative screening must begin with a complete history and physical examination. The purpose of these are not only to determine if overt evidence of prior bleeding tendencies exist but also to define which laboratory tests should be performed.

The history of prior bleeding during surgery or dental procedures is the most important feature of the examination. Circumcision, dental extraction, and tonsillectomy can each produce excessive bleeding in a patient with congenital abnormalities too subtle to produce overt bleeding. Bleeding during a biopsy procedure in an adult patient is another clue that hemostatic defects may occur.

Unusual menstrual bleeding with heavy or prolonged flow rather than breakthrough bleeding is also a relevant finding. Epistaxis follows a similar pattern of prolonged bleeding rather than increased frequency of bleeding. In patients without overt bleeding, a tendency to bruise easily should be determined. The formation of bruises on the extremities is not a reliable indicator of bleeding tendencies, since minor trauma is a highly variable occurrence. The formation of bruises on the face or trunk, however, should alert the questioner to the possible presence of a bleeding disorder.

Special attention to drug use and systemic diseases is an important feature of the review. Many pharmacological agents can produce disorders of hemostasis. In addition, the use of aspirin which is a component of many over-the-counter products, should be ascertained. In general, use of aspirin and aspirin-containing products should be discontinued at least one week before elective surgery. Anticoagulants are also used widely in our society, and particular attention should be paid to the history of coumarin-derivative use. Lastly, an attempt to elicit a valid alcohol history should be made.

Upon completion of the history, a complete physical examination must be performed on each patient. The patient should be completely disrobed and the skin inspected in its entirety. The presence of ecchymosis, purpura, and angiomata may not be noted by the patient, especially if they occur on the back, buttocks, or extremities. A rectal examination is important, with a stool guiac examination to exclude the presence of occult gastrointestinal bleeding. In addition, the mucosal membranes of the mouth and nose should be examined for the presence of telangectasias or other mucosal abnormalities. An evaluation of the lymph nodes of the neck, axillae, and groin are important, not only to exclude primary lymphatic disease, but also to identify a potential AIDS patient in those areas where the disease is prevalent. Finally, the abdomen should be examined and the liver and spleen carefully palpated for enlargement or abnormalities. The presence of ascites, dilated veins around the umbilicus, or jaundice will alert the examiner to the presence of significant liver disease.

Due to cost considerations, a complete laboratory evaluation of the hemostatic reserves is not possible for every patient. A patient without signs or symptoms of hemotologic abnormalities who is undergoing an operation that does not involve a significantly increased risk of bleeding will have only routine screening tests performed. In most hospitals, these include a complete blood count, including platelets, PT and PTT, and a chemical profile, including liver function tests.

The CBC is used to determine the presence of a quantitative defect in platelets and to exclude the presence of infection, myeloproliferative disease, and occult bleeding. This test however, does not exclude the presence of qualitative defects in platelet function. PT and PTT are tested to evaluate the extrinsic and intrinsic clotting pathways, respectively. In most instances, these tests are adequate and cost-effective when used in combination with a complete history and physical exam and when unexpected bleeding is unusual.

Any patient who is suspected of having the potential for increased bleeding based on history, physical examination, or routine laboratory examination should have more extensive laboratory tests performed, and the defects should be corrected before surgery. An extended examination should include at least a bleeding time test, a blood smear, and thrombin time test.

The bleeding time test is a procedure designed to determine the actual time it will take for an incision in the skin to stop bleeding and to reflect specifically the primary platelet function. A small incision is made through a template on the forearm after inflation of a blood pressure cuff to 40 mm Hg. The blood is then blotted every 30 seconds until bleeding has stopped (modified Ivy method). If performed under standardized conditions 60 percent of patients will stop bleeding within 5 to 6 minutes, and 95 to 98 percent within 10 minutes. The majority of qualitative defects severe enough to result in unusual surgical bleeding can be identified by this test, and a cause can then be sought.

The blood smear is a useful adjunctive test because it provides a way of identifying qualitative morphological abnormalities in platelets, RBCs and WBCs in a noninvasive manner. The presence of nucleated RBCs or premature polymorphonuclear neutrophil leukocytes (PMNs) can indicate important underlying disease processes. Platelet sizes that are outside the normal range can also indicate the presence of a qualitative defect.

The thrombin time test is performed by adding dilute thrombin to plasma and measuring the time for a clot to form. By bypassing the need for native thrombin generation, this test assesses the efficiency of the fibrinogen conversion reaction of the plasma. The test is important in defining two common clotting abnormalities unrelated to deficiencies in clotting factors: increased antithrombin activity and increased fibrinolysis. Antithrombin activity can be due to the persistence of heparin in patients who have been anticoagulated before or during surgery, or it may be due to heparin-like activity of a variety of circulating factors. Fibrinolysis increases thrombin time because fibrin split products interfere with the formation of fibrin polymers rather than by depletion of fibrinogen. It is therefore a more sensitive indicator of subclinical fibrinolysis than fibrinogen levels alone.

Diagnosis, Treatment, and Postanesthesia Implications

The above preoperative evaluation will define and allow correction of most patients' bleeding problems. Thus, the occurrence of unexpected bleeding during or after surgery is an uncommon finding. There are however two groups of patients who will bleed diffusely during or immediately after surgery. One group consists of patients who have poorly defined platelet abnormalities and who bleed after routine surgery. As noted above, qualitative defects in platelet function are not routinely examined before surgery. Those with these defects comprise the majority of patients who bleed diffusely after routine surgery. The second group consists of patients who have relatively minor preoperative defects but develop hemostatic defects as a result of the operative procedure. This group of patients will have surgery using cardiopulmonary bypass and extracorporeal circulation, massive trauma with transfusion-related defects, and prostatic surgery. In both groups, a preoperative hemostatic defect is either not expected or not present; therefore, diagnostic tests must be repeated. Diagnosis for these patients occurs either in the operating room or in the PACU soon after completion of the operation.

The preliminary finding is one of increased blood loss out of proportion to the standard for any given procedure. This may be noted during measured blood loss in the operating room, or it may be manifested by poor urine output or hypotension in the PACU. At this point, a decision must be made regarding the most likely cause of the finding. In most cases, increased blood loss during the operation is due to a failure in local hemostasis rather than a defect in hemostatic mechanisms. Bleeding from hemostatic defects is rarely limited to the operative incision itself, and a careful examination of intravenous access sites and mucous membranes will usually reveal diffuse bleeding.

In the absence of these findings defects in local hemostasis must be considered as the most likely cause. In the PACU, hypotension, due to volume depletion and third-space losses, is much more likely to occur than hemorrhage and must be excluded. Since both hemorrhage and third-space losses produce a similar spectrum of clinical signs and symptoms, it is usually the persistence of findings after appropriate volume resuscitation that indicates the presence of prolonged bleeding. If the wound edges, mucous membranes, and other sites of minor injury are involved, a hemostatic defect should be considered.

The laboratory examination and treatment of bleeding are often performed concurrently, due to the lack of time to await results, and treatment is often based on historical and subjective biases. When the diagnosis of an unexpected hemostatic defect is made, the routine laboratory screening tests are repeated and a thrombin time test and blood smear are obtained. A bleeding time test is often unreliable in the immediate postoperative period, due to peripheral vasoactive changes and the effect of anesthetic agents.

Treatment is usually mandated before the results of any laboratory tests can be obtained. In general, it follows standard formulas. Volume replacement and RBC maintenance are given the highest priority, and reoperation to augment local hemostasis is considered. Replacement of clotting factors with FFP is initiated if a potential deficiency state is suspected. Platelets are administered in the form of fresh (less than five days), cold-stored, pooled, platelet-rich plasma. When the

Normal and Abnormal Hemostasis 251

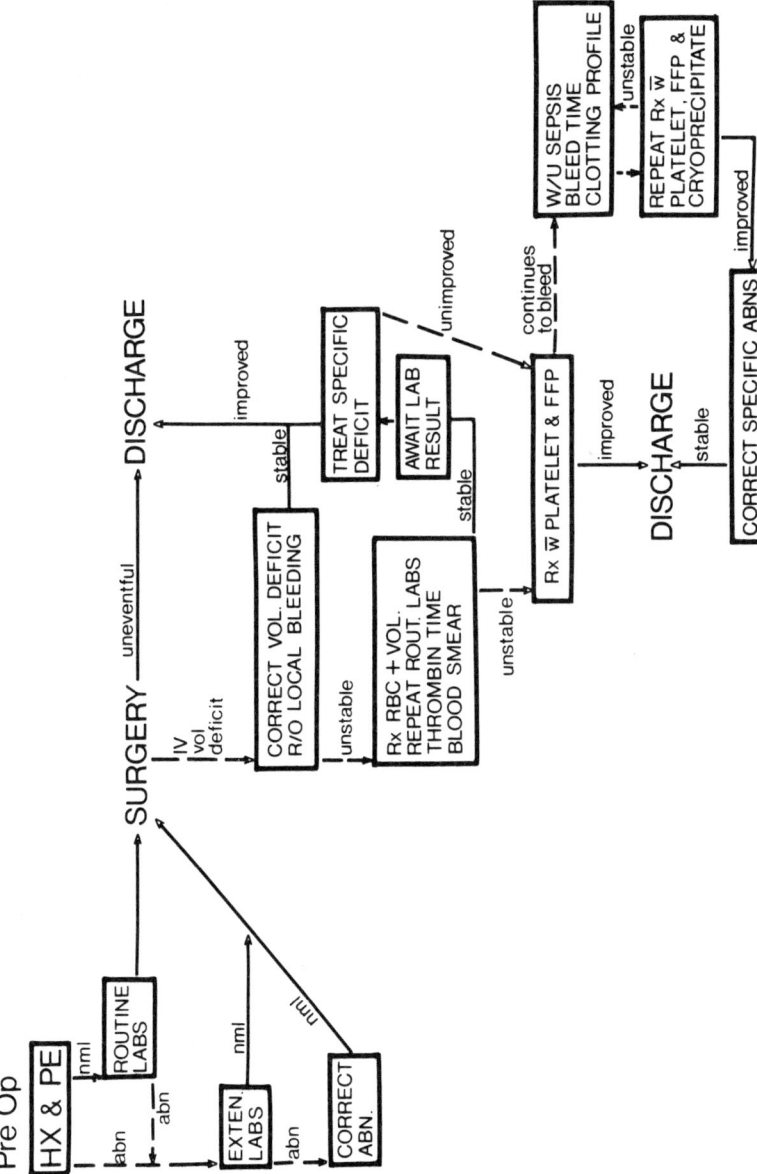

Figure 16-4 Evaluation and Treatment of the Surgical Patient with a Hemostatic Defect

results of the laboratory examination become available, attention can be directed to correction of specific abnormalities. Continued bleeding in these circumstances dictates a repetition of "shotgun" therapy. Simultaneously, reevaluation of potential causes is conducted in further laboratory testing. Figure 16-4 presents a flowsheet of one possible management schema that can be followed in the evaluation and treatment of hemostasis in the surgical patient, incorporating the concepts outlined above.

BIBLIOGRAPHY

Physiology

Altman, R., and Hemker, H. "Contact Activation in the Extrinsic Blood Clotting System." *Thrombosis et Diathesis Haemorrhagia* 18 (1967):525.

Baumgartner, H.R., Muggli, R., Tschopp T., and Turrito, V. "Platelet Adhesion, Release and Aggregation in Flowing Blood." *Thrombosis et Diathesis Haemorrhagia* 35 (1976):124.

Born, G.V.R. "Aggregation of Blood Platelets by Adenosine Diphosphate and Its Reversal." *Nature* 194 (1962):927.

Bowie, E.J., and Sharp, A.A. *Hemostasis and Thrombosis*. Boston: Butterworths, 1985.

Feinstein, M.B., and Fraser, C. "Human Platelet Secretion and Aggregation Induced by Calcium Ionophores." *Journal of General Physiology* 66 (1975):561.

Frojmovic, M.M., and Milton, J.C. "Human Platelet Size, Shape and Related Factors in Health and Disease." *Physiological Reviews* 62 (1982):185.

Fukami, M.H., and Salganikoff, L. "Human Platelet Storage Granules: A Review." *Thrombosis and Haemostasis* 38 (1979):963.

George, J.N. "Direct Assessment of Platelet Adhesion to Glass." *Blood* 40 (1972):862.

Jackson, C.M., and Nemerson, N. "Blood Coagulation." *Annual Review of Biochemistry* 49 (1980):765.

McFarlane, R.G. "Enzyme Cascades in Blood Clotting." *Nature* 202 (1964):498.

Mannucci, P.M., and Sharp, A.A. "Platelet Volume and Shape in Relation to Aggregation and Adhesion." *British Journal of Haematology* 13 (1967):604.

Ogston, D. *The Physiology of Hemostasis*. Cambridge, Mass.: Harvard University Press, 1983.

Radley, J.M., and Scurfield, G. "The Mechanism of Platelet Release." *Blood* 56 (1980):996.

Salzman, E.W. "The Events That Lead to Thrombosis." *Bulletin of the New York Academy of Medicine* 48 (1972):225.

Stahl, K., Themann, H., and Dane, W. "Ultrastructural Morphometric Investigations on Normal Human Platelets." *Haemostasis* 7 (1975):242.

Wright, I.S. "The Nomenclature of Blood Clotting Factors." *Thrombosis et Diathesis Haemorrhagia* 7 (1967):381.

Local Hemostasis

Cushing, H. "Control of Bleeding in Operations for Brain Tumor." *Annals of Surgery* 54 (1911):1.

Cushing, H., and Bovie, W.T. "Electrosurgery As an Aid to the Removal of Brain Tumors." *Surgery, Gynecology, and Obstetrics* 47 (1928):752.

Degenshein, G., Hurwitz, A., and Ribacoff, S. "Experience With Regenerated Oxidized Cellulose." *New York State Journal of Medicine* 63 (1963):2639.

Hait, M.R. "Microcrystalline Collagen: A New Hemostatic Agent." *American Journal of Surgery* 120 (1970):330.

Halstead, W.S. "The Employment of Fine Silk Sutures in Preference to Catgut and the Advantages of Transfixing Tissues and Vessels in Controlling Hemorrhage." *Journal of the American Medical Association* 60 (1913):1119.

Lupinetti, F.M., Stoney, W., Alford, W., Burrus, G., Glassford, D., Petracek, M., and Thomas, C. "Cryoprecipitate-Topical Thrombin Glue. Initial Experience in Patients Undergoing Cardiac Operations. *Therapeutic Cardiovascular Surgery* 90 (1985):502.

Matras, H. "Fibrin Seal: The State of the Art." *Journal of Oral and Maxillofacial Surgery* 43 (1985): 605.

Pilnick, S., and Steichen, F. "The Use of the Hemostatic Scalpel in Operations of the Breast." *Surgery, Gynecology, and Obstetrics* 162 (1986):589.

Rudkowski, W.J. *Disorders of Hemostasis in Surgery*. London, England: University Press, 1977.

Sawyer, P.N., and Wesolowski, A.A. "Electrical Hemostasis." *Annals of the New York Academy of Science* 115 (1964):455.

Ulin, A.W., and Gollub, S.S. *Surgical Bleeding*. New York: McGraw-Hill Book Co., 1966.

Abnormal Hemostasis

Allain, J.P. "Dose Requirements for Replacement Therapy in Hemophilia A." *Thrombosis and Haemostasis* 42 (1979):825.

Caen, J.P., Castaldi, P., Leclerc, J., Inceman, S., Larrieu, M., Probst, M., and Bernard, J. "Congenital Bleeding Disorders With Long Bleeding Times and Normal Platelet Counts: 1. Glanzman's Thrombasthenia." *American Journal of Medicine* 41 (1966):4.

Deykin, D. "Regulation of Heparin Therapy." *New England Journal of Medicine* 287 (1972):355.

Donaldson, G.W., Davies, S., Darg, A., and Richmond, J. "Coagulation Factors in Chronic Liver Disease." *Journal of Clinical Pathology* 22 (1969):199.

Kelly, D.A., and Tuddenham, E. "Hemostatic Problems in Liver Disease." *Gut* 27 (1987):339.

Kitchens, C.S. "Surgery in Hemophilia and Related Disorders. A Prospective Study of 100 Consecutive Procedures." *Medicine* 65 (1986):34.

Rappaport, S.I. "Genetic Clotting Factor Disorders." In *Introduction to Hematology*, edited by S.I. Rappaport, 345–55. New York: Harper & Row, 1971.

Ratnoff, O.D. "Disorders of Hemostasis in Hepatic Diseases." In *Diseases of the Liver*, edited by L. Schiff, 147–54. Philadelphia: J.B. Lippincott, 1969.

Rizza, C.R. "The Treatment of Hereditary and Acquired Bleeding Disorders." In *Hemostasis and Thrombosis*, edited by E.J. Bowie and A.A. Sharp, 259. London, England: Butterworth, 1985.

Rudowski, W. "Major Surgery in Hemophiliacs." *Annual Review of the College of Surgeons of England* 63 (1981):111.

Sharp, A.A. "Disorders and Treatment of Disseminated Intravascular Clotting." *British Medical Bulletin* 33 (1977):265.

Smith, W.W. "Bleeding Disorders in Surgical Patients." *Monographs in the Surgical Sciences* 1 (1964):3.

Sutor, A., Bowie, E., and Owen, C. "Effect of Aspirin, Sodium Salicylate and Acetominophen on Bleeding." *Mayo Clinic Proceedings* 46 (1972):178.

Abnormal Surgical Bleeding

Ampel, L.L., Marshal, S., and Caprini, J. "Etiology, Diagnosis and Treatment of Recovery Room Bleeding." *Heart Lung* 14 (1985):556.

Aster, R.H., chairman. *Platelet Transfusion Therapy*. Consensus Development Conference Statement. Washington, D.C.: National Institutes of Health, 1986.

Didisheim, P. "Screening Tests for Bleeding Disorders." *American Journal of Clinical Pathology* 47 (1967):622.

Harker, L.A., and Slichter, S. "The Bleeding Time As a Screening Test for Evaluation of Platelet Function." *New England Journal of Medicine* 287 (1972):155.

Harrigan, C., Lucas, C., Ledgerwood, A., Walz, D., and Mammen, E. "Serial Changes in Primary Hemostasis After Massive Transfusion." *Surgery* 98 (1985):836.

Jim, R.T.S. "A Study of the Plasma Thrombin Time." *Journal of Laboratory and Clinical Medicine* 50 (1952):45.

Levine, P.H. "Emergency Search for a Bleeding Diathesis." *Archives of Internal Medicine* 130 (1972):445.

Martin, D.J., Lucas, C., Ledgerwood, A., Hoschner, J., McGonnigal, M., and Grabow, D. "Fresh Frozen Plasma Supplement to Massive Red Blood Cell Transfusion." *Annals of Surgery* 202 (1985):505.

Morrison, F.S. "Hemorrhagic Complications in Surgery." In *Complications in Surgery and Their Management*, edited by J. Hardy, 56. Philadelphia: W.B. Saunders, 1981.

Nye, S., Graham, J., and Brinkhaus, K. "The Partial Thromboplastin Time As a Screening Test for Detection of Latent Bleeders." *American Journal of the Medical Sciences* 243 (1962):279.

Quick, A.J. "Clinical Interpretation of One-Stage Prothrombin Time." *Circulation* 24 (1961):1422.

Yardumian, D.A., Mackie, I., and Mackin, S. "Laboratory Investigation of Platelet Function: A Review of Methodology." *Journal of Clinical Pathology* 39 (1986):701.

Chapter 17

Surgical Patients with Respiratory Disease: Preventing Acute Respiratory Failure

Virginia Schwend, R.N., B.S.N.

INTRODUCTION

A tour through the PACU on any given day will show numerous examples of minor respiratory "emergencies." PACU nurses routinely meet these events: repositioning airways, inserting artifical airways, suctioning pulmonary secretions, and encouraging deep breathing or coughing. At any time, however, if the knowledge, diligence, and quick intervention of the postanesthesia nurse were lacking, the smallest complication could lead to a crisis.

This chapter focuses on patients with preexisting lung disease who, even prior to surgery, carry the risk of acute respiratory failure. For these patients especially, there is little margin for error in the diagnosis of acute respiratory failure (ARF).

A definitive diagnosis of ARF is determined by arterial blood gas analysis (ABGs) and has arbitrarily been set at a PaO_2 value less than 60 mm Hg, a percent O_2 saturation of less than 80 mm Hg, with or without the presence of hypercarbia ($Paco_2$ over 45 mm Hg).

Because acute respiratory failure occurs so readily in patients with preexisting lung disease, nursing care is directed at the *prevention* of ARF, especially in the PACU.

The prevention of ARF requires that the PACU nurse:

- understand the *settings* in which acute respiratory failure is most likely to occur in the PACU

- recognize the *nonspecific* signs and symptoms that are early indicators of impending respiratory failure
- be inquisitive enough to draw arterial blood gases when the question of respiratory failure is first introduced
- understand the preventive nursing and medical measures in ARF
- understand the patient's underlying disease process and its complications
- create and implement a care plan based on the patient's preexisting disease and postanesthesia respiratory complications

THE SETTINGS OF ACUTE RESPIRATORY FAILURE

Intraoperative Settings

The postanesthesia period carries the potential for creating acute respiratory failure in even the healthiest of patients.

Adverse Respiratory Effects

Anesthesia has many adverse respiratory effects. The most notable are hypoxia, reduced functional residual capacity, hypercarbia, increased closing volumes, disturbances in ventilation/perfusion relationships, and shunts.

Postoperative hypoxia depends on the length of time the patient undergoes anesthesia. Unlike awake patients, anesthetized individuals have a decreased ventilatory response to carbon dioxide in the presence of hypoxia. This especially occurs with halothane (Fluothane), thiopental (Pentothal), and pentobarbital (Nembutal) and, to a lesser extent, with ketamine.

General anesthesia is associated with reduced alveolar ventilation of oxygen. During spontaneous ventilation, increased anesthetic depths with any agent other than diethyl ether will cause increased alveolar carbon dioxide levels. This will decrease alveolar oxygen, and any previous FIO_2 may be inadequate. During anesthesia, an FIO_2 of at least 30 percent should be maintained to prevent hypoxia.

Due to an unknown mechanism during anesthesia, the functional residual capacity (FRC) also decreases. FRC refers to the amount of air in the lungs at the end of expiration. When the FRC falls, there will be less supportive air in the lungs, and at the end of expiration more airways will collapse, leading to less oxygen exchange. FRC is also reduced with age, obesity, and pregnancy and, most important, with a supine patient position. Sitting the patient upright will significantly increase the FRC, preventing atelectasis and hypoxia.

Anesthesia also increases closing volume. Closing volume refers to the amount of air volume left in the lungs when the airways close on exhalation. Patients with COPD have premature airway closure on exhalation, thereby trapping excess air, which increases their closing volume. Under anesthetic effects, when closing volumes rise and the functional residual lowers, the net result is areas of the lung that stay closed during part or all of the inspiration. This prevents good ventilatory exchange and leads to absorption atelectasis, whereby oxygen continues to be extracted from obstructed alveoli until they collapse.

Ventilation/perfusion abnormalities and shunt can also occur with anesthesia. When areas of the lung are not ventilated, there is less area for gas exchange and hypoxia results. Normally, due to local pulmonary vasoconstriction in the presence of hypoxia, blood is diverted from underventilated areas to areas of good ventilation. However, under anesthesia, this vasoconstriction response to hypoxia is inhibited; blood continues to flow past both underventilated areas, creating a ventilation (V)-to-perfusion (Q) mismatch, or flow past totally obstructed areas, creating a true shunt. A shunt indicates that venous blood from the right heart is moving past underventilated alveoli and back to the left heart and the general circulation. On the other hand, an unexplained increase in alveolar dead space also occurs under anesthesia, representing well-ventilated alveoli that unfortunately are underperfused.

Other intraoperative factors that may cause hypoxia or hypercarbia include:

- intubation of one mainstem bronchus
- aspiration of foreign material
- pulmonary edema—fluid overload, hypersensitivity reaction to drugs or blood products
- pulmonary emboli—blood clots, multiple transfusions, air, fat
- bronchospasms
- pneumothorax—placement of deep vein lines, high positive airway pressures, needle puncture during paravertebral block
- pulmonary collapse (rare)—absorptive atelectasis due to obstruction, altered alveolar airway surface tension
- airway obstruction—usually soft tissue of upper airway.

Hypercapnea

Hypercapnea occurs as a result of central depression of ventilation. The effects of inhalants are a lessened ventilatory drive in the presence of pCO_2 and rapid, shallow breathing. There is also an unexplained increase in alveolar dead space. Thus, along with shallower tidal volumes, the net effect is a reduced amount of functional air reaching the lungs, meaning less alveolar ventilation, and gas exchange occurs. As explained earlier, V/Q mismatches and shunts due to atelectasis allow more mixed venous blood to return unchanged back to the left side of the heart for circulation.

These effects are modified by various factors. Surgical stimulation and metabolic acidosis will increase ventilation. Narcotics will decrease the rate of breathing, but they have less of an effect on tidal volume. Many factors will contribute to increased pCO_2, including increased FIO_2, metabolic alkalosis, obesity, kyphoscoliosis, central nervous system disease, chronic lung diseases, muscle relaxants, neuromuscular diseases, flail chest, trauma to diaphragm, increased airway resistance, and decreased lung compliance.

Patients with preexisting lung disease may elect to have spinal or epidural anesthesia. However, there may be adverse respiratory effects associated with such regional anesthesia as well. Under epidural anesthesia, respiratory paralysis is rare, since anesthetic agents do not diffuse as easily in the epidural space as in the cerebrospinal fluid (CSF). The effects of high spinal anesthesia may be respiratory insufficiency and loss of the ability to cough and clear secretions. This usually represents impairment of abdominal muscles (forced exhalation) rather than direct impairment of the diaphragm or intercostals. Since high spinal anesthesia and a higher drug concentration is indicated in upper abdominal procedures, there may be paralysis of the intercostal muscles. High intercostal paralysis (C5–C6) is signaled by a feeling of suffocation and signs of motor and sensory paralysis in the arms. The patient may have suggestive dyspnea because proprioceptive sensations from abdominal and intercostal muscles are lost.

If the spinal anesthetic reaches the phrenic nerve root at C3, the diaphragmatic strength will be affected. The patient will be unable to speak and may lose consciousness. Such an event requires intubation and mechanical ventilation until the paralysis wears off.

Postoperative Settings

Hypoxia, Hypercapnea, and Acidosis

Postoperative hypoxia depends on the length of time spent under anesthesia and on the nature of the operative site. No alteration in anesthetic technique seems to change the incidence of postoperative hypoxia. The closer abdominal or thoracic surgery occurs to the diaphragm, the more severe and prolonged the hypoxia and hypoventilation will be. In various studies it has been found that the mean PaO_2 in lower abdominal procedures falls about 10 mm Hg lower than normal for about 24 hours postsurgery. After upper abdominal surgery, the amount of hypoxia is

Preventing Acute Respiratory Failure 259

greater, lasting 5 to 7 days. Hypoxia is greatest on the third day postoperatively. If a thoracic incision occurred, the fall in Pao_2 lasts anywhere from 10 to 15 days. Also, a doubling of the respiratory rate has been noted; this occurs on the second day after upper abdominal surgery. This compares with only a 10-percent increase in rate after a hernia repair.

Arterial blood continues to show venous admixtures postanesthesia, but whether this is from V/Q mismatches or shunts is uncertain. Postoperatively, functional residual capacity (FRC) continues to be below normal. The primary cause is atelectasis. Atelectasis is due to shallow breathing, immobility, depressed or absent cough reflexes, and altered ciliary clearance of secretions. Several factors raise the diaphragm level and prevent full lung expansion. These include pain, edema, obesity, wound dressings, abdominal binders, distended bowel, and packing. A supine position, as well as age, is a primary reason for a decreased FRC; thus, for the PACU nurse it is important to remember that raising the head of the bed not only increases the depth of breathing but also greatly increases FRC.

In sum, changes seen in pulmonary function testing postoperatively may include the following:

- decreased FRC—diminished with all surgeries but especially with upper abdominal surgery
- decreased TV—decreased TV by approximately 20 percent in upper abdominal surgery for at least 12 days postoperatively
- decreased VC—decreased by about 45 percent
- decreased FEV percent, the amount of air forcibly exhaled by the patient over one second
- decreased sigh rate and volume, in upper abdominal surgery but not in lower abdominal surgery

Factors that contribute to respiratory failure in the postanesthesia period can be divided into four areas, corresponding to the four parameters of the respiratory process:

1. pulmonary ventilation, or the flow of air into and out of the lungs
2. the gas diffusion of O_2 and CO_2 across the pulmonary capillary membrane
3. oxygen and carbon dioxide transportation from body tissues
4. respiratory control mechanisms that regulate respiratory rate, rhythm, and depth

Within each of these areas, the following specific problems and factors contribute to respiratory failure:

1. Problems that affect ventilation

   - obstructive pulmonary diseases
   - neuromuscular disease
   - neuromuscular blockage drugs
   - obesity
   - supine position
   - abdominal or thoracic surgery
   - ascites
   - pregnancy
   - splinting of respirations due to pain
   - pneumothorax
   - loss of chest wall stability
   - old age
   - pleural effusion
   - malnutrition

2. Problems that affect gas diffusion

   - restrictive respiratory disease
   - pulmonary edema
   - Adult Respiratory Distress Syndrome (ARDS)
   - oxygen toxicity
   - loss or impairment of surfactant
   - pulmonary embolus or microembolus
   - fat emboli
   - postcardiopulmonary bypass
   - pancreatitis
   - uremia

3. Problems of gas transport to and from cells

   - hypotensive or hemorrhagic shock
   - myocardial infarct
   - arrhythmias
   - left ventricular failure

- sickle cell anemia
- neurogenic shock
- sepsis
- Disseminated Intravascular Coagulation (DIC)
- cor pulmonale (right-sided heart failure)

4. Factors affecting respiratory control mechanisms

- high spinal or epidural anesthesia
- narcotics and sedatives
- increased intracranial pressure
- uremia

The usual signs and symptoms of ARF arise from the joint presence of hypoxia, acidosis, and hypercarbia. All three factors cause constriction of the arterial pulmonary vasculature, raising resistance to right ventricular ejection. This causes right-sided heart failure, which impairs venous return to the heart and lowers cardiac preload. Severe acidosis causes shifts in potassium from the cells to blood (hyperkalemia), leading to cardiac arrhythmias. Hypoxia causes direct myocardial damage. Acidosis affects the respiratory center and causes tachypnea. The same three factors—hypoxia, acidosis, and hypercarbia—cause cerebral vasodilation and edema, leading to increased intracranial pressure and changes in mentation.

The most common signs of hypoxia are restlessness (the first and most important signal), anxiety, and tachycardias. Other symptoms include headache, drowsiness, confusion, agitation, arrhythmias, pulmonary edema, diaphoresis, coolness, and cyanosis (a late sign, not found with significant blood loss).

Signs of hypercapnea include hypertension, flushing, dulled sensorium, and rapid, shallow respirations. In mild or early respiratory failure, tachycardia and hypertension are present. In severe or late respiratory failure, arrhythmias, bradycardia, and hypotension are present.

It cannot be emphasized enough that, in the PACU, anxiety and restlessness are assumed to be due to respiratory failure unless proven otherwise. The use of sedatives to calm a restless patient without first ruling out respiratory failure is a dangerous practice.

Some of the less common signs of respiratory failure are:

- lethargy
- irritability
- headaches

- paranoia
- confusion
- vagueness
- facetiousness
- jerky motions
- asterixis
- mydriases
- anorexia
- impaired motor function
- impaired judgment

As noted earlier, a definitive diagnosis of ARF is determined by blood gas analysis, in which the determination for ARF has been arbitrarily defined as:

$Pa_{O_2} < 60$ mm Hg % O_2 saturation $< 80\%$ with/without
$Pa_{CO_2} > 50$ mm Hg

When hypoxia is present without a rise in the Pa_{CO_2} level, the condition may be due to an interstitial disease, such as pulmonary fibrosis. In ARDS, the arterial blood gas sample will show an extremely severe hypoxia and a normal or even low level of Pa_{CO_2}, due to the patient's effort to increase minute ventilation.

Hypoxia is a constant feature in ARF. The presence of hypercarbia signals an obstructive process that may be either acute or chronic. If the pH is within normal limits, it can be assumed that the hypercarbia is due to a chronic respiratory disease state and resultant low pH compensated by bicarbonate retention. If however, the pH is acidotic and uncompensated, an acute obstructive process is at work. Any Pa_{CO_2} rise that is 5mm Hg above the baseline Pa_{CO_2} value in a patient with chronic obstruction respiratory disease signifies an acute process superimposed over the chronic abnormality.

It is notable that the treatment of ARF closely follows normal postanesthesia care of the surgical patient.

Oxygenation and Ventilation

Treatment of ARF in the PACU is aimed at improving oxygenation and ventilation, improving cardiac output and the oxygen-carrying capacity of the blood, and decreasing the patient's oxygen requirements.

Oxygenation. Oxygenation is improved by increasing the patient's FIO_2. PEEP should be instituted, if the patient's Pao_2 cannot be maintained at or above 60 mm Hg, with FIO_2 levels about 50.

Ventilation. To improve ventilation, an open airway must be established. Mechanical ventilation (Ambuing or mechanical ventilator) is used to improve the rate or depth of respirations. The action of drugs that depress the central nervous system or affect respiratory muscle function is reversed with Narcan or neostigmine.

Excessive secretions are removed from airways by

- Thinning secretions for easier expectoration through intravenous hydration. Airway drying is prevented through the use of humidified oxygen. The use of saline nebulization is of questionable value.
- Stimulating coughing and deep breathing
- Positioning the patient for drainage of affected areas, which should be percussed to move secretions toward the mainstem bronchi
- Suctioning the patient

To treat atelectasis, the following actions are taken:

- Stimulate patient to deep breathe.
- Set the tidal volume on the mechanical ventilator to about 100 cc above the normal tidal volume (normal tidal volume is about 10 cc × patient weight in kilograms).
- Set the sigh volume on the mechanical ventilator to about one and one-half times the amount of the patient's tidal volume setting. The sigh rate should be six sighs per hour.
- Position the patient as upright as possible. This drops stomach contents and allows the diaphragm to drop lower on inspiration, and allows for freer use of accessory muscles.

Cardiac Output. To improve cardiac output (for efficient distribution of oxygen from the lungs to the tissues), the patient's fluid balance should be normalized. If the venous return is low due to hypovolemia, the proper crystalloids should be infused. If the patient is fluid-overloaded, fluids should be restricted and diuretics given.

The patient's afterload is decreased by reducing systemic vascular resistance (SVR). Pain and anxiety should be treated to increase SVR. Morphine is excellent for reducing afterload. Action should be taken to prevent hyperthermia, which causes peripheral vasoconstriction and increases systemic vascular resistance. The use of systemic vasodilators, such as nitroprusside (Nipride), will reduce heart work and oxygen consumption. (Note: this requires close monitoring of blood pressure; an arterial line is indicated.)

To increase preload, the following guidelines are relevant. If the patient has a Swan-Ganz catheter, the wedge should be about 10–12 mm Hg. A wedge below this level indicates low venous return to the heart or low cardiac preload. If the patient has a CVP line, the normal CVP reading should be about 5–10 mm Hg via pressure lines or 5–15 cm H_2O pressure via a manometer. A low CVP reading indicates low venous return, while a high CVP indicates fluid overload or an obstruction process in the cardiopulmonary vascular system.

To improve cardiac contractility, positive inotropic drugs, such as digitalis, should be used. Acidosis or electrolyte imbalances should be corrected to avoid arrhythmias. An antiarrhythmic drug should be used that is appropriate to the arrhythmia present.

Oxygen-Carrying Capacity. Improvement of the oxygen-carrying capacity of the blood involves oxyhemoglobin, the major method of transporting oxygen to the tissues. Therefore, an adequate hematocrit and normal cardiac output are required to transport oxygen to the cells.

Oxygen Requirements. A decrease in oxygen requirements is the final action required in improving oxygenation and ventilation in the treatment of ARF. In effect, this means reducing the same factors that previously raised oxygen requirements:

- increased work of breathing
- pain
- anxiety
- shivering
- tachycardia
- fever

Other Respiratory Complications

Postanesthesia nursing care also concerns itself with the "prevention" of other respiratory complications arising in the postoperative period, for example:

- aspiration pneumonia
- pulmonary infections
- pulmonary embolism
- microembolisms of lung circulation.

Prevention of aspiration pneumonia is accomplished by positioning the patient in a full side-lying position, with the face directed toward the bed. Suction equipment should be readily available to suction the mouth (not the throat) of the vomiting patient. If nausea and vomiting persist, an antiemetic, that is, hydroxyzinc (Vistaril), promethazine (Phenergan), or prochlorperizine (Compazine), should be given unless further sedation of the patient is contraindicated.

Prevention of pulmonary infections through sterile suctioning techniques and chest physiotherapy is designed to clear the lungs of retained secretions, which are a medium for bacterial growth.

Prevention of pulmonary emboli begins in the PACU. Persons at special risk for pulmonary emboli are anyone over age 40 and, especially, the very elderly or injured. Also at risk are patients with factors that favor venous thrombosis. These factors include stasis, venous injury, an increase in blood coagulability, and disease. Factors that may be present in postanesthesia patients are prolonged bedrest or immobilization, obesity, advanced age, burns, any surgery (but especially on lower extremities, pelvis, abdomen, or thorax), fractures or injuries to legs or pelvis, malignancies, chronic lung disease (cor pulmonale), heart disease, diabetes mellitus, history of thrombus formation or vascular insufficiency, infectious processes, hypovolemia, or sluggish circulation.

Patients in the PACU should be turned and repositioned at least every two hours. If immobilized, they should have passive range of motion done, especially on the lower extremities, where over 75 percent of embolized thrombi originate. The legs of postanesthesia patients should be raised 15 degrees or more in order to improve venous return to the heart from the great veins of the legs. Patients should be kept well-hydrated in order to prevent increased blood viscosity and platelet clumping. Patients with a history of a thromboembolic disorder often have sequential compression boots placed over their lower extremities during operative procedures. This treatment should continue throughout postanesthesia recovery and until the patient is ambulating well.

At least 90 to 95 percent of pulmonary emboli originate in veins of the legs or pelvis and travel through the great veins back to the heart, entering the lungs. Signs and symptoms are severe dyspnea (90 to 95 percent), cough (40 to 70 percent), chest pain (20 to 50 percent), and hemoptysis (10 to 25 percent). The physical exam will show tachypnea, tachycardia, anxiety, rales, hypotension, cyanosis, atrial arrhythmias, diaphoresis, and pedal edema (secondary to right-sided heart failure). Severe cases of right-sided heart failure will show anginal pain, mental confusion, increased jugular venous distension, pulmonary or tricuspid valve insufficiency, and a pulsating liver (indicating a poor prognosis). ABGs will show a decreased po_2 and a lower than normal pco_2 (due to the patient's tachypnea). Treatment concerns itself with the support of vital signs and the prevention of further emboli (see Table 17-1).

Table 17-1 Treatment of Pulmonary Emboli

Treatment	Purpose
Oxygen	To treat hypoxia
Vasopressors	To improve circulating failure
Heparin	To prevent the clot from enlarging; given via IV drip initially, then as oral anticoagulant after four to seven days
Narcotics	For anginal pain and anxiety
Digitalization	To improve right-sided heart failure
IV fluids	To counteract shock
Thrombolytic agents	Urokinase or streptokinase to dissolve the present clot
Embolectomy	Emergency surgical removal of the clot

Prevention of lung microembolization is largely the responsibility of the anesthesiologist and the PACU nurse who hangs blood or blood products. All blood contains microaggregates of cells and cellular debris. Usually when introduced into the veins, no obstruction is caused by the debris until the blood reaches the microcirculation of the lungs, the circulation found around the alveoli. It is here that circulation is obstructed, causing wasted ventilation. The alveoli are being ventilated, but no gas exchange occurs, leading to hypoxemia and pulmonary hypertension.

To treat this, blood units should be hung with micropore filters. Extra fine filters are available to prevent the transfusion of significant amounts of cellular debris.

PULMONARY DISEASES

Classification

Lung diseases can be divided into two major groups: (1) obstructive and (2) restrictive. The specific diseases in each group are shown below.

1. Obstructive lung diseases

    - Chronic obstructive pulmonary disease (COPD), including bronchitis, and emphysema
    - Asthma

- Cystic fibrosis
- Bronchiectasis

2. Restrictive lung diseases

- Fibrotic diseases, including diffuse interstitial pulmonary fibrosis, sarcoidosis, and hypersensitivity pneumonia
- Collagen diseases, including scleroderma, lupus erythmatosis, and rheumatoid arthritis
- Diseases of the pleura, including pneumothorax, pleural effusion, and pleural thickening
- diseases of the thoracic cage, including scoliosis and ankylosing spondylitis
- Neuromuscular diseases, including amyotrophic lateral sclerosis, multiple sclerosis, myasthenia gravis, and Guillain-Barré syndrome

Other pulmonary disorders include pulmonary edema, morbid obesity/Pickwickian syndrome, pulmonary embolic disorders, and anemias (sickle cell diseases).

Obstructive Lung Diseases

Pathophysiology

Obstructive lung diseases are characterized by resistance to airflow into and out of the lung, due to disorders arising (1) inside the lumen of the airway, as with retained secretions; (2) in the airway walls, as with bronchospasms due to bronchiolar smooth muscle contractions, or (3) in the peribronchial regions of the lung, as with tumors compressing on the bronchus.

To visualize the disorders inherent in obstructive lung diseases, it is necessary to review the anatomy of the lower respiratory airways. The trachea bifurcates in the area just behind the angle of Louis (where the manubrium and sternum meet) to become the right and left mainstem bronchi. These in turn become the lobar (secondary) bronchi, which further divide into two to five segmental (tertiary) bronchi. This branching process continues down until the terminal bronchioles. Until this point they are considered the conducting airways. Beyond this point, there is the acinus or functional portion of the airway. In the above conducting zone, air is transported, but there is no gas exchange. The volume of air in this area is about 150 cc (or 1 cc per pound of body weight) and is considered dead space volume. In the area below the terminal bronchioles, there are alveolar outcroppings found in the airway walls where gas exchange can occur. Airways where gas exchange occurs are considered functional. These airways are called the respiratory bronchioles; they lead directly into the alveolar duct, which is an airway completely lined with alveoli. This, in turn, opens into the alveolar atrium, which leads to the alveolus, a collection of alveoli.

As the bronchi branch and become progressively smaller (below 1 mm in diameter), they lose their cartilaginous rings and can collapse. The cartilaginous bronchioles are lined with a pseudostratified ciliated columnar epithelium interspersed with goblet cells. The goblet cells secrete mucus and work in concert with the cilia, which undulate in a coordinated pattern. Ciliary action passes secretions upward through the laryngeal opening. The cilia are very sensitive; for example, smoking can paralyze the cilia temporarily, and chronic infections can destroy cilia permanently.

The more distal bronchioles have fewer goblet cells, which are replaced by special cuboidal cells that are thought to secrete surfactant. Under the mucosal cells are two helical tracts of smooth muscle fibers that cross over each other in opposite directions. Dilation or contraction of these muscles widens or constricts the diameter of the airways. Elastin bands within the bronchiolar walls also contribute to the normal elastic recoil of the lungs commencing on exhalation.

There are about 200 to 600 million alveoli in the normal lung. The acinar area makes up most of the lung. Its volume is about 3000 cc. The entire functional surface area is from 40 to 100 square meters. It is directly related to body length, and the amount of functional surface decreases 5 percent per decade of age.

Chronic Obstructive Pulmonary Disease

Chronic obstructive pulmonary disease (COPD) is a collective term that usually includes the disease states of emphysema and chronic bronchitis. It is common for patients to have varying amounts of both diseases at the same time; and it is difficult for the physician to distinguish just how much of each is present, since dyspnea on exertion is a major feature of both. At times, asthma or bronchiectasis are also present; thus, the term COPD sometimes includes asthma and bronchiectasis as well. For purposes of our discussion, these various diseases are treated separately.

Emphysema. Emphysema is more common in men than women (a ratio of 4:1), with the highest incidence occurring after age 50. It is strongly associated statistically with cigarette smoking. It is currently believed (not proven) that, during smoking, elastolytic enzymes are released in the lung and break down the elastin fibers in the pulmonary parenchyma. It is known that there are rare individuals in the population (less than one in two thousand) who are severely deficient in alpha 1-antitrypsin, a molecule that inhibits elastolytic enzymes. These persons, male or female, easily develop emphysema, whether they smoke or not. Smoking, then, may either inhibit alpha 1-antitrypsin or it may release extra elastolytic enzymes and allow them to operate unchecked. Environmental pollutants have also been implicated in the disease.

The definitive diagnosis of emphysema can be made only at autopsy. Emphysema involves gradual destruction of the acinus. It causes dilation of the airways distal to the terminal bronchioles because of the progressive destruction of alveolar walls due to elastolytic enzymes. As walls are destroyed, the clusters of alveoli merge, and the patient will have increased dead space to fill on inhalation. Loss of gas diffusion area occurs with the loss of alveolar walls and the accompanying destruction of capillaries. Alveolar walls collapse easily without elastic support and trap air on exhalation. The pressure of the trapped air leads to further alveolar dilation, rupture, and destruction.

Collapsed airways also increase airway resistance on exhalation. Emphysemics show severely reduced expiratory flow rates. This increases the work of exhaling. Usually, in the "pure" emphysemic patient, arterial blood gas values are normal at rest. The patient raises minute volume to compensate for the loss of gas exchange area. The "pure" emphysemic patient has even been described as the "pink puffer." However, on exertion, the chronic, severe emphysemic will become exceedingly dyspneic.

There are several types of emphysema. The most common are centrilobular and panlobular. Centrilobular, or centriacinar, emphysema is the type closely associated with smokers and bronchitis. In its milder stages, no apparent dysfunction is found. It involves enlargement of the proximal portions of the acinus, the terminal bronchioles, and the respiratory bronchioles. The damaged areas occur most often in the upper lobes and superior segments of the lower lobes. Dysfunction becomes apparent usually at about 40 to 50 years of age. As the disease progresses, the areas of disorder spread downwards.

Panlobular, or panacinar, emphysema involves the entire acinus uniformly. It is usually worse in the inferior and anterior portions of the lungs. It is closely associated with familial emphysemics who possess the alpha-1 antitrypsin deficiency. The disorder usually begins to manifest itself by age 40 and often occurs without a cough.

Chronic Bronchitis. The most important feature of chronic bronchitis is excessive mucus production in the bronchial tree. This clinical assessment is subjective; for diagnostic purposes, "excessive" is considered to be expectoration occurring on most days for at least three months in the year for two consecutive years.

Mild forms of chronic bronchitis show no changes on x-ray or in pulmonary function tests. Pathological changes are all related to airway narrowing. These include:

- hypertrophy of mucus-secreting cells (goblet cells) in the large bronchi
- chronic increase in mucus production and excessive amounts of mucus in airways
- occasional mucus plugs
- chronic inflammatory changes in smaller airways, causing edematous narrowing of the airway, cellular infiltration, and loss of cilia (decreased mucociliary clearance)
- excessive granulation tissue, causing airway stenosis
- fibrosis of tissue around the airways
- hypertrophy and hyperreactivity of bronchial smooth muscle

There may also be pulmonary hypertension due to chronic hypoxia (cor pulmonale). Chronic bronchitics have difficulty clearing their airways of mucus and foreign matter, making them an excellent source of bacterial infection. The major features of the disease thus create a vicious cycle.

COPD—Type A and Type B. As noted earlier, COPD is usually a manifestation of two disease entities; rarely do emphysema or chronic bronchitis occur singularly. However, two COPD patients may present with varying combinations of these diseases; hence, there is a wide array of clinical COPD. Yet, two extreme types of COPD can be distinguished: Type A and Type B.

Type A: "The pink puffer." This is characteristic of a man in his mid-50s who has had increasing shortness of breath for about three to four years. A cough may be absent or present and productive of a small amount of white sputum. On physical examination, the patient has a thin cachectic build and a history of weight loss. Chest examination shows an overexpanded chest, quiet breath sounds, and no adventitious sounds, except for late expiratory wheezes. A chest x-ray shows hyperlucent and overexpanded lungs, the cardiac silhouette is narrow and small, there is an increased anteroposterior diameter of the chest (barrel chest), and the diaphragm is flattened. The patient is tachypneic and uses pursed-lip breathing, and the sternocleidomastoid muscles are hypertrophied.

Emphysemics usually maintain normal ABG values by increasing their minute ventilation. With dyspnea, the arterial blood gases show only moderate hypoxia; the Pao_2 is usually greater than 55 mm Hg, and the $Paco_2$ is usually normal. Along with loss of alveolar space, there is loss of capillary space. Blood continues to pass mostly ventilated areas, so there is less of a V/Q (ventilation-to-perfusion) mismatch than expected.

In pulmonary function tests, lung volumes are normal or increased. The increase results when increased dead space must be filled. Because of the obstructive elements, flow rates, especially expiratory flow rates, are markedly decreased. The patient will show no improvement in flow rates with bronchodilators, unlike asthmatics or chronic bronchitics.

Type B: "The blue bloater." The blue bloater shows less dyspnea than the emphysemic patient. There is no generalized destruction of capillaries; therefore, venous-mixed blood passes by unventilated alveoli, creating a right-to-left shunt. About 10 percent of patients have hypoxemia with a Pao_2 of less than 55 mm Hg. This, along with polycythemia (the hematocrit may be as high as 55 percent) and cor pulmonale, gives this disorder its name, blue bloater. The chronic hypoxia and resultant polycythemia cause viscous blood. Together, they cause pulmonary hypertension, which creates an increased workload on the right heart and leads to right-sided heart failure (cor pulmonale). On x-ray, the heart and the pulmonary vessels are enlarged.

Through various tests, blue bloaters are found to have lost dry weight. However, because of cor pulmonale and resultant fluid retention, they may appear to have gained weight.

Auscultation shows early inspiratory crackles and a variety of high- to low-pitched inspiratory and expiratory wheezes. The lower-pitched wheezes can be eliminated through coughing. Bronchitis patients generally have more reactive airways. Bronchodilators will improve smooth muscle constriction.

Hypercapnea ($Paco_2$ more than 45 mm Hg) does occur, but the ensuing respiratory acidosis is compensated by retention of bicarbonate (base) ions by the kidneys. The pH, then, is normal.

The general profile of the COPD patients shows a male city-dweller who is poor and smokes. Two-thirds of COPD cases start at ages 30 to 40 years with a chronic, productive cough, repeated colds, and deep-chest infections, progressing to dyspnea on exertion.

The sequelae of COPD in its severest form include the following:

- enlargement of airspaces distal to the terminal bronchioles and increased dead space
- loss of elastic fibers around airways, causing airway collapse; premature airway closure during exhalation; CO_2 retention; and increased work of breathing
- areas of interstitial and alveolar fibrosis due to chronic pneumonias and decreasing lung compliance and lung volumes, adding to the work of breathing
- capillary and alveolar wall destruction, leading to loss of area for gas exchange
- pulmonary hypertension due to fibrosis-constricted pulmonary vessels and chronic hypoxia

- cor pulmonale (right-sided heart failure) as a result of pulmonary hypertension

A small number of COPD patients have retained large blood levels of carbon dioxide for chronic periods. Over time, respiratory acidosis is compensated by bicarbonate ion retention in the kidneys and blood pH is normal. However, hypoxia has supplanted hypercapnea as the central stimulus to breathe. The administration of supplemental oxygen to these patients may shut off their respiratory drive. The resultant hypoventilation causes CO_2 retention to become "CO_2 narcosis," worsening ventilatory failure and precipitating an arrest. Supplemental oxygen is not contraindicated in these patients when their percent O_2 saturation is less than 80 percent. Low flow rates of oxygen (1–2 liters/minute) via nasal prongs or face mask if tolerated; 24–28 percent oxygen concentrations via Venturi masks should not depress respiration if the Pa_{O_2} is kept about 60 mm Hg. This should ensure a percent O_2 saturation of about 90 percent—enough oxygenation to meet metabolic needs. Adequate treatment of hypoxia will also prevent pulmonary hypertension and its sequelae.

Many COPD patients are on continuous low-flow oxygen therapy at home. However, in the PACU, during supplemental oxygen therapy, the nurse should be cognizant of the risk of respiratory depression. Monitoring arterial blood gases (ABGs) during oxygen therapy is essential to prevent a rise in po_2 to more than 60 mm Hg and resultant respiratory depression. ABGs should also be monitored during mechanical ventilation to prevent respiratory alkalosis and depression of the respiratory drive.

For COPD patients, death may eventually occur from acute respiratory failure, cor pulmonale, pneumonia, bronchitis, pulmonary emboli, or peptic ulcer disease (extreme blood loss).

Anesthesia Considerations in COPD. In the preoperative phase, the anesthesiologist should determine the severity of the disease by a thorough history and examination, pulmonary function tests, and arterial blood gas analysis. If any factors contributing to the disease can be reversed, such as infectious processes, they should be treated first, before the patient goes to surgery.

The presence of dyspnea, cough, sputum production, or decreased exercise tolerance are all indicators of the need for pulmonary function tests. The ratio of FEV (1.0) (forced expiratory volume measured over one second) to vital capacity should be greater than 50 percent, or the patient's ability to cough and clear secretions will be impaired and risk of acute respiratory failure will be increased. It is unusual for carbon dioxide retention to occur until the ratio of FEV (1.0) to vital capacity is less than 35 percent.

If cor pulmonale is present preoperatively, with mean pulmonary artery pressures of more than 20 mm Hg, it will be aggravated by hypoxia. Preoperatively, it should be treated with arterial oxygenation and correction of acidosis. Diuretics and positive ionotropic drugs relieve some of the vascular congestion of cor pulmonale; but the primary defect, pulmonary hypertension, is due to hypoxia and acidemia, which lead to vasoconstriction and the loss of pulmonary capillaries, causing increased pulmonary vascular resistance.

Because infections, evidenced by purulent sputum, contribute to respiratory failure, they should be treated with the appropriate antibiotics. Secretions should be removed by hydration (to thin secretions) and chest physiotherapy. Adequate hydration and the reversal of hypokalemia will help treat muscle weakness, which could impair the work of breathing.

Preoperatively, the patient should be taught pursed-lip breathing. The objective is to control exhalation so that it is slowed and prolonged. The patient should be taught to cough and clear secretions properly. The preoperative goals are to increase expiratory flow rates, decrease sputum production, and lower $Paco_2$ levels to normal or baseline levels. Expiratory wheezes should be diminished or absent.

Regional anesthesia is considered ideal for lower abdominal procedures that do not breach the peritoneum and for procedures that involve the extremities. Regional anesthetic agents should not produce sensory anesthesia about thoracic 6 (T_6), since, at this level or above, the ability of the patient to clear secretions is impaired. If sedatives are needed, they should be carefully titrated so that the patient's minute ventilation remains adequate.

General anesthesia with a volatile agent is also considered safe, since during emergence the body can quickly eliminate the agent through applied hyperventilation. This will minimize any depressant effects postoperatively. Holathane, enflurane, and isoflurane are considered agents of choice. The problem in using nitrous oxide (N_2O) stems from its propensity to expand in enclosed body cavities. In emphysemics, N_2O might expand in the bullae (lung cavities formed by breakdown of bullar walls and a tension pneumothorax). N_2O also limits inspired oxygen concentrations (diffusion hypoxia), which may aggravate the condition of patients with pulmonary hypertension and cause an increase in the right-to-left shunting of pulmonary circulation. High inspired oxygen should be used on emergence.

Narcotics cause respiratory depression, and they have a more prolonged duration of action than volatile gases. Therefore, their risk of causing postoperative depression is higher. They should be used judiciously. Another drawback to narcotic-type anesthesia is that it includes the use of nitrous oxide.

The bronchodilating effects of deep general anesthesia are beneficial to COPD patients with hypertrophy of bronchial smooth muscle and hyperreactive airways.

It should be remembered that the increased work of breathing in obstructive airway diseases requires adequate muscle strength. If possible, long-acting muscle relaxants should not be used. If used, mechanical ventilation should be continued well into the recovery period to permit the patient to be adequately tested for muscle strength prior to extubation.

During long procedures, mechanical ventilation should be used intraoperatively and considered for postoperative use. Larger tidal volumes (10–15 cc/kg) with slow peak inspiratory flow rates will ensure that all functional airspaces are reached. A slower respiratory rate (6–10 breaths/minute) will prevent hyperventilation and dangerous respiratory alkalosis. The slower respiratory rate will also allow increased time between respirations when intrathoracic pressures will be lower and venous return to the heart will be enhanced. Most important, a slower rate will give more time for exhalation. PEEP (positive end expiratory pressure) may aggravate air trapping and is generally contraindicated for patients with bullous diseases, such as emphysema. Peak inspiratory pressures should also be kept low so as not to rupture weakened alveolar walls.

Upon arrival in the PACU, the patient may be intubated for immediate placement on the ventilator until extubation criteria have been met (see above discussion regarding mechanical ventilation). The same ventilator guidelines apply postoperatively as applied intraoperatively (that is, slowed, deep respirations with low peak inspiratory pressures).

Arterial blood gases are closely monitored during the weaning process as minute ventilation is decreased. For patients with chronic carbon dioxide retention, minute ventilation should be adjusted so that the patient does not hyperventilate and raise pH. The patient's Pa_{CO_2} levels should be at preoperative baseline values indicated by a normal pH.

The hypoxic respiratory drive is maintained by keeping arterial oxygen levels at about 60 mm Hg. If this drive is depressed, the resultant hypoventilation may confuse attempts to assess the patient's readiness to be extubated. The weaning goal is to return the patient to baseline ABG levels. Sedatives and narcotics should be very carefully titrated pre- and postextubation to prevent respiratory depression.

Postanesthesia care includes careful observation for signs of respiratory failure in the patient with COPD. The following are signs of respiratory failure in patients with COPD:

1. Altered mentation

    - anxiety and restlessness (early)
    - confusion

- fatigue
- lethargy
- coma

2. Labored breathing

   - gasping inspirations
   - prolonged, forced exhalations
   - asynchrony of thoracic and abdominal muscles
   - use of abdominal muscles during expiration, and even on inspiration
   - use of accessory muscles of the neck
   - intercostal retractions
   - patient struggling to sit upright and forward, with arms held away from body (tripod position)

3. Air trapping

   - relatively immobile chest
   - diminished breath sounds
   - diminished airflow during exhalation
   - tympanic percussion note (rule out possible pneumothorax)

4. Ausculatory findings

   - diminished breath sounds
   - basilar rales early on inspiration
   - scattered high- and low-pitched wheezes, especially on exhalation
   - right ventricular gallop (louder on inspiration: signals right-sided heart failure)

5. Arterial blood gases

   - $Pao_2 < 40$ mm Hg with supplemental oxygen
   - $Paco_2 > 65$ mm Hg and rising
   - pH < 7.25 and falling, signaling acute respiratory failure in the chronic patient

6. Signs of right-sided heart failure

- cyanosis
- increased pulmonary arterial pressures
- decreased cardiac output
- jugular venous distention
- hepatic engorgement
- peripheral edema

7. Dysrhythmias—due to hypercapnea, acidosis hypoxia, and right ventricular engorgement
8. Hypertension (early) or hypotension (late)—due to hypercapnea, acidosis hypoxia, and dysrhythmias

Two conditions in the lungs of COPD patients are reversible: (1) the clearance of excessive secretions (see Table 17-2) and (2) improvement of airway size (see Table 17-3). These objectives, along with treatment of pulmonary hypertension, cor pulmonale (see Table 17-4), and decreasing oxygen demands (see Table 17-5), are the major goals in caring for the patient in the PACU.

Asthma

Asthma is characterized by acute episodes of airway obstruction. Most patients (about 65 percent) develop the disease before the age of five, and it occurs twice as often in males as in females. The obstructions are caused by bronchial smooth muscle constriction, inflammation and edema of the airway mucosa, hypertrophied mucous glands, abnormally thick and tenacious mucus, and infiltrates made up of eosinophils. The sputum may be scant and white, but it may appear purulent when eosinophils are present. The patient may sometimes expectorate sputum with mucus plugs called Curschmann's spirals. Ordinarily, all of these changes are reversible. However, if asthma is frequent and long lasting (hours to days), changes similar to those in emphysema may eventually occur.

Bronchospasms. Bronchospasms are due to increased tone in the circular smooth muscle of the large bronchi or smaller bronchioles. There are two mechanisms of action that create bronchospasms: abnormal neurogenic effects and chemical mediator effects (for example, histamine and SRS-A).

Abnormal Neurogenic Effects. During fight or flight, beta receptors or bronchiolar smooth muscles are stimulated to produce adenylcyclase. This enzyme

Table 17-2 Improvement of Airway Size

Action	Rationale
1. Allow patient to sit upright and even slightly forward.	• Stomach contents fall due to gravity, which allows patient's diaphragm to drop, increasing intrathoracic space during inspiration. • Sitting forward allows for freer use of accessory muscles.
2. Encourage slow, deep, pursed-lip breathing.	• Slower, deep respirations allow all possible lung spaces to be filled and increase diameter of the bronchioles. • Pursed-lip breathing prevents floppy air passages from collapsing or narrowing prematurely on exhalation.
3. Give bronchodilators (parenteral aminophylline, and nebulized (or parenteral) adrenergic agonists).	• This will increase the diameter of bronchioles, especially if an asthmatic component of the disease is present. • Theophylline (Accurbron) will also increase the respiratory drive and improve minute ventilation.
4. Give steroids (IV or aerosol)	• Steroids decrease inflammation around airways. Caution: Patients on chronic steriod use may require increased dosages postoperatively due to the stress of surgery.

converts ATP (adenosine triphosphate) to cAMP (cyclic 3' 5' Adenosine Monophosphate). The intracellular messenger enzyme cAMP is essential for producing dilation of the airway, that is, a favorable response to the fight-or-flight stimulus. A lack of or a defect in adenylcyclase will cause less production of cAMP and less dilation of bronchial smooth muscle. This represents a partial beta-receptor blockade, which manifests itself as hyperirritability of the bronchial tree in response to various stimuli.

Chemical Mediator Effects. Most asthmatics have a genetic predisposition to be sensitized to environmental allergens. When such patients inhale a substance (antigen) to which they are hypersensitive, abnormally high amounts of IgE (immunoglobulin) are produced. These antibodies, bound to mast cells and basophils in the lung interstitium, react to the specific antigen and release both histamine and SRS-A. Histamine causes the mucous membrane to excrete excessive amounts of mucus. Goblet cells then secrete very thick, viscous mucus that is

Table 17-3 Clearing Airways of Excessive Secretions

Action	Rationale
1. Adequately hydrate the patient.	• Intraoperatively, the patient may not have fluid needs met. The endotracheal tube bypasses the normal humidification system of the upper airway, and anesthetic agents have a drying effect on airways. • Adequate IV hydration is very effective in thinning secretions, making it easier for the patient to expel mucoid secretions. • Humidified oxygen should be applied only to prevent further drying of airways.
2. Encourage deep breathing.	• The airways widen on deep inspiration and narrow on expiration, causing a "milking" action that raises secretions up along the airways.
3. Encourage coughing.	• The usual sharp, forceful cough is generally effective only in the larger airways. • The cascade cough is a series of short, multiple coughs, each at a succeedingly lower volume during one exhalation. • The patient should take deep breaths, then cascade the cough until the patient feels there is no air left.
4. Do postural drainage.	• The nurse should auscultate the lungs to search for consolidation or collapse of airways (diminished breath sounds) or the presence of secretions (rales, rhonchi, or wheezes). • The lungs are like a closed jar half-filled with water. In all positions, air in the jar rises to the top, while water settles in the most dependent area. Generally, due to patient intolerance, postsurgical positions in the PACU are limited to supine and sitting, upright supine/flat, or side-lying/flat. • Lung areas to be drained are positioned up, which always helps to increase ventilation to that area.

Table 17-4 Treatment of Pulmonary Hypertension

Action	Rationale
1. Use of supplemental oxygen	• Correction of alveolar hypoxia will reduce pulmonary vasoconstriction and lower pulmonary vascular resistance and pressure.
2. Use of diurectics	• Used cautiously, diuretics will lower preload and right ventricular congestion.
3. Improvement of airway size and secretion clearance	• Improvement of ventilation and the use of supplemental oxygen are the major actions to reduce pulmonary hypertension. • Improved ventilation corrects respiratory acidosis, another cause of vasoconstriction in the lungs.
4. Use of vasodilator drugs	• Vasodilator drugs are of questionable use. Drugs like nifedipine, a calcium channel blocker, may reduce pulmonary artery pressures. Patients should have pulmonary artery pressures monitored during treatment.
5. Use of digitalis	• Digitalis is given to improve myocardial contractility in order to overcome vascular resistance and improve cardiac output. • Digitalis may be contraindicated because it causes dysrhythmias.

difficult to expectorate. Coughing may not be effective in clearing the mucus. SRS-A attaches to specific receptor sites of the smaller bronchi and causes swelling of the smooth muscle and airways there. In addition, SRS-A triggers the release of prostaglandins, which enhances the effects of histamine in the lungs.

At this point, the signs and symptoms are dyspnea, high-pitched wheezes, and coarse rales or rhonchi. As the episode progresses, on inhalation, the narrowed airways will still open slightly to allow for passage of air to the alveoli, but on expiration the swollen air passages will close off prematurely before the acini can empty most of the air. This causes air trapping. When this occurs, the symptoms are a barrel chest, hyperresonance, and a prolonged expiratory phase. Mucus may begin filling the lung bases and inhibit ventilation to large areas. Blood will be shunted to other more ventilated areas of the lungs, but this maneuver still cannot compensate enough. Further hypoxia and respiratory acidosis are the results.

Table 17-5 Decreasing Patient's Oxygen Demands

Action	Rationale
1. Clear airways of secretions and improve airway diameter.	• This will decrease the workload of breathing and decrease the patient's oxygen needs.
2. Treat pain cautiously.	• Pain alone stimulates an increased respiratory rate, which increases the work of breathing.
3. Correct hypothermia.	• Shivering raises the metabolic rate and increases oxygen consumption.
4. Reduce fever.	• Fever raises the metabolic rate and oxygen needs.
5. Calm patient's anxiety.	• Anxiety is another stimulus to hyperventilation, raising O_2 consumption.

The major effects of an asthmatic attack are airway narrowing, increased airway resistance, dyspnea, and wheezing. The results are hyperinflation, gas exchange defects, and increased respiratory work.

Asthma may occur suddenly, but often the asthmatic episode takes days. Some impending signs are "tightness in the chest," increased wheezing, cough, some sputum expectoration, and nocturnal dyspnea. Those with IgE-mediated asthma should have specimens of blood IgE levels drawn. The normal total blood eosinophil count (usually less than $50/mmL^3$) will begin rising. During active asthma, the count may rise above $300/mmL^3$. ABGs are a good clue to the severity of the attack. In the milder stages, initially, the pO_2 and pCO_2 will be normal. At this point, the minute volume will be increased due to mediated reflexes arising from chemical stimuli to sensory receptors in the airway. As the attack progresses, hypoxia will occur first.

The precipitating factors in asthma may be:

- exposure to allergens
- infections
- exercise (especially in cold temperatures)
- aspirin ingestion
- anxiety (not itself a cause but can trigger episodes in persons with the disease)

Treatment. Medication, rather than environmental manipulation, is the primary method of treatment in asthma. The patient can never be fully protected from the environment; there may be more than one environmental factor that is causing the asthmatic attacks. Yet, dietary counseling and immunotherapy (allergy shots) may help prevent food allergies or some allergic reactions to the environment.

It is much easier to prevent than to treat asthma, and the patient is usually on a prophylactic drug regimen. To monitor the benefits of each drug, medications are added to the patient's regimen in a stepwise fashion. Oral theophylline (Accurbron), a bronchodilator, is started first. Levels are monitored both to achieve an adequate therapeutic level and to prevent excessive side effects. The usual serum therapeutic range is 10–20 μg/mL. If theophylline alone is sufficient, oral or inhalant beta-adrenergic agonists—terbutaline (Brethine), isoetharine (Bronkosol), epinephrine (Adrenalin), or metaproterenol (Alupent)—are added to increase the amount of cAMP, which is needed for its bronchodilatory effects. Later, cromolyn (Intal) sodium, which inhibits the allergic response in asthma, or adrenal corticosteroids, which limit inflammatory changes and enhance the production of cAMP, may be added.

It is best not to undertreat. Patients are taught to increase their inhalant medication during exacerbations. If adverse reactions occur, patients are advised not to stop medications, but to inform their physician of the side effects (unless of course the side effects are particularly severe).

Preoperative Assessment. Preoperatively, the history should establish the events that precipitate the attacks, the frequency and severity of the attacks and the medications used to treat the bronchospastic episodes. The patient should be examined for active presence of the disease: rising IgE blood levels, ABG changes, wheezes or rales, and complaints of dyspnea or cough. The patient should be given pulmonary function tests both before and after bronchodilatory therapy. Between episodes of bronchospasms, the patient's lungs are essentially normal, and pulmonary function tests will reflect this. During episodes of bronchospasm, however, the patient will have a prolonged expiratory phase, and the rates of residual volume to total lung capacity will be increased, reflecting air trapping. These symptoms are reversible with bronchodilator therapy, which distinguishes asthma from most other obstructive diseases.

Preoperative Treatment. Preoperatively, bronchodilators not only dilate and open airways but also facilitate drainage of secretions. Adequate systemic hydration will thin secretions making them easier to expectorate. Chest physiotherapy and postural drainage are aimed at clearing the airway of mucus, especially if ambulation is not possible. Decreased mucus in airways will help prevent an infection, which itself is a precipitating factor in the asthmatic episode.

The patient's usual bronchodilator drugs should be continued up until the time of induction of anesthesia. If the history reveals severe or frequent asthmatic events, an aminophylline drip may be started preoperatively and then be continued throughout all phases of surgery and postanesthesia recovery.

Preoperative Medication. There appears to be no preferred regimen of preoperative medications. However, there are cautions to be considered with some commonly used drugs. Anticholinergic medications, such as atropine, may dry secretions excessively, making expectoration more difficult. Morphine, a histamine-releaser, does not usually cause bronchoconstrictions in doses normally ordered preoperatively; but, as a narcotic, it may produce undesired respiratory depression. Codeine is a cough suppressant and should be used cautiously with asthmatics with excessively thick and copious secretions.

Anesthetic Considerations. If it is possible, regional anesthesia should be chosen rather than general anesthesia. Cold humidified gases and an endotracheal tube constitute foreign material in the respiratory tree, and they are powerful bronchoconstricting stimuli. When general anesthesia is necessary, however, the major goal of the anesthesiologist is to totally depress hyperreactive airway reflexes with selected anesthetic agents.

Induction. Thiopental (Pentothal), a short-acting barbiturate, when given alone is insufficient for totally depressing airway reflexes. Ketamine (Ketalar) has sympathomimetic effects that inhibit bronchoconstriction and has been suggested as a good induction agent. Although succinylcholine (Anectine) causes histamine release, there does not appear to be a significant increase in airway resistance with its use.

Once the patient is unconscious, the lungs are ventilated with a volatile agent in order to increase the patient's depth of anesthesia and further depress airway reflexes prior to intubation. Unfortunately, halothane (Fluothane), which has potent bronchodilating effects, can cause cardiac arrhythmias when administered in the presence of a beta-adrenergic agonist or aminophylline. Enflurane (Ethrane) and isoflurane (Forane) do not normally cause arrhythmias; thus, they are more appropriate choices.

Another method of reducing airway resistance is to give lidocaine, 1–2 mg/kg, in an intravenous bolus immediately prior to intubation. Topical administration of lidocaine intratracheally is another method. Although the introduction of cold solution itself may trigger bronchospasms, the anesthesiologist may elect to maintain a lidocaine drip for continuous depression of airway reflexes rather than use volatile anesthetics, which may in any case be contraindicated in a patient with a low cardiac reserve.

Maintenance. As with COPD patients, maintenance should be continued with volatile agents, which can dissipate quickly postoperatively, rather than with narcotics, which may cause continued respiratory depression during recovery. D-tubocurarine causes histamine release sufficient to produce increased airway resistance; therefore, other nondepolarizing neuromuscular blockade drugs—such as pancuronium (Pavulon), metocurine (Metubine), atracurium (Tracrium), or vencuronium (Narcuron)—are preferred.

Mechanical ventilation should provide adequate oxygenation and ventilation during maintenance. In general, PEEP is contraindicated because of its potential for increasing air trapping and lung hyperinflation in patients with narrowed airways. As with COPD patients, in order to distribute ventilation most efficiently, a slower-than-normal inspiratory flow rate is used. Slowed breath rates are used to allow more time for complete passive exhalation, and tidal volumes may be increased somewhat above normal volume in order to guarantee the patient's normal minute ventilation. Humidification of breaths delivered by mechanical ventilation can help prevent excessive drying of mucus in airways due to anesthetic agents.

Note that excessive cold humidification may itself trigger laryngospasms. The warmth of humidified gases is very important in preventing bronchospasms, especially in patients with a history of exercise-induced asthma, in which cold air is an important precipitating factor. However, the best method for thinning secretions is through adequate parenteral hydration with crystalloid fluids.

Another effect of general anesthesia is to reduce hepatic blood flow, which prevents the usual hepatic clearance and deactivation of aminophylline. Intraoperatively, therefore, the therapeutic drip rate of aminophylline should be lowered by one-third to prevent such toxic side effects as arrhythmias, tachycardia, or hypotension.

Emergence. In order to prevent bronchospasms, the endotracheal tube should be removed before the patient emerges from deep anesthesia. Since this is not always advisable, an alternative method is to give lidocaine intravenously to obtund airway reflexes until the patient emerges and criteria to extubate can be fully assessed.

Postoperative Phase. Occasionally, patients with a history of asthma enter the PACU still intubated with airway reflexes obtunded by anesthetic agents and without an aminophylline drip. At this stage, patients without asthmatic-induced airway resistance may be placed on a T-piece or mechanical respiratory support. The lungs of these patients should be continuously monitored for the advent of wheezing and hypoventilation, since bronchospasms can start suddenly as the patient emerges from deep anesthesia. In our PACU we have found that Bronkosol (isoetharine), given via nebulizer at the first sign of wheezing, is usually sufficient to halt bronchospasms. The patient then continues to emerge and is safely extubated without further problems, since the endotracheal tube is no longer present.

Should bronchospasms persist, the most important treatments are aminophylline and corticosteroids. When the patient is awake, impending signs of an asthmatic episode may be a complaint of tightness in the chest, wheezing, coughing, and an increased respiratory rate. Those with IgE-mediated asthma will show a rise in their blood eosinophil count from the normal 50 mmL^3 to above 300 mmL^3 during the active asthmatic attack.

ABGs are a vital clue to the severity of an attack. In the milder states, the po_2 and pco_2 will be normal. The pco_2 may be even lower than normal, since at this stage the patient has increased minute volume. This may be due to vagally mediated reflexes possibly arising from chemical stimuli to sensory receptors in the airways. As the attack progresses, hypoxia occurs first because mixed venous blood continues to flow past obstructed alveoli, although the amount is diminished somewhat due to hypoxic-induced pulmonary vasoconstriction. As areas of obstruction become more numerous due to increased edema, secretions, and mucus plugs, the pCO$_2$ will rise and blood pH will fall.

The following specific signs of an impending asthmatic episode should be considered in the postoperative nursing assessment:

1. Signs of obstruction

   - prolonged expiratory phase (> four seconds)
   - diminished breath sounds
   - faint, high-pitched wheezes
   - thickened sputum/coarse rales
   - intercostal and neck retractions

2. Signs of increased work with breathing

   - rapid shallow breathing
   - use of accessory muscles (neck, shoulders, abdomen)
   - flaring nostrils
   - exercise intolerance/fatigue

3. Signs of overinflation of the lungs

   - widened intercostal spaces
   - low, poorly moving diaphragm
   - decreased lateral expansion of chest
   - hyperresonance to percussion
   - increased lung translucency on chest x-ray

4. Increased thoracic pressures—pulsus paradoxus (a fall in systolic pressure during inspiration), due to depressed cardiac output on inspiration
5. Other cardiovascular changes

    - tachycardia and hypertension (early signs due to anxiety and hypoxia)
    - bradycardia, arrhythmias, and hypotension (late signs due to extreme hypoxia and both respiratory and metabolic acidosis)
    - cyanosis

6. Behavior changes

    - anxiety and restlessness (initially)
    - confusion or panic (later)
    - fatigue (even later), a dangerous sign, indicating that the patient's ability to oxygenate blood is inadequate to meet the oxygen needs demanded by the increased work of breathing

7. Indications of impending respiratory arrest

    - obvious exhaustion
    - decreased level of consciousness, silent chest
    - FEV < 0.5 percent
    - VC < 1 liter (in adults)
    - no bronchodilator response
    - pneumomediastinum (evidence of barotrauma)

As with COPD patients, the goals of treatment are to support the work of breathing, to widen narrowed air passages, and to clear the lungs of secretions. The specific steps and their rationale in the treatment of patients with asthma are listed in Table 17-6.

Restrictive Lung Diseases

Restrictive lung diseases are the second category of chronic lung diseases. Restrictive disorders are those in which the patient has difficulty in expanding the lung, due either to intrinsic lung tissue disorders, as in interstitial fibrosis, or to factors outside the lung tissues, as in kyphoscoliosis or myasthenia gravis. Unlike

Table 17-6 Prophylactic Treatment Measures for the Patient with Asthma

Steps in Nursing Care	Rationale
1. Keep atmosphere calm.	• This decreases the patient's anxiety and oxygenation needs.
2. Give oxygen support.	• The amount of oxygen needed to help the increased work of breathing is based on ABG analysis.
3. Allow patients to position themselves.	• This gives the patient a feeling of control. Indeed, the patient is often the best judge of which position works best. In general, the position should be upright.
4. Give bronchodilators.	• Bronchodilators widen airways. Drugs are the mainstay of therapeutic intervention in asthma. It is best to overmedicate rather than undermedicate during asthmatic episodes.
5. Give corticosteroids.	• Corticosteroids reduce inflammation and edema of airways.
6. Thin retained secretions (follow orders to hydrate patient with IV fluids. The advantages of saline nebulizer treatments are debatable; monitor intake and output accurately); encourage patient to cough.	• Secretions are a major cause of the obstruction. Hyperventilation dries secretions in the airways and leads to significant loss of hydration. Thinned secretions are more easily expectorated, which reduces the work of breathing.
7. Avoid oversedation or overuse of narcotics.	• Although anxiety is present, it is in response to hypoxia, not the cause of the attack. Treatment of severe pain is appropriate for decreasing oxygen needs. Also, if the operative site is near the diaphragm, the patient may hypoventilate due to splinting. However, remember that it is necessary to keep the patient as alert as possible and to avoid respiratory depression.
8. Monitor ABGs.	• ABGs are valuable clues to the patient's status and response to treatment.
9. Monitor FEV, 1.0 percent and vital capacity.	• Obstructions cause a decrease in the percentage of forced expiratory volume. Obstructive disorders like asthma will also decrease the vital capacity.
10. Give chest physical therapy.	• This clears airways of secretions. The nurse should assess the patient's energy levels and ability to ventilate the lungs. Physical therapy should be undertaken only when the patient's po_2 is > 60 mm Hg (see chest physiotherapy method under nursing measures for COPD).

the situation in COPD, the resistance to airflow in the airways is unimpeded. However, mixed restrictive and obstructive diseases can and do occur.

Diffuse Interstitial Pulmonary Fibrosis

The etiology of diffuse interstitial pulmonary fibrosis is unknown. It is uncommon, mostly affecting adults in late middle age. The suspected cause is air immunological reaction to interstitial lung tissue. Initially, inflammation and thickening of the interstitium around the alveolar walls occur. There is infiltration of plasma cells and lymphocytes into the area. Later, fibroblasts appear and lay down thick collagen fibers. This creates the restriction to lung expansion characteristic of the disease. Fibrous tissue reduces the distensibility of the lung, so lung volumes are small. It takes a large inspiratory force to affect normal volumes in patients with the disease. Patients breathe shallowly and rapidly in order to increase their minute volume without greatly increasing the work of breathing.

On exhalation, as the lung recoils, the terminal airways do not collapse, as in COPD; rather, they remain dilated due to retraction of elastic fibers on the terminal airways. The lung takes on a "honey-combed" appearance because of the thick walled and dilated terminal and respiratory bronchioles. On inspiration there is little resistance to airflow, but lung volumes are reduced because of the difficulty in expanding the lungs beyond low volume. There may also be a cellular exudate in the alveoli formed by macrophages and mononuclear cells, called desquamation. The onset of the disease is usually insidious, but there is an acute form called the Hamman-Rich syndrome.

The signs and symptoms of pulmonary fibrosis are dyspnea (especially with exercise); rapid, shallow breathing; irritating, productive cough; cyanosis (worsens with exercise); and finger clubbing (common). Auscultatory findings show diffuse bilateral fine rales, heard especially at the end of inspiration. Chest x-rays show a "ground-glass" haziness, especially at the base of the lungs. Patchy shadows near the diaphragm indicate atelectasis, since shallow breathing means less ventilation to dependent lung areas. Later, the chest x-ray will show the honey-comb appearance described earlier.

Pulmonary hypertension occurs when the pulmonary capillary bed is destroyed by fibrosis and scarring. Local pulmonary hypoxia causes increased vasoconstriction and, eventually, hypertrophy of the pulmonary vascular smooth muscle. This, in turn, leads to cor pulmonale and a decreased cardiac output. Arterial blood gases show hypoxia and a decreased mixed venous oxygen saturation; the peripheral circulation is sluggish and the tissues extract more than the normal amount of oxygen off the red blood cells (cyanosis and clubbing).

Pulmonary function tests reveal that all lung volumes are reduced, but the relative proportions of each correspond to normal lung volume relationships. At any given volume, the lung will show maximum elastic recoil. Increased recoil means that inspiratory volumes are low and exhalation time is shorter, unlike the situation in COPD patients. Because of the reduced vital capacity, patients with diffuse interstitial pulmonary fibrosis have a weaker cough response and often develop frequent respiratory infections. Eventually, they may develop the lung changes seen in patients with COPD.

Treatment and Anesthetic Care

ABGs. In the early stages of restrictive lung disease, hypoxemia is mild at rest and increased with exercise. At later stages, significant hypoxia will be present, even at rest. P_{CO_2} levels will be normal at rest, or even lower than normal if the resting respiratory rate is high. If hypoxia is extreme and chronic, the patient will have an underlying acidosis compensated by bicarbonate retention. Exercise creates a dramatic fall in P_{O_2}, with a milder climb in P_{CO_2}. Cyanosis is clearly visible during exercise.

Earlier, it was believed that ABG disorders are caused by the thicker alveolar walls presenting a barrier to gas diffusion, especially the diffusion of oxygen (since CO_2 diffuses across the normal alveolar capillary membrane 20 times more easily than oxygen). During exercise, the transit time for red blood cells passing the alveoli is quickened, leading to less oxygen binding to the hemoglobin molecule. Newer theories suggest that the problem of gas exchange is due to ventilation/perfusion abnormalities as well. Because of shallower breathing, there is less ventilation to lung bases where the larger amount of lung circulation is found. On the other hand, fibrotic destruction of capillaries creates alveolar dead space (ventilated alveoli with little perfusion).

Preoperatively, the patient should be assessed as to the severity of the restrictive lung disease. Any reversible factors such as infection are treated. The lungs should be well-cleared of secretions, and the patient should be taught deep breathing and coughing techniques. If dyspnea is present, preoperative pulmonary function tests should be done and ABGs drawn. When vital capacity is reduced to below 15 cc kg (normal is 70 cc kg) or the P_{CO_2} is higher than normal at rest, the risk of postoperative complications is high.

In general, restrictive lung diseases do not require a unique choice of agents to be used during anesthesia. However, drugs should be chosen that will not depress respirations in the recovery phase. Controlled ventilation should certainly be used intraoperatively, and it should also be considered postoperatively if the patient demonstrates poor ventilatory ability prior to surgery. The ventilator's peak inspiratory pressures can be expected to be higher than normal (20–30 cm H_2O).

Since the patient's lungs will be poorly compliant, the patient should emerge fully from anesthesia and be assessed for normal extubation criteria prior to the endotracheal tube removal.

Preventing Acute Respiratory Failure   289

Extubation/Postventilation Requirements. In our PACU, the extubation/postventilation requirements are assessed when the patient has been on T-piece or CPAP successfully for at least 20 minutes. For patients with restrictive lung diseases and on mechanical ventilation, the following extubation/postventilation requirements apply:

1. Increased level of consciousness

   - awake and alert
   - responsive to simple commands
   - presence of laryngeal and pharyngeal reflexes

2. Normal arterial blood gases

   - $po_2 > 60$ mm Hg with patient on FIo_2 of 40 percent
   - $pco_2 < 45$ mm Hg
   - pH 7.35–7.45

3. Normal respiratory rate and pattern

   - respiratory rate of 12–24/minute
   - regular pattern of respirations

4. Adequate respiratory volume measurements

   - TV $\geq$ 5 cc kg (normal: 7–20 cc kg)
   - vital capacity $\geq$ 15 cc kg (normal: 70 cc kg, taken by respirometer attached to ET tube)

5. Adequate muscle strength

   - strong, sustained hand grips ($\geq$ 5–7 sec.)
   - lifts head easily
   - opens eyes wide
   - demonstrates negative inspiratory force (IF) > 20 cm H_2O through use of the IF meter attached to ET tube

Postanesthesia Care. Postanesthesia nursing care should include administering O_2, sitting the patient upright as much as possible, encouraging deep breathing often, and assisting the patient to cough. It should be remembered that age, lack of patient effort, pain, residual anesthetic effects and obesity all combine to reduce further lung capacity in patients with restrictive lung disease. The nurse should also be aware of the factors that increase oxygen consumption in these patients.

BIBLIOGRAPHY

Bordow, Richard A., and Moser, Kenneth M. "Chronic Obstructive Pulmonary Disease: Management." In *Manual of Clinical Problems in Pulmonary Medicine*, edited by Richard A. Bordow and Kenneth M. Moser, 199–204. Boston: Little, Brown & Co., 1985.

Glauser, Frederick L. *Signs and Symptoms in Pulmonary Medicine*. Philadelphia: J.B. Lippincott, 1983.

Guenter, Clarance A., and Welch, Martin H. "Obstructive Diseases." In *Pulmonary Medicine*, 2d ed, 664–793. Philadelphia: J.B. Lippincott, 1982.

LoSasso, Alvin M., Gibbs, Phillip S., and Moorthy, M. "Recognition and Management of Respiratory Failure, Restrictive Pulmonary Disease, and Chronic Obstructive Pulmonary Disease." In *Anesthesia and Co-Existing Disease*, edited by Robert K. Stoelting and Stephen F. Dierdorf. New York: Churchill Livingstone, 1983.

Moser, Kenneth M. "Acute Hypercapnic Respiratory Failure." In *Manual of Clinical Problems in Pulmonary Medicine*, edited by Richard A. Bordow and Kenneth M. Moser, 227–231. Boston: Little, Brown & Co., 1985.

Moser, Kenneth M., and Bordow, Richard A. "Chronic Obstructive Pulmonary Diseases: Definition, Epidemiology and Pathology." In *Manual of Clinical Problems in Pulmonary Medicine*, edited by Richard A. Bordow and Kenneth M. Moser, 191–195. Boston: Little, Brown & Co., 1985.

Ramsdell, Joe W. "Asthma: Clinical Presentation and Diagnosis." In *Manual of Clinical Problems in Pulmonary Medicine*, edited by Richard A. Bordow and Kenneth M. Moser, 184. Boston: Little, Brown & Co., 1985.

Ramsdell, Joe W. "Asthma Management." In *Manual of Clinical Problems in Pulmonary Medicine*, edited by Richard A. Bordow and Kenneth M. Moser, 188–191. Boston: Little, Brown & Co., 1985.

Sexton, Dorothy L. *Chronic Obstructive Pulmonary Disease: Care of the Child and Adult*. St. Louis, Mo.: C.V. Mosby, 1981.

Spagnolo, Samuel V., and Medinger, Ann. "Acute Respiratory Failure in the Patient with Chronic Airflow Obstruction." *Handbook of Pulmonary Emergencies*, 151–177. New York: Plenum Publishing Co. 1986.

Traver, Gayle A., ed. *Respiratory Nursing: The Science and the Art*. New York: John Wiley & Sons, 1982.

West, John B. *Pulmonary Pathophysiology: The Essentials*, 2d ed. Baltimore, Md: Williams & Wilkins, 1982.

Wyper, S., "Pulmonary Embolism: Hazard of Immobilization." In *Combating Cardiovascular Diseases Skillfully*, 1978 Nursing Skills Book edited by Helen Hamilton, 133–140. Horsham, Pa.: Intermed Communications, 1978.

Chapter 18

Surgical Patients with Infectious Diseases

Lawrence C. Madoff, M.D.

GENERAL CONSIDERATIONS

Infectious diseases—those caused by bacteria, viruses, fungi, and parasites—are the most common illnesses in humans. Antibiotics, public health measures, and vaccination have made great progress in combating these diseases, but they remain major problems today. In addition, the growing use of immunosuppression to allow organ transplantation has created a new realm of unusual infections. Indeed, the emergence of a new infectious disease, acquired immune deficiency syndrome (AIDS), has become one of the most important public health issues of our era.

In caring for surgical patients, an understanding of infectious diseases is particularly important, for a number of reasons. First, surgery is frequently performed to treat or diagnose an infectious process. Second, infections are the most common complications of surgical procedures. Third, patients with infections can, in some cases, transmit these infections to other patients or to those caring for them. Finally, the hospital environment can expose the patient to additional risk of infection.

CRITICAL ASPECTS OF INFECTIOUS DISEASE

The present discussion centers on three aspects of infectious disease that are of critical importance in the perioperative patient: (1) the care of a patient with a preexisting infection, (2) the etiology and prevention of infections occurring as a result of surgery, and (3) the control and prevention of transmission of infection among patients and hospital personnel.

Patients with Preexisting Infection

It is important to remember that many surgical procedures are performed precisely because the patient has an infection that requires more than antimicrobial therapy. Abscesses, for example, are infections that are walled off from their surroundings by a thick connective-tissue membrane. Antibiotics penetrate very poorly into abscesses; and, except in certain specialized situations, the generally accepted treatment is incision and drainage. The perforation of an abdominal organ—for example, the appendix or gallbladder—results in spillage of gram-negative and anaerobic bacteria into the peritoneal cavity, causing peritonitis. This catastrophe requires surgery in order to correct the underlying defect; antibiotics alone would be unsuccessful in treating this serious infection. Infections of prosthetic devices, such as prosthetic heart valves or joints, often fail to be cured by even prolonged antibiotic therapy and thus require surgical removal.

On other occasions, surgery is performed in order to diagnose an infectious process. Examples are open-lung biopsy in a patient with an unknown pulmonary infection and brain biopsy in a patient with suspected herpes simplex encephalitis.

Whenever surgery is performed on a patient with an infection, the physiological changes caused by infection need to be considered. The most common manifestations of infection are fever and tachycardia. Fever in turn results in increased insensible fluid loss and an increased fluid requirement. Other manifestations of infection are specific to the site of infection. Pneumonia results in impaired gas exchange and may cause hypoxia. Infection in the central nervous system—meningitis, encephalitis, or brain abscess—may result in impaired consciousness, focal neurological defects, or lower seizure threshold.

Many local infections are capable of invading the bloodstream and causing bacterial sepsis. This serious infection induces a number of physiological changes that may be critically important in the immediate postoperative period. Signs of sepsis include fever, shaking chills (rigors), increased respiratory rate, and hypotension. Laboratory findings include elevated white blood cell count with a "left shift" (increased numbers of polymorphonuclear cells and bands) and a respiratory alkalosis with a metabolic acidosis (lowering of both pCO_2 and HCO_3). Bacterial infection of the blood may result in the septic shock syndrome leading to severe, refractory hypotension, anuric renal failure, acute respiratory distress syndrome (ARDS), disseminated intravascular coagulation (DIC), or high-output cardiac failure.

A complete discussion of the pathophysiology and management of septic shock is beyond the scope of this chapter. However, a few points bear mentioning here. It is important in bacterial sepsis to attempt to make an etiological diagnosis. At least two sets of blood cultures should be obtained whenever a blood-borne bacterial infection is suspected. These should be obtained aseptically from a peripheral site (not through an intravascular line), and each should be drawn at least 15 minutes apart. Cultures of any other possible sites of infection—such as urine, sputum, and body cavity drainage—should also be obtained. All cultures should be obtained prior to initiating antibiotic therapy. Obviously, in life-threatening infection antimicrobial therapy must be instituted before the results of cultures are known.

The choice of antibiotics to be used is dictated by a number of factors, including the age and underlying immune status of the host and the suspected site of primary infection. When a skin source is suspected, therapy is directed against the usual skin flora, especially gram-positive bacteria. Thus, a penicillinase-resistant penicillin, such as oxacillin sodium, is often used. When an intraabdominal source is suspected, antibiotic coverage is directed against the bowel flora. Since the bowel contains a diverse pool of organisms, including both gram-negative aerobes and anaerobes as well as some gram positives, two or more antibiotics are often used together. A commonly used regimen in this setting is the use of an aminoglycoside, such as gentamicin (Garamycin) (to cover gram-negative aerobic rods), and an agent active against anaerobes, such as clindamycin (Cleocin), metronidazole (Flagyl), or cefoxitin (Mefoxin).

Supportive management of bacterial sepsis is directed at correcting the physiological aberrations mentioned earlier. The deficit in effective circulating volume is corrected by aggressive fluid and electrolyte replacement. Inotropic agents, such as dopamine (Intropin), and pressors, such as norepinephrine, are used to support the blood pressure and maintain circulation to the brain and kidneys. Endotracheal intubation is continued; and high concentrations of oxygen, along with positive end expiratory pressure (PEEP), is used to overcome the effects of ARDS. Blood products, such as platelets and fresh frozen plasma, are sometimes used to attempt to reduce bleeding caused by DIC.

Infections Occurring As a Result of Surgery

Infections are the most common complications of surgery. Perhaps the most obvious way in which the surgical patient is put at risk of infection is by the disruption of the normal physical barriers to infection. The protective barrier of skin is violated by the surgical incision. Intravenous catheters provide a portal directly from the environment to the bloodstream. Urinary catheters contaminate the normally sterile bladder. Endotracheal tubes allow the oral flora to pass into the lower respiratory tract. The surgery itself (for example, bowel surgery) may allow the normal bowel flora to enter an area, such as the peritoneum, where it becomes pathogenic. The placement of artificial devices, such as permanent venous access catheters or prosthetic joints, sets up an area that is not easily accessible to the body's immune system and therefore can become a nidus of infection.

As discussed in the preceding section, surgery is often performed at a time when a patient has a serious infection, and the disruption of barriers can lead to further spread of infection. In addition, surgery itself is a major stress that may further reduce the body's ability to clear pathogenic organisms. The use of prophylactic antibiotics (discussed later) may, paradoxically, promote infection by altering the host's normal bacterial flora and allowing the overgrowth of pathogens.

Postoperative infections may not become evident until many days after surgery, but steps to prevent them should begin even before surgery. A number of factors increase the risk of postsurgical infection: the length of surgery, emergency surgery, "contaminated" or "dirty" surgery, and underlying immune defect in the host. Some techniques, such as strict asepsis and the use of prophylactic antibiotics, are useful in preventing many types of infection.

Common Postoperative Infections

In the following sections, the most common postoperative infections are described; and some of the factors that contribute to their occurrence, the pathogenic organisms that frequently cause them, and the steps that may be taken to minimize the risk of their occurrence are examined.

Urinary Tract Infection. Urinary tract infection (UTI) is the most common postoperative infection. The most common causative organisms are enteric gram-negative rods, for example, *Escherichia coli*. Undoubtedly, the largest single factor contributing to UTIs in hospitalized patients is the use of in-dwelling bladder catheters. The risk of infection increases with the length of time the catheter is left in place, with a nearly 100-percent risk of infection if the catheter is left in place for two weeks. Strict aseptic technique in insertion and removal of the catheter as soon as feasible will minimize the risk of UTI.

Pneumonia. A number of factors contribute to the development of pulmonary infection in the postoperative period. The placement of an endotracheal tube almost immediately results in contamination of the normally sterile lower respiratory tract by mouth flora. In nonhospitalized patients, the mouth flora consist of gram-positive cocci, such as streptococci, and anaerobic organisms, such as peptostreptococci.

Hospitalized patients and patients who are chronically ill are usually colonized by gram-negative organisms. Abdominal or thoracic surgery impair the patient's ability to cough effectively, and lingering effects of anesthesia may impair consciousness and allow the aspiration of oral or even gastric contents. Minimizing the use of endotracheal intubation and limiting its duration, as well as ensuring that the patient is fully awake before extubation, are important steps in preventing postoperative pneumonia. Aggressive respiratory therapy postoperatively may also decrease the risk of pneumonia.

Bacteremia. Bacteremia can complicate infection at a number of sites, most commonly in the peritoneum, intraabdominal abscesses, wounds, and the lungs or urinary tract or at vascular catheters. Prevention of bacteremia depends on prevention and prompt treatment of the localized infections. Vascular catheter infection can be prevented by careful, aseptic insertion and by frequent (at least every 72 hours) changing of access sites. In one study, it has been suggested that particulate filters may prevent phlebitis related to IV lines.[1] Perhaps this will reduce the incidence of bacteremia from these lines as well.

Central venous access lines are a frequent source of infection. These sites should be carefully monitored for signs of infection, and lines should be removed promptly if redness or exudate appears. Catheter tips should be sent for culture whenever they are removed from a febrile patient.

Intraabdominal Infection. Peritonitis or abdominal abscess may complicate any intraabdominal surgery. This may be due to spillage of bowel contents at the time of surgery or to other complicating factors. Organisms involved are usually gram-negative enteric bacteria, anaerobes, and occasionally enterococci (Group D streptococci). The use of perioperative prophylactic antibiotics (discussed below) may be the most important factor (beyond careful surgical technique) in preventing and promptly treating these infections.

Wound Infection. Many wounds become contaminated, but the development of infection depends on host factors as well. Careful aseptic technique and the use of preoperative antiseptics minimize the risk of these infections, as do prophylactic antibiotics. The usual organisms involved in wound infections are the skin flora, usually gram-positive aerobes like *Staphylococcus aureus* and *streptococci*. Occasionally, the wound may become contaminated with abdominal contents; in such cases, gram-negative organisms play a role. More serious infections of wounds may involve anaerobes, such as clostridium, and can be life threatening. Maintenance of a clean wound with sterile dressings in the immediate postoperative setting is important in the prevention of wound infections.

Transfusion-Related Infection. Blood products may contain a number of potential pathogens, including cytomegalovirus, viral hepatitis (both Type B and Type non-A, non-B), and, in rare cases, bacteria or parasites, such as malaria.

Blood is now routinely screened for hepatitis Type B virus and HIV (the AIDS virus).

Fever

Virtually all patients develop a fever postoperatively. Clearly, however, not all postoperative fever represents infection. Atalectasis, drugs, thromboembolism, and pancreatitis are all common causes of noninfectious postoperative fever. It is only when fever persists for longer than three days or when it recurs after an initial afebrile period that a search for infection should begin.

Prophylaxis

One of the most powerful weapons in the surgeon's armamentarium to prevent postoperative infection is the use of prophylactic antibiotics. "Prophylactic" refers to the fact that these antibiotics are used in the absence of established infection in an effort to prevent infection from occurring. A large number of prospective studies, involving a variety of different surgical procedures, have documented the benefit of antibiotics in the prevention of postoperative sepsis and wound infection.

An antibiotic, often a cephalosporin, is given as a single dose just prior to surgery. A critical factor here is the presence of high levels of antibiotic in the tissue at the time of initial incision. The choice of antibiotic is dictated by the location and type of surgery and the related potential pathogens that cause infection. For example, in orthopedic surgery, *Staphylococcus aureus* and *S. epidermidis* are frequent causes of infection and therefore an antibiotic active against these organisms, such as cefazolin (Ancef) or vancomycin (Vancocin) is most frequently used. In abdominal surgery, where enteric gram-negative and anaerobic bacteria are the likely pathogens, an antibiotic combination, such as clindamycin (Cleocin) and gentamicin (Garamycin), is used. During lengthy operations, it is sometimes necessary to give an additional dose of antibiotics to maintain high levels in tissue.

In "dirty" surgery—for example, surgery for a ruptured viscus or a contaminated laceration—antibiotics are sometimes continued for several days postoperatively. This should not be considered prophylaxis, since it actually represents treatment of a presumptive infection.

A second kind of antimicrobial prophylaxis is bowel decontamination. This is done as a preparation for colorectal surgery where spillage of bowel contents is considered possible. An oral combination of antibiotics—for example, erythromycin and neomycin—is given the day preceding surgery in order to reduce the bacterial load of the large intestine. Studies have not yet determined whether this type of regimen is best used alone or with a parenteral antibiotic combination.

It should be stressed that there is potential hazard in the use of any antimicrobial agent. All antimicrobials carry the risk of adverse reactions, including allergic phenomena. In addition, there is the risk of superinfection with resistant organisms. Enterococci, for example, are resistant to all of the cephalosporins and may cause wound infections or sepsis following surgery. Pseudomembranous colitis, a diarrhea caused by *Clostridium difficile*, has been reported as an occasional complication of nearly every antibiotic in current use. Nor do prophylactic antibiotics compensate for poor surgical technique, improper asepsis, or careless wound management.

In Table 18-1, commonly used regimens currently implemented for surgical prophylaxis are listed.

Controlling the Spread of Infection

Isolation Guidelines

Many infections, as noted above, are endogenous, that is, caused by microorganisms that inhabit the body of the host. Infection results when the relationship between the host and the flora is altered. Other infections are exogenous, resulting from the invasion by a pathogenic organism of a susceptible host. The field of infection control is concerned with the prevention of these exogenous infections. The hospital setting provides an environment in which there is frequent close contact between patients and hospital personnel. In addition, many of the normal barriers to infection have been breached, and a growing number of patients are immunosuppressed, either by disease or by medication designed to allow organ transplantation. Special precautions are necessary to prevent the spread of infection among patients and between patients and health care workers.

The rational use of isolation guidelines requires an understanding of the several mechanisms by which exogenous infections are spread. Contact transmission is the direct person-to-person spread of an infectious agent, for example, the acquisition by a nurse of herpetic whitlow from a herpetic lesion on a patient's lip. In common-vehicle-spread infection, an inanimate object—food, water, blood products, or equipment—becomes contaminated and capable of spreading infection to a number of susceptible hosts. An outbreak of salmonellosis from a hospital cafeteria is an example of this type of transmission. In airborne transmission, the pathogenic agent is spread through the air from source to recipient. Agents vary in the distance they can be spread, in part depending on the droplet size in which the microorganism is carried. Streptococcal infection is spread by droplets produced by coughing, generally over a short (less than one meter) distance. Varicella and tuberculosis are examples of airborne infection that can occur over a much greater

Table 18-1 Prevention of Wound Infection and Sepsis in Surgical Patients

Nature of Operation	Likely Pathogens	Recommended Drugs	Adult Dosage Before Surgery[a]
Clean			
Cardiovascular			
Prosthetic valve and other open-heart surgery, pacemaker implantation[b]	Staphylococcus epidermidis, S. aureus, Corynebacterium sp., enteric gram-negative bacilli, fungi	Cefazolin or vancomycin[c]	1 gram IV
Arterial reconstructive surgery involving the abdominal aorta, a prosthesis, or a groin incision	S. aureus, S. epidermidis, enteric gram-negative bacilli	Cefazolin or vancomycin[c]	1 gram IM/IV 1 gram IV
Orthopedic			
Total joint replacement, internal fixation of proximal femoral fracture	S. aureus, S. epidermidis	Cefazolin or vancomycin[c]	1 gram IM/IV 1 gram IM/IV
Clean-Contaminated			
Head and neck			
Entering oral cavity or pharynx	S. aureus, streptococci, oral anaerobes	Cefazolin	1 gram IM/IV
Gastroduodenal	Enteric gram-negative gram-positive cocci	High risk or gastric bypass only: cefazolin	1 gram IM/IV
Biliary tract	Enteric gram-negative bacilli, Group D strep, clostridia	High risk only: cefazolin	1 gram IM/IV
Colorectal	Enteric gram-negative bacilli, anaerobic bacteria, Group D streptococci	Oral: neomycin plus erythromycin base	1 gram of each at 1:00 P.M., 2:00 P.M., and 11:00 P.M. the day before the operation[d]

Table 18-1 continued

Nature of Operation	Likely Pathogens	Recommended drugs	Adult Dosage Before Surgery[a]
		Parenteral: cefoxitin or clindamycin plus gentamicin or tobramycin	1 gram IV 600 mg IV 1.5 mg/kg IM/IV
Appendectomy	Enteric gram-negative bacilli, anaerobic bacteria	Cefoxitin	1 gram IM/IV
Vaginal or abdominal hysterectomy	Enteric gram-negative bacilli, anaerobes, Group B and D streptococci	Cefazolin	1 gram IV
Cesarean section	Same as for hysterectomy	High risk only: cefazolin	1 gram IV after cord clamping
Abortion	Same as for hysterectomy	First trimester in patients with pelvic inflammatory disease: aqueous penicillin G	1 million units IV
		Second trimester: cefazolin	1 gram IM/IV
"Dirty" Ruptured viscus	Enteric gram-negative bacilli, anaerobes, Group D streptococci	Clindamycin plus Gentamicin or tobramycin or cefoxitin with/without gentamicin or tobramycin	600 mg IV q6h 1.5 mg/kg q8h IV 1 gram q 4-8h IV 1.5 mg/kg q8h IM/IV
Traumatic wound	S. aureus, Group A strep, clostridia, Pasteurella multocida[e]	Cefazolin	1 gram q8h IM/IV

[a]Parenteral prophylactic antimicrobials for clean and clean-contaminated surgery can be given as a single dose just before the operation. For prolonged operations, additional intraoperative doses should be given q4-8h for the duration of the procedure. For dirty surgery, therapy should usually be continued for 5–10 days.
[b]Prophylaxis not needed for pacemaker implantation in centers with low incidence of infection.
[c]For hospitals in which methicilin-resistant S. aureus and S. epidermidis frequently cause wound infections after these procedures.
[d]After appropriate diet and catharsis (R.L. Nichols, *Principles and Practice of Infectious Diseases*, ed. G.L. Mandell, et al., 2d ed. [New York: John Wiley & Sons, 1985], 1641).
[e]With dog or cat bites.

Source: Reprinted from *The Medical Letter on Drugs and Therapeutics*, Vol. 27, No. 703, p. 108, with permission of The Medical Letter, Inc., © 1985.

distance. Vector-borne transmission implies insect carriage of infection and is less important in hospital infections in this country.

Infection control guidelines are usually decided upon by a hospital infection control committee or hospital epidemiologist. Guidelines are provided by the CDC in its publication *Isolation Techniques for Use in Hospitals.* Nurses in many hospitals, especially critical-care nurses, can institute isolation procedures without a physician's order.

The isolation guidelines presented below are typical of those in many hospitals and are consistent with CDC guidelines. Health care workers should always check with the infection control nurse or hospital epidemiologist concerning the precautions at their particular hospital. It should also be noted that the PACU, like other special care units, represents a special case, in that, in the PACU, private rooms are frequently not available. Thus, modifications of the following guidelines may be necessary in order to accommodate a particular situation. For example, except with certain highly infectious diseases, a cubicle may be substituted for a private room.

Contact Isolation. Contact isolation is designed to prevent the transmission of infections spread primarily by direct contact. Examples of patients in this category are newborns with conjunctival gonococcal disease, *Herpes simplex* virus (HSV), or *Staphylococcus aureus.* Also included in this group are patients with Group A streptococcal infection, staphylococcal pneumonia, disseminated HSV, bacteria that are resistant to multiple antibiotics, pediculosis, scabies, and rubella. In addition, pediatric patients with acute respiratory infections or pharyngitis are often included in this category. Precautions include the use of a private room where available, strict handwashing, masks, gowns (if soiling is likely), and gloves (for direct contact).

Respiratory Isolation. Respiratory isolation is designed to control infections that are spread primarily via airborne transmission. These diseases include measles, *Hemophilus influenza,* epiglottitis, meningitis, pneumonia, meningococcal disease, mumps, and pertussis. Active tuberculosis (where there is chest x-ray or microbiological evidence of active disease) also may be included in this group. Precautions for this group include the use of private room, masks at all times, and strict handwashing, but gloves and gowns are not generally required.

Enteric Precautions. Enteric precautions are used when the patient is infected with one of the enteric pathogens present in stool. These include *Salmonella, Shigella, Campylobacter,* toxigenic *Escherichia coli, Yersinia,* hepatitis A, *Giardia,* amoeba, cryptosporidium, *Clostridium difficile,* and pathogenic vibrios. These agents are spread by the fecal-oral route. Prevention of the spread of the infections requires the use of gowns whenever soiling is likely and the use of gloves whenever there is likely to be contact with contaminated material. Private room and mask are generally not required.

Blood and Body Fluid Precautions. Blood and body fluid precautions are for agents that are present in blood and body fluid but generally are infective only when in contact with blood or mucous membranes of the recipient. These agents include HIV (AIDS virus), hepatitis B virus, and malaria. Patients with non-A, non-B hepatitis, Jakob-Creutzfeld disease, leptospirosis, or primary or secondary syphilis should also be included in this category.

The precautions call for the use of gloves when handling blood or body secretions and the separate disposal of needles (without cutting, bending, or recapping) in a prominently labeled, puncture-proof container. They also call for the cleaning of blood spills with a dilute solution of sodium hypochlorite (5.25-percent diluted 1:10 in water).

Drainage and Secretion Precautions. Drainage and secretion precautions are designed to prevent the spread of purulent drainage material from an infected body site. Precautions include the use of gloves for direct contact with contaminated sites and the use of gowns if soiling is likely. Strict handwashing is emphasized.

Strict Isolation. Strict isolation is a rarely used precaution for certain highly contagious or virulent infections that are spread both by air and by contact. These diseases include Lassa fever (and other viral hemorrhagic fevers), pneumonic plague, smallpox, varicella (chickenpox), and zoster in an immunocompromised host. Strict isolation requires a private room with the door kept closed and masks, gloves, and gowns for all who enter the room.

Reverse Isolation. In contrast to the above types of isolation precautions, reverse isolation is designed to prevent the spread of infection from the environment to an unusually susceptible host. Patients in this category might be neutropenic (deficient in circulating neutrophils), either from disease or treatment, or they might be immunosuppressed, either by disease (for example, AIDS or hypogammaglobulinemia) or by drugs used to prevent transplant rejection or to treat autoimmune disease. Precautions in this category are somewhat controversial—some institutions stress only careful handwashing, whereas other hospitals require strict isolation with laminar airflow rooms, which allow the passage only of highly filtered air.

Infectious Hazards for PACU Personnel

Health care workers are continuously exposed to patients, their secretions, and their excretions, and are therefore at increased risk for acquiring infections. In addition, they are at risk for transmitting infections to their families, other patients, and, in the case of pregnant women, to their patients' fetuses. The isolation precautions described in the preceding section help protect the hospital staff as well as other patients. In this section, infections that are transmissible in the hospital environment and relevant precautions to prevent their acquisition are considered. A list of common infectious diseases encountered by PACU personnel, as well as by other hospital employees, is presented in Table 18-2.

Because of their increased risk of exposure to infectious diseases, health care workers should be especially careful with regard to their vaccination status. Immunization for a number of important infectious diseases are available. PACU staff who have contact with blood (perform phlebotomy, start IVs, and so on) should be immunized against hepatitis B. This currently requires a series of three deltoid injections and is provided by the employee health service in many hospitals. This immunization is greater than 90-percent effective in healthy individuals, lasts for several years, and has been shown not to transmit HIV (AIDS virus). Immunization against influenza is also recommended on an annual basis for all employees with extensive patient contact. Persons with patient contact should be certain that they are immune to measles, rubella, and mumps. If in doubt, immunity can be determined by blood tests, and vaccination against these viral illnesses should be obtained. Health care workers should know their immune status to chickenpox, making them aware of whether or not exposure to patients with chickenpox or zoster is safe. If a nonimmune employee is exposed to chickenpox, the use of varicella-zoster immune globulin (VZIG) should be considered.

Of particular concern to hospital workers is the needlestick injury, which carries with it the risk of exposure to a number of blood-borne infections. Hospital staff who are exposed to a contaminated or unknown needle injury should report such exposure promptly to their employee health department. The hepatitis B status of both the source and the recipient should be determined. If the source is positive for hepatitis B antigen and the recipient is nonimmune, the recipient should receive hyperimmune globulin and a vaccination series against hepatitis B should be initiated. If the source is negative for hepatitis B, some experts would still recommend treatment of the recipient with immune serum globulin in an effort to reduce the risk of non-A, non-B hepatitis. Employees who carry hepatitis B should be counseled and should wear gloves during patient contact.

A related issue that has caused considerable concern, and in some cases panic, involves the patient with the acquired immune deficiency syndrome (AIDS). The high concern is obviously due to the seriousness of this infection, which uniformly results in the death of its victims. Hospital personnel should be reassured that there is negligible risk of acquiring AIDS in the health care setting. The HIV appears to be transmissible only by sexual contact, transfusion of contaminated blood products (which are now routinely screened for antibody to the virus), or by sharing of

Table 18-2 Infectious Diseases Encountered by PACU Personnel and Other Hospital Employees

Infectious Agent	Incubation Period	Period of Communicability	General Precautions	Diagnostic Tests	Vaccines or Prophylaxis
Hepatitis B	6 to 24 weeks	While HBsAg positive	Blood precautions for patients; HBsAg positive personnel are informed, counseled to wear gloves, but not usually removed from work unless chronically ill.	HBsAg = acute or chronic infection or carrier; HBeAg = increased infectivity; anti-HB = immunity; anti-HB = acute, chronic[c] or previous infection	Passive prophylaxis HBIG 0.06 mg/kg body weight for HBsAg-positive needlesticks. Repeat at 1 month if not vaccinated; active prophylaxis hepatitis B vaccine, 20– μg doses at 0, 1, and 6 months
Non-A, non-B hepatitis	3 to 18 weeks	Unknown	Same as for hepatitis B	None available	No therapy, or possibly ISG (0.06 mg/kg body weight) for needlestick injuries
Hepatitis A	2 to 7 weeks	2 to 3 weeks before jaundice until 7 days after onset of jaundice	Stool precautions for patients; good handwashing by employees; remove from work for 7 days after onset of jaundice.	Anti-HAV IgM (acute), IgG (immune)	ISG 0.02 mL/kg
Rubella (German measles)	14 to 21 days	7 days before to 5 days after onset of rash	Employee history is unreliable; respiratory isolation for patients; remove infected	HA to screen HAI (fourfold rise) to diagnose acute disease	Rubella vaccine; women should not conceive for 3 months after vaccination.

Table 18-2 continued

Infectious Agent	Incubation Period	Period of Communicability	General Precautions	Diagnostic Tests	Vaccines or Prophylaxis
			employee from work for period of communicability.		
Rubeola (measles)	Adults 8 to 15 days; from the onset of catarrhal stage to 4 days after onset of rash	5 to 21 days after exposure	Respiratory isolation for patients; employee history is reliable; exposed susceptible employees should be removed from work 5 to 21 days after exposure.	Usually not necessary	Measles vaccine ISG, 0.25 mL/kg, may be helpful for exposed patients and personnel.
Mumps	12 to 26 days	7 days before to 9 days after parotitis	Respiratory isolation for patients; positive history is reliable; if negative may still be immune; employee usually removed from work for period of communicability.	Usually not necessary	Mumps vaccine
Influenza	1 to 3 days	1 day before to 5 days after clinical onset	Respiratory precautions for patients; remove employees from work for period of communicability.	CF and HAI antibody tests available; viral isolation possible	Influenza vaccine is given yearly; amantidine, 100 mg, orally twice a day is effective prophylaxis against influenza A.

Disease	Incubation	Infectious period	Precautions	Diagnosis	Prophylaxis
Varicella-zoster (chickenpox)	Usually 14 to 21 days after exposure	10 to 21 days after exposure	Patients with chickenpox require strict isolation; patients with localized herpes zoster are placed on contact precautions: history of chickenpox is reliable; exposed susceptible employees should not work; infectious employees are removed until lesions dry and crust; employees with localized herpes zoster should cover lesions and not care for high risk patients.	FAMA most sensitive test; false-negative tests occur with CF	VZIG may attenuate or prevent disease, should be given to high-risk patients and considered for personnel.
Herpes simplex (herpatic whitlow)	Variable	Until lesions crust over	Employee history is suggestive; employees should use gloves when caring for infected patients; infected employees should avoid contact with immunosuppressed patients or neonates.	Not helpful; viral culture available	None
Acquired immunodeficiency syndrome	6 months to 2 years	Unknown	Blood, secretion, and excretion precautions are standard; additional precautions	HTLV-III or LAV antibody tests available	None

Table 18-2 continued

Infectious Agent	Incubation Period	Period of Communicability	General Precautions	Diagnostic Tests	Vaccines or Prophylaxis
Tuberculosis	Usual 3 to 5 weeks; range: 2 to 8 weeks	Until 3 consecutive sputa are free of tubercle bacilli or the patient is on adequate therapy for 2 weeks	Evaluate contacts & monitor employees with PPD skin test; respiratory precautions for patients; ventilation UV lights in high risk areas.	Tuberculin skin tests; acid fast smears; cultures	Isoniazid prophylaxis indicated; BCG not recommended depend on the patient's illness.
Meningococcal meningitis	Variable: 1 to 10 days	Variable	Close prolonged exposure required for transmission (mouth-to-mouth resuscitation or prolonged exposure to infected secretions).	Culture on blood or chocolate agar	Rifampin, 600 mg, orally twice a day for 2 days (sulfonamide, if sensitive); vaccine against meningococcal groups A, C, Y, and W135 available
Salmonella, Shigella, Campylobacter	Variable: 1 to 5 days	While organism is present in stool (days to weeks)	Enteric precautions for patients; employees should be removed while symptomatic; employees with salmonella should not have contact with high-risk patients.	Culture on selected agar or broth	Antibiotic treatment for selected or severely ill

Staphylococcus aureus	Variable: 4 to 10 days	During skin infection or as a nasal "disseminator"	Patients placed on contact precautions; infected personnel should be evaluated by employee health service and may be removed from work.	Culture on blood agar	Topical or oral antibiotics are sometimes used to treat carriers
Scabies	Days to weeks	Until mites or eggs are destroyed	Patients should be isolated until treated.	None	Topical lindane as directed. All clothes and bedding should be decontaminated by washing in hot, soapy water.

Note: HBsAG = hepatitis B surface antigen; HBIG = hepatitis B immune globulin; HBeAg = hepatitis B e antigen; anti-HBs = antibody to HBsAg; anti-HBc = antibody to hepatitis B core antigen; ISG = immune serum globulin; HAV = hepatitis A; HAI = hemagglutination inhibition antibody; CF = complement fixation; FAMA-fluorescent antibody membrane antigen; VZIG = varicella zoster immune globulin; HTLV-III = human T cell lymphotropic virus type III; LAV = lymphadenopathy associated virus; PPD = purified protein derivative; BCG = bacille Calmette-Guerin; UV = ultraviolet.

Source: Reprinted from *Annals of Internal Medicine*, Vol. 102, No. 5, pp. 664–665, with permission of American College of Physicians, © 1985.

contaminated needles. Although transmission by accidental needlestick has been reported, it is an extraordinarily rare event. In more than 1,500 health care workers who have sustained needlestick injuries or direct exposure to potentially infectious secretions, only 3 have become HIV seropositive. In contrast, transmission of hepatitis B occurs between 6 and 30 percent of the time. Thus, although appropriate precautions should be taken to prevent the nosocomial transmission of AIDS, patients with this illness deserve the same compassionate care as any other patient.

It has been estimated that between one and three million Americans have been exposed to HIV and are potentially infectious. Those exposed increasingly are found outside the defined risk groups. The most prudent approach would be to assume that all blood is potentially contaminated and should be handled accordingly.

Tuberculosis (TB) is another disease for which health care workers are at risk. Although the incidence of this disease has declined steadily in recent decades, there is still a substantial incidence, especially in the elderly. In addition to the precautions taken with known active diseases, workers should be screened periodically for exposure to TB with skin tests. Certain patients with a new positive PPD skin test, generally those under 35 or with impaired immunity, should take isoniazid daily for one year in order to prevent the development of active disease.

Cytomegalovirus and rubella present special problems to the pregnant woman because of their association with congenital malformations. Women intending to become pregnant should receive rubella vaccination if they are not already immune, and they should delay pregnancy until three months after vaccination. Pregnant women should be aware of their immune status with regard to cytomegalovirus. If not immune, they should avoid contact with patients with known CMV infection or who are at high risk for infection. High-risk groups include immunosuppressed patients and organ transplant recipients.

NOTES

1. Falchuk, K.H., Peterson, L., and McNeil, B.J., "Microparticulate-Induced Phlebitis: Its prevention by In-line filtration." *New England Journal of Medicine* 312, no. 2 (1985):78–82.

BIBLIOGRAPHY

"Antimicrobial Prophylaxis for Surgery." *Medical Letter* 27 (1985):105–108.

Brachman, P. "Transmission and Principles of Control." In *Principles and Practice of Infectious Diseases*, 2d ed. edited by G. Mandell, R.G. Douglas, and J.E. Bennett, 102. New York: John Wiley & Sons, 1985.

Cohn, I., and Bornside, G.H. "Infections." In *Principles of Surgery*, edited by S.I. Schwartz, 14th ed., 165. New York: McGraw-Hill Book Co., 1984.

Centers for Disease Control. *Isolation Techniques for Use in Hospitals*. Washington, D.C.: Author, 1975.

Chodak, G.W., and Plaut, M.E. "Use of Systemic Antibiotics for Prophylaxis in Surgery." *Archives of Surgery* 112 (1977):326–334.

Garner, J.S., and Simmons, B.P. "Isolation Precautions." In *Hospital Infections*, edited by J.V. Bennett and P.S. Brachman, 2d ed., 143–150. Boston: Little, Brown & Co., 1986.

Gleckman, R.A. "Unusual Infections Following Abdominal Surgery." In *Manual of Clinical Problems in Infectious Disease*, edited by N.M. Gantz, R.A. Gleckman, R.B. Brown, and A.L. Esposito, 2d ed., 255–260. Boston: Little, Brown & Co., 1986.

Health and Public Policy Committee, American College of Physicians and the Infectious Diseases Society of America. "Acquired Immunodeficiency Syndrome." *Annals of Internal Medicine* 104 (1986):575–581.

Laurence, J. "Tracking the Transmission of HTLV-III Infection." *Infections in Medicine* (November/December 1986):575–581.

Patterson, W.B., Craven, D.E., Schwartz, D.A., Nardell, E.A., Kasmer, J., and Nobel, J. "Occupational Hazards to Hospital Personnel." *Annals of Internal Medicine* 102 (1982):658–680.

Pitcher, W.D., and Musher, D.M. "Critical Importance of Early Diagnosis and Treatment of Intra-Abdominal Infection." *Archives of Surgery* 117 (1982):382.

Chapter 19

Surgical Patients with Coronary Artery Disease

Mary Ellen Luczun, R.N., M.S.N.

GENERAL CONSIDERATIONS

Twenty years ago, individuals suffering a myocardial infarction at home were likely to die before reaching the hospital. Those who were fortunate enough to obtain medical attention were still in danger of succumbing to undetected lethal arrhythmias.

In recent years, advanced medical technology has brightened this picture considerably. Today, the life expectancy for this segment of the population is considerably increased. Research findings, sophisticated diagnostic techniques, newer drugs, better equipment, CPR, emergency medical services (EMS), and cardiac care units have all contributed to this result. Patients with heart disease now have the benefits of early detection, rapid entry into the health care system, and effective treatment, options that were simply not available in the past.

In light of these advances, it is not uncommon for these patients to require either emergency or elective surgery at some point. PACU nurses can, therefore, expect to be caring for such patients on a regular basis.

PATHOPHYSIOLOGY

The major cause of heart disease appears to be the development of obliterative atherosclerotic lesions within the coronary arteries that serve to narrow or obstruct

---

The author would like to thank Dr. Martin Post, assistant professor of medicine, the New York Hospital–Cornell Medical Center, for his kind assistance in the preparation of this chapter.

these vital vessels.[1] Contributing factors include genetic predisposition, familial history, certain personality traits (Type A), professional stresses, hypertension, deficient diet, and cigarette smoking.

Lack of oxygenated blood supply to the heart produces changes in structure that ultimately interfere with function. Coronary insufficiency, angina pectoris, and myocardial infarction are the consequences of arteriosclerotic heart disease. Angina represents inadequate blood flow to the myocardium or an imbalance between myocardial oxygen supply and demand. Infarction means death of cardiac muscle. Although the pathophysiology of myocardial infarction is only partially understood, the major variables seem to be thrombosis, hemorrhage into an atherosclerotic plaque, and coronary arterial spasm. All of these events will produce further compromise of an already compromised blood flow.

The basic disturbance in function, then, is an imbalance between myocardial oxygen supply and demand. In other words, the oxygen needs or demands of the myocardium may, at times, exceed the blood supply that can be delivered. Exertional angina is a symptom of this imbalance. The normal myocardium is able to maintain a balance at rest and during exercise or stress. Stenosed coronary arteries, in contrast, cannot meet increased demands for oxygen as adequately as they can at rest. When oxygen supply is reduced, ischemia follows. Factors influencing oxygen supply are, therefore, the adequacy of coronary arterial blood flow, myocardial metabolic demands, heart rate, blood pressure (afterload), and the oxygen-carrying capacity of the blood (hemoglobin level).

In addition to those patients with documented coronary artery disease (CAD), there is also a high-risk subgroup: those who have CAD but show no signs of the disease. Patients with a known history of CAD can be managed in the perioperative period; patients with no discernible symptoms, however, pose a special problem. A significant amount of CAD may indeed be present in this high-risk subgroup, and, for this reason, they should be treated as if that were, in fact, the case.

The following are considered to be risk factors associated with CAD:

- genetic factors
- ECG abnormalities
- hypertension
- heavy cigarette smoking
- diabetes
- lipid abnormalities
- sedentary life style

- personal stress
- high-caloric, high-fat diet
- obesity

ANATOMY AND PHYSIOLOGY

Every organ in the body receives its blood supply from the heart. The quality of this blood supply is directly related to the ability of the heart muscle to contract adequately. It is vital, therefore, that the heart receive its own blood supply; this is accomplished during diastole. The coronary arteries perform this function. Both right and left arteries arise from the aortic sinuses of the ascending aorta.

The right coronary artery arises in the right aortic sinus and passes into the coronary sulcus. It then follows the sulcus around to the diaphragmatic surface of the heart. This configuration forms half of a circle or crown around the heart. The left coronary artery arises in the left posterior aortic sinus and divides into the anterior descending and circumflex branches completing the remaining half of the circle (see Figure 19-1).

PREOPERATIVE EVALUATION

The preoperative evaluation, a mandatory procedure for all surgical patients, may well mean the difference between life and death for cardiac patients. These patients may be classified in three categories:

1. those who have not suffered a myocardial infarction
2. those who have previously had a myocardial infarction
3. those who have undergone coronary artery bypass surgery

Of these groups, patients who have not experienced angina or myocardial infarction (the high-risk subgroup) pose the biggest problem in predicting both operative and postoperative outcomes. This is because the absence of such manifestations makes it difficult to assess the extent of preexisting cardiac disease. Thus, individuals presenting with a significant number of risk factors (cigarette smoking, obesity, lipid abnormalities, and so on) warrant very careful assessment indeed.

The risk of perioperative reinfarction for patients who have had myocardial infarctions is about 30 percent for infarctions sustained 0–3 months preoperative-

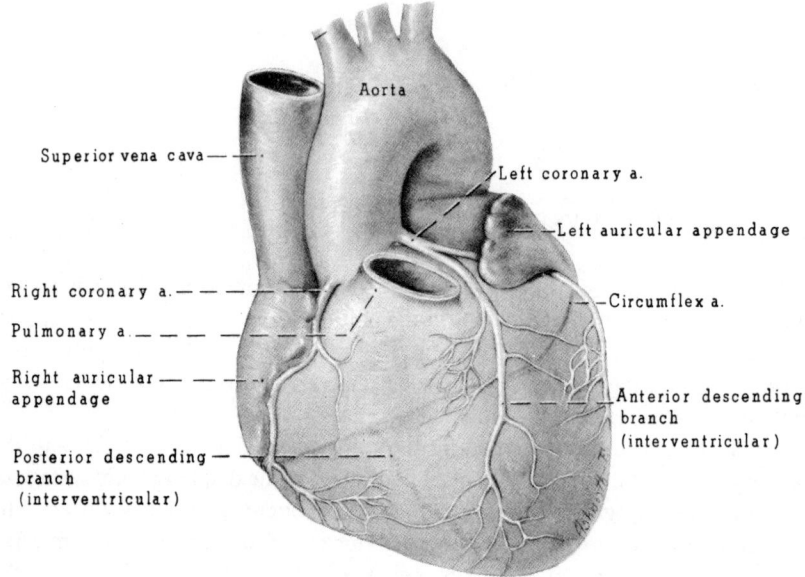

Figure 19-1 Coronary Arteries Supplying the Heart. *Source:* Reprinted from *Structure and Function in Man,* 4th ed., by S.W. Jacob, C.A. Francone, and W.J. Lossow, p. 350, with permission of W.B. Saunders Company, © 1978.

---

ly and about 15 percent for those sustained 3–6 months preoperatively.[2] Some sources believe that mortality from a recurrent myocardial infarction occurring in the perioperative period approaches 50 percent.[3] In any event, surgery and anesthesia place these patients at greater risk of reinfarction, more so in fact than patients who have already suffered repeated myocardial infarctions not complicated by surgery.

Patients who have undergone prior coronary artery bypass surgery appear to be the safest group. Their incidence of reinfarction is near zero.[4] Bypass surgery serves a protective function: It is a safeguard against future myocardial infarctions. Beyond this, the surgery itself represents a previous test of survival. Individuals who did not experience a myocardial infarction following cardiac surgery are not likely to experience one during subsequent perioperative periods. The preoperative assessment parameters for patients with CAD or associated risk factors may be summarized as follows:

1. history of previous myocardial infarction
2. pattern of angina-exertional (stable) versus unstable (angina at rest)

- When does angina occur (associated with exercise and/or stress)?
- Is pain relieved by nitroglycerin?
- How long does the pain last?
- How severe is the pain?
- How frequent are the attacks?
- Does pain occur at rest (unstable angina)?

3. past ECG tracings (resting and with exercise)
4. stress test results
5. signs of congestive heart failure (further evaluation may be indicated)

- orthopnea
- paroxysmal nocturnal dyspnea
- distended jugular veins
- S3 gallop with rales

6. preoperative ECG (all suspicious tracings must be followed up)
7. chest x-ray
8. blood work (in particular, CBC and digoxin and potassium levels)

Other considerations in the preoperative evaluation of patients with CAD include:

- continuation of beta blocker and calcium channel blocking agents
- discontinuance of aspirin therapy two weeks preoperatively
- discontinuance of anticoagulant therapy in time to allow the prothrombin time to approach within 20 percent of the normal value

ANESTHETIC CONSIDERATIONS

The goal of anesthesia is to prevent myocardial ischemia during the surgical procedure. Particular care must be taken to keep hemodynamic changes to a minimum, thereby avoiding an imbalance between myocardial oxygen supply and demand. Myocardial oxygen consumption is affected by myocardial wall tension, heart rate, BP or afterload, and contractility. The object is to manipulate these variables to ensure decreased myocardial oxygen consumption. It must be remembered that, as myocardial oxygen demands increase, diseased coronary arteries may not be able to supply enough blood.

The anesthesiologist uses specific maneuvers to lower left ventricular end diastolic volume. In doing so, wall tension is decreased, and the left ventricle ejects more blood, leaving less behind. The end result is a decrease in myocardial oxygen consumption. Decreasing the heart rate is another vital factor in decreasing myocardial oxygen consumption.

In addition to lowering myocardial oxygen consumption, the anesthesiologist must be attentive to oxygen supply. Again, a decreased heart rate is indicated, allowing for maximal coronary filling. Coronary perfusion is increased by increasing the aortic diastolic pressure while decreasing the left ventricular end-diastolic pressure. This technique ensures optimal perfusion of the coronary arteries and assists in maintaining the balance between supply and demand. Under these circumstances, the incidence of myocardial ischemia is greatly reduced.

Hypotension is best avoided intraoperatively. Low blood pressure means poor coronary perfusion, and this will naturally upset the balance between oxygen supply and demand. In this instance, as in others that threaten to cause myocardial ischemia, the treatment must be aggressive. Specific problems and intervention modalities in the treatment of myocardial ischemia are shown in Table 19-1.

At present, there is no evidence to suggest superiority of regional anesthesia over general anesthesia. Both techniques, however, have inherent disadvantages for patients with CAD. In each case, left ventricular function will dictate the choice of the agent as well as the administration of narcotics.

Table 19-1 Prevention and Treatment of Myocardial Ischemia

Problem	Intervention
1. Tachycardia	• Increase anesthetic agent. • Check for hypovolemia.
2. Increased blood pressure	• Increase anesthetic agent • Give vasodilator, such as nitroprusside (Nipride).
3. Decreased blood pressure	• Give an alpha antagonist, such as phenylephrine (Neo-Synephrine), but only if decreased blood pressure is due to vasodilation.
4. Evidence of ischemia: Increased pulmonary artery pressure Increased pulmonary capillary wedge pressure ST segment depression (late sign)	• Give nitroglycerin. • Decrease fluid intake.

One of the chief advantages of regional anesthesia is in its blockage of both efferent and afferent nerve conduction, thereby suppressing the release of catecholamines. It is also comforting to know that the patient is awake and able to communicate with the anesthesiologist throughout the procedure. Unfortunately, these are probably the only advantages of regional anesthesia. Sympathetic blockade all too often results in hypotension, which can lead to inadequate coronary perfusion, ischemia, and infarction. Increasing IV fluids to counteract this fall in blood pressure is not advisable, especially since fluid overload can occur in the PACU as vascular tone returns.

In the case of general anesthesia, the type will vary depending on left ventricular function. Patients who have CAD may or may not have left ventricular dysfunction; preoperative evaluation will provide this information. This is a crucial assessment parameter in terms of the choice of anesthetic agent.

Patients who have normal left ventricular function can receive most inhalation agents. These agents depress myocardial contractility, thereby decreasing myocardial oxygen consumption, a desirable feature for such patients. Sympathetic stimulation is also decreased, which is another benefit. The only exception to these benefits is in the use of isoflurane (Forane), which appears to "steal" oxygenated blood supply from the diseased portion of the myocardium and deliver it to healthy areas. Isoflurane does this, it seems, by constricting the intima of affected vessels while dilating the normal ones.

Patients with left ventricular dysfunction are not candidates for myocardial depression. Pump integrity cannot be compromised for this group; hence, oxygen requirements must be balanced in other ways.

Intravenous narcotics offer a higher margin of safety. Narcotics in titrated doses provide a stable heart rate, blood pressure, and filling pressure in the absence of major surgical stimuli. They also suppress the release of catecholamines. Fentanyl (Sublimaze), in particular, provides excellent short-term hemodynamic stability, especially during intubation. Should additional anesthesia be required, nitrous oxide is preferable, since it reduces oxygen consumption by the myocardium.

POSTANESTHESIA CARE

Practically speaking, PACU care of patients with CAD is no different than that rendered to other postoperative patients. Yet, though the principles are the same, observation must be intensified. Unlike patients with healthy coronary arteries, patients with CAD cannot adequately tolerate any imbalance between oxygen supply and demand. With such patients, the major goal in the PACU is, therefore, the same as that in the preoperative and intraoperative phases: the prevention of myocardial ischemia. The strategy necessary to achieve this goal is to decrease myocardial oxygen consumption while ensuring an optimal supply of oxygenated blood to the heart.

The combination of impeccable airway assessment and promotion of adequate ventilation combats hypoxemia, a condition that can lead to myocardial ischemia. Patients who have undergone thoracic or high abdominal procedures will require very cautious assessment. Hypoventilation in response to pain is all too common for these individuals, the potential danger being hypoxemia.

If pain is the problem, the intravenous titration of narcotics is indicated. Before beginning titration, however, a state of preexisting hypoxia (a chief cause of restlessness) must be ruled out. The most precise method of titration involves assessment of expiratory pause.[5] This pause occurs at the end of expiration just prior to the next inspiration. The presence of pain will shorten this pause. Small titrated doses of narcotic given at intervals of three to five minutes will produce a gradual lengthening of the expiratory pause. As this happens, the patient will display signs of pain relief.

Adequate pause generally corresponds to a pupil size of 1–2 mm in diameter. In addition to pupil size, however, pain relief is also reflected by patient verbalization of other concerns, such as thirst, the need for an extra blanket, the desire to see family members, and so forth. Dr. Van Poznak regards these concerns as being representative of psychological pain, the type of pain that narcotics cannot alleviate.[6]

At this point, a tranquilizer, such as promethazine (Phenergan), may be indicated—again, in titrated doses. Safe pain control is a must for all patients, but the benefits are particularly desirable for patients with CAD. A calm and comfortable patient is less likely to experience increases in myocardial oxygen demands.

Other assessment parameters include blood pressure, pulse, intake and output, ECG monitoring, and pulmonary artery (PA) and pulmonary capillary wedge pressure (PCWP) measurements (if a Swan-Ganz catheter is in place). In the absence of a Swan-Ganz catheter, a central line should be utilized, and central venous pressure (CVP) should be monitored very closely.

Hypotension may lead to inadequate coronary perfusion, causing myocardial ischemia or infarction. Blood pressure readings below what is considered normal for the patient must be reported and treated promptly.

Postoperative bleeding represents two problems: ischemia and decreased oxygen-carrying capacity of the blood (decreased supply). A return trip to the operating room may be warranted and, if indicated, blood replacement with packed cells (to avoid volume overload) must be ordered. Tachycardia must be carefully assessed, since an increased heart rate increases myocardial oxygen demand while decreasing diastolic time necessary for adequate filling of the coronary arteries. Both oxygen demand and supply are affected by increased heart rates, a situation requiring rapid treatment.

Not all patients with CAD will have a Swan-Ganz catheter. Those undergoing thoracic and high abdominal procedures, however, are prime candidates. A Swan-Ganz catheter affords the earliest possible detection of ischemia and left-sided heart failure, an invaluable adjunct for monitoring these patients. Any increase in pulmonary artery pressure reflects ischemia. Measures to reverse this condition can then be instituted before the situation becomes critical. Similarly, an increase in pulmonary capillary wedge pressure (PCWP) will alert the heart care team to any impending left-sided heart failure.

It should be evident that every possible effort must be made to provide a favorable balance between myocardial oxygen supply and demand. As we have seen, standard PACU protocol contributes substantially to this effort. Surgery and anesthesia are stressful events for all patients. The key concept to bear in mind is that patients with CAD are extremely vulnerable to stress. The increased metabolic demands of tissues following surgical trauma, for instance, causes cardiac output to increase, thereby increasing oxygen demands that lead to ischemia and infarction. Cardiac disease may prevent an increase in cardiac output sufficient to meet those demands, the outcome being congestive heart failure. Postoperative infections also increase oxygen demand.

PACU nurse specialists will be able, as a result of astute observations, to see patients with CAD through the crucial, immediately postoperative hours. Knowledge of oxygen supply and demand will optimize the benefits of basic PACU techniques. For example, keeping these patients comfortable, pain-free, and warm is an excellent way to decrease oxygen demand. Along with hemodynamic monitoring, body temperature must be frequently assessed. Again, an increase in temperature increases heart rate, a situation that will upset the balance between oxygen supply and demand. Finally, strict aseptic technique is the first line of defense in infection prevention. In all these ways, the entire array of elements of PACU nursing will be able to ensure a favorable prognosis for patients with CAD.

NOTES

1. J. Luckman and K. Creason Sorenson, *Medical-Surgical Nursing: A Psychophysiologic Approach*, 2d ed. (Philadelphia: W.B. Saunders, 1980), 839.

2. J.H. Tinker, "Preoperative Assessment of the Adult with Cardiac Disease," in *Manual of Cardiac Anesthesia*, ed. S.J. Thomas (New York: Churchill Livingstone, 1984), 153.

3. W.H. Bellows and L.A. Newberg, "Anesthesia and Cardiac Disease," in *Clinical Anesthesia Procedures of the Massachusetts General Hospital*, ed. P.W. Lebowitz, L.A. Newberg, and M.T. Gillette, 2d ed. (Boston: Little, Brown & Co., 1982), 378.

4. J.H. Tinker, "Preoperative Assessment of the Adult with Cardiac Disease," in *Manual of Cardiac Anesthesia*, ed. S.J. Thomas (New York: Churchill Livingstone, 1984), 153.
5. A. Van Poznak, "The Role of Respiratory Patterns in the Treatment of Pain and Anxiety," in *Postanesthesia Nursing: A Comprehensive Guide*, M.E. Luczun (Rockville, Md: Aspen Publishers, 1984), 66–69.
6. *Ibid.*, p. 67.

BIBLIOGRAPHY

Bellows, W.H. and Newberg, L.A. "Anesthesia and Cardiac Disease." In Lebowitz, P.W., Newberg, L.A., and Gillette, M.T., eds. *Clinical Anesthesia Procedures of the Massachusetts General Hospital*, 376–381. Boston: Little, Brown & Co., 1982.

Carnes, G.D. "Understanding the Cardiac Patient's Behavior." *American Journal of Nursing* (June 1971): 1187.

Foster, E.D. "Risk of Non-Cardiac Operations in Patients with Defined Coronary Disease: The Coronary Artery Surgery Study (CASS) Registry Experience." *Annals of Thoracic Surgery* 41 (January 1986): 42–50.

Friedman, M., and Rosenman, R.H. *Type A Behavior and Your Heart*. Greenwich, Conn.: Fawcett Publishers, 1974.

Froelicher, V.F., and Altwood, J.E. "Interpretation and Use of Tests." *Cardiac Disease: A Logical Approach Considering DRG's*, 25–37, 158. Chicago: Yearbook Publishers, 1986.

Goldman, L., Caldera, D.L., and Nussbaum, S.R. "Multifactorial Index of Cardiac Risk in Noncardiac Surgical Procedures. *New England Journal of Medicine* 297 (1977): 845.

Hillis, L.D., Firth, B.G., and Willerson, J.T. "Non-Cardiac Surgery in Patients with Coronary Artery Disease." *Manual of Clinical Problems in Cardiology*, 2d ed., 360–362. Boston: Little, Brown & Co., 1984.

Jeffery, C.C., Kunsman, J., and Cullen, D.J. "The Usefulness of the Goldman Cardiac Risk Index." *Anesthesiology* 57 (1982): A–443.

Kapriva, C.J., Brown, A.C.D., and Pappas, G. "Hemodynamics during General Anesthesia in Patients Receiving Propranolol." *Anesthesiology* 48 (1978): 28.

Levy, R.S. "Hyperlipidemia: From Trial and Error Toward Scientific Precision." *Consultant* 7 (October 1978): 32.

Mahar, L.J., Steen, P.A., and Tinker, J.H. "Perioperative MI in Patients with Coronary Artery Disease With and Without Aorto-Coronary Artery Bypass Grafts." *Journal of Thoracic Cardiovascular Surgery* 76 (1978): 533.

Mangnano, D.T., Hedgcock, M.L.D., and Wisneski, R.S. "Non-Invasive Prediction of Left Ventricular Dysfunction in Coronary Artery Disase." *Anesthesiology* 57 (1982): A–21.

Oliver, M.F. "Prevention of Coronary Artery Disease—Propaganda, Promises, Problems and Prospects." *Circulation* 73 (January 1986): 1–9.

Steelman, R.B. "About Arteriosclerotic Heart Disease." *Consultant* 18 (June 1978): 143.

Steen, P.A., Tinker, J.H., and Tarkan, S. "MI Reinfarction after Anesthesia and Surgery." *Journal of the American Medical Association* 239 (1978): 2566.

Tarkan, S., Moffitt, E.A., and Taylor, W.F. "MI After General Anesthesia." *Journal of the American Medical Association* 220 (1972): 1451.

Tinker, J.H. "Preoperative Assessment of the Adult with Cardiac Disease." In *Manual of Cardiac Anesthesia*, edited by Stephen J. Thomas, 153. New York: Churchill Livingstone, 1984.

Chapter 20

Quality Nursing Care of Older Adults

Marjorie A. Miller, R.N., M.S.N., A.N.P.

INTRODUCTION

Current publicity about the aging population of the United States (11 percent of the population is over 65 years of age) must give nurses in acute care facilities a sense of déjà vu. Nurses know from personal experience that older adults constitute an increasing proportion of those they care for. They also know that, compared with younger adults, older adults often do not heal as rapidly after surgery or an acute medical illness and are more apt to have complications. The reasons for these differences cannot be stated simply or with complete satisfaction. However, this chapter presents what is known about the physical changes in aging, the implications of these changes for the nursing care of older adults, the areas of concern for the nurse as a result of these changes, and, lastly, some of the subtle influences on nursing care of the older adult.

GENERAL CONCEPTS ABOUT THE AGING PROCESS

Recent research has given us increased knowledge about the process of aging, though much still remains unknown. One important advance has been made: the recognition that the aging process is different from the pathological processes that may affect an older adult. There are certain illnesses to which older adults are prone, just as there are certain illnesses to which young children are prone. That aging is a process separate from the diseases affecting an older person seems simple and obvious, but it is a concept that is still not recognized by much of the population. Nurses in particular must not confuse these two processes; such confusion encourages lack of concern for the minor problems older persons may have—"What can you expect; you're 72 years old and stiff knees aren't so bad"—when, in fact, a more complete medical evaluation might lead to therapy for those "stiff knees." The lack of concern for "minor" problems is particularly apt to occur (understandably) in a busy acute care setting, and nurses must guard against the attitudes that lead to it.

Other facts about the aging process should be kept in mind:

- There is great individuality in how fast one ages. One 78-year-old may look and act much younger than another.
- There is great individuality as to which area of the body is most affected by the aging diminution of function. One 75-year-old may have decreased cardiac reserve, another may have decreased body water reserve, while a third may have neither of these.
- Age 75 seems to be a cut-off point, beyond which many (but not all) persons begin to show the effects of the decrease in function of aging organs.

What conclusions can be drawn at this point for the busy nurse caring for older adults in an acute care setting? The primary conclusion is *not to presume* incompetent physical function on the basis of the *age* of the person. Rather, objective indicators of physiological function should be used as a basis for action. Clear support for the use of such indicators is found in the Baltimore Longitudinal Study of Aging, which shows that, although many older adults do show the normal physical changes of aging, many do not.[1] A detailed listing of these changes is presented in Table 20-1.

Research has also demonstrated that certain basic tissue changes with aging are common to all organs of the body:

- There is a gradual decrease in the number of cells as one ages, for example, nephrons, neurons, liver cells. This contributes to the loss of function of an organ.
- There is a gradual loss of elastic fibers in tissues. Thus, wrinkles appear in the skin, lung compliance decreases, arteries are more rigid.
- There is an increase in rigidity of connective tissue fibers, due to increased cross-linking of collagen fibers (the structural cell of connective tissue). This makes arteries less capable of complying with blood volume changes.

Table 20-1 Normal Physical Changes With Age

1. Cardiovascular system
    Heart
    - Decreased cardiac muscle mass
    - Decreased cardiac output
    - Decreased cardiac reserve

    Arteries
    - Increased fibrosis
    - Decreased elasticity

    Blood
    - Little change in components (hematocrit and biochemical and cell composition)

2. Respiratory system
    - Increased size of alveoli
    - Decreased elasticity
    - Decreased compliance
    - Decreased vital capacity
    - Increased residual volume
    - Decreased respiratory reserve

3. Nervous system
    Brain
    - Slight decrease in size of brain
    - Altered sleep pattern: increased frequency of Stage 1 sleep
    - No change in intelligence
    - Learning speed slower

    Nerves
    - Decreased perception of pain
    - Decreased vibratory perception in feet
    - Slowed reflexes, especially in lower extremities

    Special senses
    - Decreased sense of smell
    - Decreased taste perception
    - Decreased hearing sense, particularly high tones

    Eye
    - Decreased visual acuity (presbyopia)
    - Decreased speed of dark adaptation
    - Slowed accommodation
    - Near convergence of eyes impaired
    - Difficulty in discriminating blue color from green
    - Lens becomes more firm and yellowish
    - Pupils decrease in size
    - Cornea loses luster
    - Decreased tear formation

4. Musculoskeletal system
    Bones
    - Decrease in density
    - Vertebral body collapses, leading to kyphosis

Table 20-1 continued

Joints	• Movement is "stiffer"
Muscles	• Decrease in muscle mass (without use)
General	• Decreased flexibility of movement
	• Decreased arm swing
5. Gastrointestinal system	
Mouth	• Decreased number of tongue papillae
	• Salivary gland secretion is decreased
	• Taste sensation may be decreased
	• Teeth may be missing
Stomach and colon	• Peristalsis is slowed
	• Absorption of nutrients is unchanged (calcium and iron absorption continue to be difficult)
Liver	• Decrease in albumin synthesis rate
6. Kidney	• Glomerular filtration rate decreased
	• Plasma flow decreased
	• Fluid balance affected by decreased muscle mass
	• Decreased fluid reserve
7. Endocrine System	• Triiodothyronine level decreased after 60 years of age
	• TSH and T4 levels and function are normal
	• Ovarian hormones decreased after menopause
	• Testerone secretion decreased slightly
	• BMR decreased slightly
	• Decreased ability to maintain normal body temperature when exposed to extreme heat or cold
8. Immune system	• Decrease in T cell function
	• Ability to form antibodies is maintained if prior immunity established
9. Skin, Hair, Nails	
Skin	• Decreased layer of subcutaneous fat
	• Decreased elasticity of skin and decreased turgor
	• Spotty overgrowth of keratin cells causes "senile keratoses"
	• Decrease in sweat gland secretion
Hair	• Decreased formation of pigment granules in hair follicles, causing gray hair
Nails	• Longitudinal ridges caused by irregular nail formation
10. Psychological Status	• Little change

These tissue changes certainly have a direct bearing on the physical changes with age listed in Table 20-1. With fewer functioning cells the organ obviously is less competent.

AREAS OF CONCERN

The physical changes listed in Table 20-1 have a direct impact on the nursing care of older adults. Several areas of concern have been identified:

- general response to stress
- temperature regulation
- fluid balance
- respiratory function
- medication response
- confusion and agitation
- teaching
- territoriality
- multiple and chronic illnesses

General Response to Stress

The general response to a stressful event is influenced by many of the physical changes of aging. In responding to stress, the individual calls on the competency of many organs—heart, lungs, kidney, endocrine glands, the immune system, and perhaps temperature control centers. If the competency of one or several of these is decreased, the effect of the decrease is directly on the general ability to respond to stress. Figure 20-1 illustrates the effect of age on the ability to survive the stress of being burned. In terms of survival, older adults clearly do less well than younger adults, even at the 10-percent body surface burn level. Nurses, of course, cannot know what the general level of reserve competency is in an older patient; and, as we have seen, one cannot depend on age per se as a guide. Therefore, nurses must be alert to the *possibility* of decreased reserve and to the need for supportive measures. Nurses who are alert to minor changes in physiological functioning can often prevent serious deterioration of the physical status.

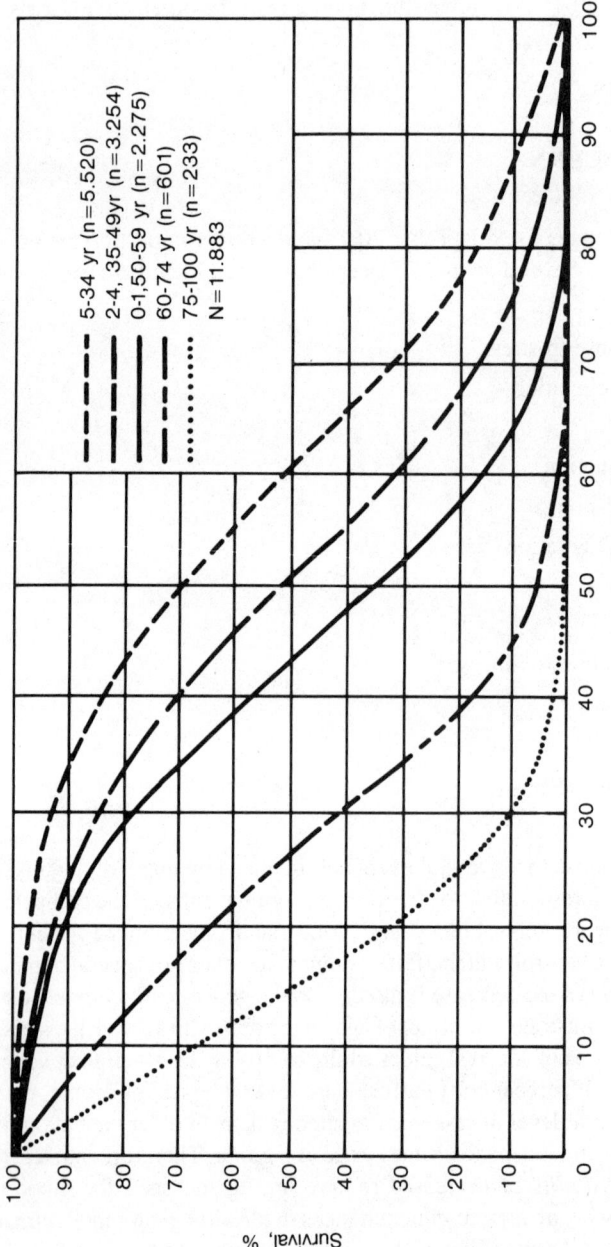

Figure 20-1 Survival of Patients as a Function of Total Percentage of Body Surface Burned and Age. *Source:* Reprinted from *Journal of the American Medical Association*, Vol. 236, p. 1944, with permission of the American Medical Association, © 1976.

Temperature Regulation

Temperature regulation in older adults does not seem to be as efficient as in younger adults. All nurses have had the experience of entering the room of an older adult that seems uncomfortably warm, yet the older person is quite comfortable. It is also known that the older age group is subject to hypothermia. Nurses caring for older adults in the hospital must be sensitive to the ambient temperature of the room and have extra blankets available.

Another aspect of temperature regulation is fever in response to an infection. Medical personnel count on the degree of fever as a signal indicating how serious the infection may be. Again, older adults may not have the elevation of temperature or the white count elevation that younger adults have. In this respect, it is easier to misjudge the severity of illness in older adults unless the nurse is alert, thoughtful, and watchful.

Fluid Balance

Fluid balance is a vital concern in all patients. It is of even more concern in older adults, however, because of the decrease in lean body mass, which decreases the reserve water in the body (see Figure 20-2). The loss of this reserve water makes excessive water loss, such as sweating on a hot day, a hazard for older adults. A

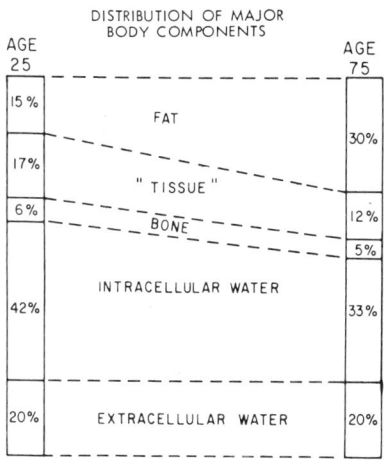

Figure 20-2 Changes in the Distribution of Major Body Components with Age. *Source:* Reprinted with permission from the American Geriatrics Society, "Speculation on Vascular Changes with Age" by R. Goldman, *Journal of the American Geriatrics Society*, Vol. 18, p. 766, © 1970.

similar hazard is involved in lack of water intake (NPO prior to tests). The lack of oral fluid intake must be made up by intravenous fluids.

Potential problems may also arise in a decreased flexibility of the arterial system, in an often-impaired cardiac action, and in decreased renal competency. A less flexible cardiovascular system responds to changing amounts of blood volume with difficulty. The blood pressure is an obvious indication of this difficulty in accommodating to volume changes. It increases when volume is too great and decreases when it is too small. A severe response to fluid increase may be pulmonary edema. Monitoring of intravenous flow rates and amounts will avoid the serious effects of blood volume changes in older adults.

A severe response to decreased volume is failure of urine flow. It should be remembered that adequate urine formation is required to regulate and maintain electrolyte balance.

The subject of intravenous fluid administration should remind the nurse that older adults have a decreased subcutaneous fat layer beneath the skin, as well as a thinner skin layer. As a result, the superficial veins are more obvious, but they have less firm support surrounding them. When one is trying to give IV medications or start an IV, these veins "roll" away from the needle tip. Therefore, it is well to allow extra time for these activities and to be mentally prepared for the extra effort.

Respiratory Function

Aging effects on the respiratory system have a great impact on a patient recovering from an anesthetic. Decreased lung compliance and vital capacity—the increased dead space—as well as the depressant effect of the anesthetic agent on pulmonary ciliary action, make the older adult a prime candidate for pneumonia. To encourage adequate lung ventilation by deep breathing or the use of "blow bottles" requires all of the interpersonal and professional skills of the nurse; and the nurse must be convinced that this procedure is vital for the older patient. A younger patient might be excused with a slightly shortened time for deep breathing; the older adult *must* follow the exact procedure.

Medication Response

Medication prescription and administration for older adults necessitate careful nursing judgment and patient advocacy. Medical personnel are in the habit of writing routine orders that include the usual adult doses for drugs; they often overlook the fact that Mrs. Jones is 68, that Mr. Smith is 75, and therefore the drug dose should be somewhat less than the usual amount. A motto to follow in prescribing for older adults is to "start low and go slow." The usual rule is to give one-half the adult dose to begin with, then increase it by a small amount each day until the optimum dose is reached.

Nurses are familiar with the fact that older adults respond excessively to sedatives and narcotics. They have all had experiences with patients who, after one dose of sleeping medication, slept 10 hours, then were lethargic and drowsy for another 10 or 12 hours. Why does this occur? The reason is that, in the older patient, the glomerular filtration is decreased and the liver function may also be somewhat depressed. These organs, the liver and the kidneys, are the excretory organs for medications; they remove drugs from the bloodstream. Because of aging changes, older adults have difficulty removing drugs from the bloodstream, and the drug effect continues unabated. Toxic symptoms occur with greater frequency in older adults, and nurses must be on the lookout for these.

Advocacy is a significant role of the nurse in regard to medication. Older adults often are taking several medications. The greater the number of different medications, the greater the likelihood of drug interaction and undesirable side effects. Nurses must bring the age of the patient to the attention of the one writing the orders. In such case, they may suggest a lower dose; when the number of drugs is very high, they may suggest that perhaps some could be eliminated. In giving medications, the nurse must use careful judgment as to the amount and frequency and must also assess the effectiveness of the medication. Finally, the nurse must look carefully for side effects (unusual side effects are more common in the elderly), as well as toxic symptoms.

Confusion and Agitation

The confused patient is not unknown to nurses. Acute confusion frequently accompanies high fever, pain, sedation, multiple medications, and the multiple and confusing sights and sounds of a PACU. It is important to distinguish between two types of confusion: (1) acute confusion (delirium) and (2) chronic confusion (dementia). Acute confusion is short-term, lasting only a few days, often for only a part of each day. In contrast, chronic confusion is long-term and deteriorating.

Acute confusion rarely becomes chronic. It is seen most often in older adults (men more than women), in those living alone or without close friends or relatives to visit, and in those who are confined to a restricted space with no familiar objects. There are two key characteristics of acute confusion: (1) A cause can usually be identified (linked to pain or medication), and (2) the nurse can usually calmly reorient the person as to location and who the nurse is.

Treatment should be aimed at the cause of the acute confusion, for example, the medication or pain. The nurse should tell the patient what the confusion is caused by and state that the confused state may return but that, when the patient improves in a day or two, the confusion will no longer be there. Acute confusion, though short-term, is distressing to the patient and family. Therefore, reassurances are most important. It is unkind to permit patients to remain confused, with no attempt at reorientation.

Confusion most often occurs at night when staffing is low; hence it is often difficult to have someone stay with the confused patient. Keeping the room quiet, with minimal light, encourages normal sleeping. Having a friend or relative stay with the confused person also helps. The sight of someone who is well-known is helpful and reassuring to the confused person.

Agitation may accompany confusion. The agitated person is suffering from a sense of loss of control. Like confusion, agitation is best dealt with immediately by displaying a calm manner and soft voice, indicating that the nurse is in control. It is natural for the nurse to be annoyed when an agitated patient tries to get out of bed, disconnects IV tubes and catheters, and talks in a loud voice. However, it is important not to demonstrate the annoyance by talking loudly and angrily. Rather it is best to help the person calm down and to determine, if possible, what the problem is. Putting an arm around the agitated person's shoulder is also reassuring and calming.

In this connection, it should be noted that older adults seldom present with the classic picture of a disease. Because of this, the nurse must be "suspicious" of minor and vague symptoms about which an older patient may complain. Sudden feelings of fatigue or a lack of desire to do usual activities may in fact be early symptoms of a serious illness. One report of persons presenting with confusion in a hospital emergency department during a three-month period found three types of causes: urinary tract infections, pneumonia, other *acute* causes. Sudden confusion in a usually clear thinking person thus should not be dismissed with the thought that the person is 82 years old and confusion is to be expected. The confusion may be masking symptoms of a serious illness. Careful concern for the symptoms' meanings and careful patient evaluation may prevent serious deterioration.

The single most important thing to remember about acute confusion and agitation is that there is a cause that can usually be identified and that must be treated. The nurse must, by talking, help the person become calm and oriented. Sedation and restraints are not the answer, although relief of postoperative pain should of course be achieved.

Teaching

Teaching is an important part of nursing care, for both young and old. However, judgment must be exercised in determining the depth of teaching to be done when the person is acutely ill. There is little that is unique in technique in teaching older adults; one learns as well at 70 years as at 20 (barring brain damage). However, special teaching methods may need to be devised for the hard-of-hearing or those with impaired vision, though these conditions are not unique to the older adult.

Older adults take somewhat longer to learn a technique, and they also are more concerned with having a reason to learn. They often do not try hard on tests when they do not see a reason for trying. Yet, in nursing the reason is often very obvious; the person with diabetes readily sees the need to learn insulin injection, the cardiac patient recognizes the need to learn about diet. In these circumstances, older adults, given adequate time, can learn difficult procedures, even home dialysis, and they can also be brought to accept the need for preoperative teaching.

Territoriality

Territoriality is involved in the care of all age groups, including those over 65 years of age. Wanting to take a cane on the stretcher while being transported to x-ray, when no walking will occur, is an indication of territoriality. Patients need a sense of territorial possession in order to feel comfortable in a setting. They need something or some area that "belongs" to them, not to the medical staff. The desire to take a religious article to the PACU is an example. Unfortunately, the concept of territoriality is frequently disregarded in many areas of hospital care. Nurses need to be conscious of territorial clues and be ready to communicate their awareness to their coworkers.

Multiple and Chronic Illnesses

Older adults entering a hospital often have more than one chronic illness, in addition to the particular acute problem precipitating hospitalization. In such cases, the nurse must keep these other chronic problems in mind and take appropriate steps to prevent their regression. Unless specific attention is paid to such chronic conditions, an acute problem of any sort (such as surgery) can lead to their deterioration. The physician should provide the required attention to these related chronic problems, but they often also become a matter of nursing and advocacy.

Summary

In all these areas of concern in the nursing care of older adults, a general summarizing statement might be this: Watchful waiting, careful assessment, and patient advocacy are the keys to quality nursing care of the older adult.

Consider the following case example of an older adult who suffered an acute illness: Mr. Jackson, 75 years old, came to the emergency department one evening to consult about his rectal bleeding, which, as it turned out, was due to hemorrhoids. Unfortunately, Mr. Jackson had a cardiac arrest while being examined, but he was easily resuscitated by a thump on the chest. He was admitted to a medical unit for observation (in the days before CCUs) and was doing well until the night he fell as he was climbing over the side-rails to go to the bathroom. A cervical fracture resulted and he was placed on bedrest. He then developed pneumonia, which required a tracheostomy for adequate suctioning of lung secretions. A gram-negative septicemia ensued, with vasopressors required to maintain the blood pressure. At one point, he had IV lines in three extremities (antibiotics, vasopressors, and "keep open") and a Foley catheter to straight drainage; he required frequent tracheostomy suctioning, turning q2h, and frequent blood pressure monitoring. He was poorly responsive. But he eventually improved and was discharged. Mr. Jackson is an inspiration and also a lesson for nurses. In spite of age-related changes developed during 75 years of living, Mr. Jackson had the strength to recuperate from the acute illness and the hospital-acquired complications.

SUBTLE INFLUENCES ON NURSING CARE OF OLDER ADULTS

Principles and Attitudes

In addition to the physical changes of aging and the specific medical problems affecting aging adults, more subtle factors can impinge on the nursing care of such persons. These factors involve personal attitudes of the nurse that have been internalized, such as the nurse's philosophy of nursing care, attitudes toward older adults, and intuition.

A philosophy of nursing care of older adults should include the principles that older adults:

- deserve to make decisions about their own medical care, to accept or to refuse care; if competent, they should not have someone else making decisions for them.
- deserve to be treated with respect as sensible adults, not as stereotypes.
- deserve to have access to medical care and should not be refused it on the basis of age.

In short, older adults deserve to be treated just as other adults are treated. In fact, older patients often do not receive the rights they deserve. Too often, older adults are told by a physician, "For someone of your age, I do not recommend surgery." In such cases, the *age* should not be the basis of the medical decision; the *health status* should be the basis.

Consider the following case: A 68-year-old woman presented with severe and painful arthritis of one hip that was incapacitating. Her orthopedist told her the only solution would be a total hip replacement. However, her physical condition was such (obesity, poor cardiac status) that he could give her only a 50-50 chance of surviving surgery. The woman agreed to the surgery against the wishes of her family members, who were fearful of her death. She felt that "life was not worth living this way." She said, "I have had a good life; if the Lord wants to take me, He will; if not, I will make it." She came through the surgery and is walking today.

This illustrates what care of the older adult should be: presenting the person with the facts, based on health status (not age), and letting the person make the decision. Children and spouses should not be making the decisions about care without consulting the person involved (unless the person is incompetent). In such situations, the nurse must be an advocate:

- for the patient, supporting the patient in making the decision to accept or refuse treatment
- with spouses and children, offering support and, encouraging them to let the patient make the final decision
- with physicians, encouraging them to present the facts to the patient (as well as family members) and offering support to the physician when the patient refuses care.

Nurses are in a difficult situation when patients refuse care. At such times, it is most important that nurses are clear in their own minds about their philosophy of care of the older adult. Do they truly believe that older adults should have the right to refuse care? If they do, their corresponding support and guidance will help them find answers to other related questions.

The Bias of Ageism

We have used the term *older adult* to refer to those 65 years of age and older because this term specifically assumes that they are indeed adults, with the rights of all other adults. Most older adults are not senile, and they should be treated with respect. Thus, nurses must be continually alert to how they are responding to older adults. Do they treat 70-year-olds the same way as 40-year-olds when the patients ask a confusing question? If nurses are alert to their reactions, they will become aware of their true feelings about older adults.

Nurses, like other members of society, normally adopt the prevailing attitudes of the day. One of the biases in today's society is exemplified by the term *ageism*, meaning, a bias against the elderly because they are old. (The term was coined by Robert Butler, the first director of the National Institute on Aging.[2]) How can nurses avoid this bias against older adults? Here are some helpful ideas:

- Be aware that the bias of ageism is prevalent.
- Deliberately avoid adopting the bias.
- Examine your feelings and actions toward older adults.
- Treat older adults as individuals not stereotypes.

The bottom line is: Do we believe that older adults have value?

Nurses are influenced in their attitude toward older adults by those they care for. Nurses care for sick adults of necessity; healthy people do not come to the hospital for nursing care. But there are of course many older adults who have never been in a hospital—a fact that many nurses might find hard to believe. Nurses see older adults with dementia and come to think that this is a usual part of aging. Yet only two to four percent of those over 65 years of age develop Alzheimer's disease, the major cause of dementia. It would be more sensible to develop our ideas about aging by looking at the older adults in our families and among our friends—among the many adults who remain relatively healthy. In short, because our attitudes are developed unconsciously (they are caught, not taught), we must make an effort to become consciously aware of those attitudes with regard to the individuals we care for, and especially with regard to aging adults.

The Use of Intuition

Another subtle, yet significant, influence on nursing care stems from the use of intuition. As nurses, we must struggle to objectify our assessment and judgments of patients. Yet there is a realm of judgment and assessment that is beyond objectivity. This is the realm that is based on previous experience. It gives us our sense that "something is not right" with a patient. This is intuition, and we must pay attention to it.

Intuition may come into play with patients of any age, but it is particularly important with older adults because they frequently do not have the usual symptoms of an illness. Coworkers of course expect nurses to be as objective as possible in their reporting, but nurses should also be sure that their intuitive sense of the situation is being considered.

When coworkers or family members remark that they are concerned about an older adult because that person does not seem to be acting normally, the nurse must try to elicit more objective data. But even if such data are not immediately available, it is important not to minimize the remark. The nurse must continue to be vigilant in monitoring the person in order to pick up further clues on the condition as it develops.

Many older adults have outlived their friends and spouses, and perhaps even their children. The nurse may be the only one to demonstrate caring concern for such people—to show that they are important and that someone cares what happens to them. Unfortunately, in some nursing areas, "tender, loving care," once an integral part of nursing, has become a forgotten phrase—not consciously rejected, but at least forgotten. Today, those caring for older adults must consciously resurrect that phrase and once more apply it liberally.

T. Franklin Williams, the present director of the National Institute on Aging, calls geriatric medicine the "fruition of the clinician."[3] The same term may be applied to nursing—to those nurses who have become experts in quality care of older adults. Their skilled care is indeed the "fruition of clinical nursing."

A REAL-LIFE EXPERIENCE IN CARING FOR THE AGED

The following reprint relates a loving, caring nursing experience with a healthy elderly adult who suffered a fall that sent her to a coronary care unit.

Mabel, You Don't Belong Here*

Ms. Mabel Maye Harrison, a hospital is no place for you!

After 91 years your back is so bent that I tower head and shoulders above you although I am only five feet tall. Your wizened face, spindly legs, skinny arms, and spidery fingers make us fear that you'll disintegrate if exposed to the air too long. Yet how sharp your mind is.

Wobbling around with a cane almost up to your chin, you've managed 30 years of perfect attendance at the race track. The racing forms and receipts in your purse show your favorites to the date of your admission.

Source: Reprinted from *American Journal of Nursing*, Vol. 73, No. 12, p. 2059, with permission of American Journal of Nursing Company, © 1973.

"I don't win as much as I used to," you admit. "It's probably my eyesight that's going. After all, it's not as if I were still 70." Right on, Ms. Harrison!

A fall brought you to the hospital from the hotel you've called home for 40 years, and an isolated episode of premature ventricular contractions sent you to the coronary care unit. How disgusted you are with CCU nurses and doctors for making you miss your beloved horse races.

"The maid waxed the floor too much—there's nothing wrong with my heart," you insist.

It turns out that you are right. Your left shoulder and arm pain is due to your sprained shoulder, but the purplish black blotches which cover that side make you look battered and pathetic. You've never had angina nor broken a bone in your life.

You don't ask for much, but you know exactly what will make you comfortable. "Hand me my cane!" you bark. "And don't call me Mrs. Harrison. My name is Miss Mabel Maye Harrison." You badger each of us for reassurance that you are going to be all right. "I've got so much to live for . . . and just think of the hotel gossip I'm missing, not to mention the races!"

You hate the telemetry box hung like a medallion around your neck. "I feel like a cat that's going to be drowned," you grumble, and stoop over so far to prove your point that you barely reach my waist. Now the box is attached to your handbag which you never allow more than a foot away from you.

Five days after admission, you are ready for discharge to your hotel. Grudgingly and reluctantly, you have come to accept us. The "Service" in the cardiac intensive care unit is "pretty good," you allow, and as long as you can watch television you'll put up with all of that blood pressure and cardiogram "nonsense."

You have flatly refused suggestions to move to a senior citizens apartment complex. Give up the races and the nightly dinners at the Post and Coach Restaurant? NEVER! For you, a spinster who supported her parents through two world wars, New York City streets and subways present no peril.

You laboriously inch your way into the clothes before discharge. You have come to enjoy the assistance you have received because you seemed so fragile, but now you are finally convinced that I'm only watching in order to assess your level of independence in dressing. You do well.

"I'm foxy," you confide, showing the cotton purse pinned to your ancient lace girdle. "I keep most of my money for the track here and just a dollar or so in my handbag in case I have to give something to a mugger."

Being transported in a wheelchair frightens and infuriates you. "No college boy is going to push me around!" you announce. "Medications? Why? WHY?"

We all hesitate to send you home alone, although we know the competent visiting nurse and occupational therapist will be seeing you tomorrow. One moment you are "absolutely unable" to use your bruised arm. The next moment you are busily fluffing up your gray hair with the same arm. "I've got to look good for the gang back at the hotel—have to brush my hair straight up. It gives me more height that way."

In parting, you inform us that you are going out to dinner tonight as usual. Only the top of your brushed-up hair is visible over the back of your wheelchair as you disappear through the double doors of the CCU. "It's a lucky thing!" you call back, "I'll be in time for my beauty parlor appointment."

Slim chance our visiting nurse has of finding you home tomorrow if the races are on. (When the visiting nurse did visit Mabel Harrison, she found this note taped to the door: "Sorry I'm not home. Went to have my whiskers waxed off—M. Harrison.")

I think of the woman who shared your hospital room. At 60, she has walled herself within her apartment and trembles at the mention of going for a walk. Like a timid deer, she is startled whenever someone enters the room. She clutches at us for comfort and sits with her hand on her pulse, "always waiting for the palpitations to come." She has lived through only the first thousand deaths she must face before her eyes close forever on the faded pictures of her dead family.

In the few days we knew you, Ms. Harrison, your spunk and spirit became symbols of strength, independence, and beauty in old age. God bless you, Miss Mabel Maye Harrison, and hit the Daily Double tomorrow!

NOTES

1. Schock, Nathan (ed). *Normal Human Aging: The Baltimore Longitudinal Study of Aging.* (Washington, D.C.: Department of Health and Human Services, National Institute on Aging, 1984), p. 207.
2. Butler, Robert N. "Age-ism: Another Form of Bigotry." *Gerontologist,* 9 (1969):243.
3. Williams, Franklin T. "Geriatrics: The Fruition of the Clinician." *Gerontologist,* 26 (1986):349.

BIBLIOGRAPHY

Benner, Patricia, and Tanner, Christine. "Clinical Judgment: How Expert Nurses Use Intuition." *American Journal of Nursing* 87 (1987):23–31.

Butler, Robert N. "Age-ism: Another Form of Bigotry." *Gerontologist* 9 (1969):243–249.

Demmerle, Barbara. "Care of the Acutely Ill: General Nursing Care." *Geriatric Nursing* 3 (1982):316–321.

Ebersole, Priscilla, and Hess, Patricia. *Toward Health Aging,* 2d ed. St. Louis, Mo.: C.V. Mosby, 1985.

Feller, I., Flora, J.D., Jr., and Bawol, R. "Baseline Therapy for Burned Patients." *Journal of the American Medical Association* 2361 (1976):1943–1947.

Fulmer, Terry, et al. "Nursing Guidelines for the Use of Restraints in Non-Psychiatric Settings." *Journal of Gerontological Nursing* 9 (1983):180–181.

Goldman, R. "Speculations on Vascular Changes With Age." *Journal of the American Geriatrics Society* 18 (1970):765–779.

National Center for Health Statistics. *Health: United States, 1985.* Washington, D.C.: U.S. Department of Health and Human Services, 1986.

Reichel, William, ed. *Clinical Aspects of Aging*, 2d ed. Baltimore, Md.: Williams & Wilkins, 1983.

Santora, Gladys. "Communicating better with the elderly." *Nursing Life* 6 (1986):24–27.

Schock, Nathan, ed. *Normal Human Aging: Baltimore Longitudinal Study of Aging.* Washington, D.C.: Department of Health and Human Services, National Institute on Aging, 1984.

Steel, Knight, et al. "Iatrogenic Illness on a General Medical Service at a University Hospital." *New England Journal of Medicine* 304 (1982):638–642.

Williams, T. Franklin. "Geriatrics: The Fruition of the Clinician." *Gerontologist* 26 (1986): 345–349.

Wolanin, Mary Opal, and Phillips, Linda R.F. "Emergency Care for Clients Who Are Acutely Confused." In *Confusion* 101–108. St. Louis, Mo.: C.V. Mosby, 1981.

Part IV
Taking Care of Ourselves

Chapter 21

Stress Management Techniques for PACU Nurse Practitioners

Mary Ellen Luczun, R.N, M.S.N.

THE MEANING OF STRESS

Stress is the nonspecific response of the body to any demand, whether it is caused by, or results in, pleasant or unpleasant conditions.[1] A stressor can be viewed as an agent or factor that challenges the adaptive capacity of an individual.[2] Stressors, therefore, can increase the need to perform adaptive functions necessary to restore normality. Since stress is a syndrome and results in groups of changes, not just a single reaction, the response is considered nonspecific.[3] The adaptive mechanisms utilized are, thus, quite independent of the activity that stimulated them. No two persons will react to a given stressor in the same way.

Stressors themselves are not necessarily good or bad. Rather, it is how we choose to interpret them that heralds the stress syndrome. Suppose you were working well into the night, trying to finish a report due the next morning, when your typewriter either runs out of ribbon or breaks down completely. The stressor—a malfunctioning typewriter in this case—is simply that—no more and no less. How will you react? Your perception of the event will undoubtedly color your response:

It is 3:00 A.M. You have waited until the last minute to finish the report. The stores are obviously closed. Repairmen do not take 24-hour call. Your neighbor does not have a typewriter (nor would you care to wake your neighbor up at such an hour in any case). But you must have this report for a 10:00 A.M. meeting; you may already be in trouble with your boss. Yet, you are not going to get any sleep worrying about this, you can do nothing at the moment, and you are going to be so nervous by the time you reach the meeting that your presentation will result in humiliation.

This is a very stressful situation indeed! The question is: How will you adapt to it? Perhaps you can make some arrangements with a typist in the morning or arrive at work early and type it yourself. Whatever you do, the whole scenario represents an inconvenience, and it will require you to adopt some problem-solving techniques.

Selye considers such an event "the stress of living," which is not of itself physical.[4] It exists in the mind of the individual who perceives it, as *it affects that particular individual*. The same situation under different circumstances may have produced a different outcome. Perhaps it was 8:00 P.M., not 3:00 A.M.; you had another ribbon, or the stores were open if you did not; or you had a neighbor with a typewriter (in the event yours was broken). In this alternative situation, if you knew you could have the report typed before the meeting, the entire event would have been only a minor inconvenience.

STRESS IS ALL AROUND US

The world in which we live is an ever-changing environment, characterized by rapid technology that threatens to limit our capacity to adapt. Tradition has been challenged, and in many cases dispensed with, in favor of newer and more sophisticated methods. The sense of the familiar is fading fast, and it is being replaced by a sense of an unfamiliar and strange, if not totally alien, environment. The result is that we worry a lot, which is a form of low-level stress. The nuclear arms race, overpopulation, crime, racism, terrorism, and a deteriorating ecology are all issues of concern. On a more personal level, we worry about contracting AIDS or other forms of sexually transmitted disease, or developing cancer or heart disease. We are concerned about being overweight, alcohol and drug abuse, smoking and its effects on nonsmokers, eating the right foods, cholesterol intake, and high blood pressure. And we fret over relationship problems—the state of our marriage, career responsibilities versus responsibilities in the home, our children, our aging parents, or our own midlife crises.

We are assaulted by stress from all directions, but the stress we experience in our immediate environment has the potential of being the most damaging. This is the type of stress that can be prolonged and can eventually compromise adaptive energy resources. Depending on where you live, the act of getting to work becomes stressful. You wait for a bus or subway only to experience delays due to traffic or congestion. In addition, you are battling crowds of people, sometimes in rain or snow or extreme heat, and experience noise levels that can drive you insane—all before you even arrive at work. Then, once on the job, the only thing you may have to look forward to is eight hours of more stress.

STRESS AND THE NURSING PROFESSION

When asked about their use of the word *stress,* most nurses describe combinations of unpleasant situations and unpleasant personal experiences.[5] Yet, although we tend to view stress as a negative experience, we also recognize that it is necessary, and even desirable. Desirable stress can in fact be pleasant, in that it serves to interest or excite. Once overstimulation occurs, however, it becomes unpleasant and is associated with anxiousness and irritability. At another level, understimulation is characterized by boredom and frustration. In short, both too much and too little stress can be detrimental.

Despite all the literature on stress and its effects, many nurses are still wary about admitting that it exists within themselves. This may be due to the nurse's tradition; that is, nurses are supposed to be strong and to be a model for others. Being strong, however, entails the ability to face one's feelings. All too often, the person who functions as if nothing is wrong is avoiding direct confrontation and, in that sense, is exhibiting weakness.

In fact, we all perceive stress in certain situations; indeed, we would be abnormal if we did not. There are three ways we can cope with perceived stress:[6]

1. Develop the skills of noticing the negative signs of stress.
2. Build the skills needed to develop an improved positive state of health.
3. Achieve the right balance between the amount of stressful pressure and our individual resources for dealing with it.

It is important to note that this protocol must be highly individualized. One nurse may view a certain form of stress as being understimulating, while another nurse may be overstimulated by the same event. Again, it is not the stressor, per se, that matters, but how the individual reacts to it.

REACTIONS TO STRESS

Stress can trigger or worsen anxiety, chronic exhaustion, nausea, palpitations, headaches, and insomnia. It can make a person edgey, irritable, hostile, or depressed. Lack of concentration, indecision, confusion, and obsession can all be accompanied by stress. Prolonged stress can lead to such problems as angina and heart disease.

Consider the special stress of being in a job you hate. Perhaps it is not the job alone but also the individuals you are forced to interact with. Day after day, additional responsibilities are taking their toll on you, while others always seem to escape or are just not pulling their weight. If you are a perfectionist, beware; you may end up with more than your fair share—after all, you are so capable! The sad part of this situation is that the ascription of responsibility does not always confer authority.

Lack of appreciation for your efforts can be particularly deadly because it erodes your confidence and batters your self-esteem. In time, you may have to think about looking for a new job. Yet, although this is one possible solution, it is not the only alternative. Despite the bleak nature of a given situation, there are always alternative choices, which we will explore later in the chapter. Learning to identify your needs and to take responsibility for yourself is a powerful weapon for diffusing stress.

STRESS IN THE PACU

Stressors are rampant in the PACU. Nurses working in this area are constantly being challenged to adapt—usually on a minute-to-minute basis. PACU nursing as a specialty is expanding as it accommodates to rapidly accelerating technology. Ambulatory PACU settings are placing additional professional responsibilities upon the nurse's shoulders in the form of patient and family discharge teaching. On any given day, PACU nurses will experience a substantial array of stress-producing events, ranging from mild inconveniences to life-threatening crises. How many times in the course of an eight-hour shift does a PACU nurse:

- answer the phone
- fight with the lab technician
- page the surgeon
- attempt to restrain restless patients
- empty drainage
- return patients to their rooms
- receive a "cool reception" from floor nurses
- change a dressing
- put on an oxygen mask
- maintain an airway
- chart
- run for an emesis basin

- troubleshoot a malfunctioning respirator
- insert an airway
- order a chest x-ray

And all this in the course of a relatively quiet day! Added to this is the stress of respiratory and cardiac arrests, bleeding problems, and other medical disasters that can and do occur. Is it any wonder the PACU nurse often experiences tension and frustration?

Working in the PACU is indeed stressful, but most PACU nurses would probably agree that it involves the stimulating type of stress. There is an enormous satisfaction to be gained from performing up to par. It is actually quite exhilarating to go home at the end of each day knowing you can cope with any PACU problem that is hurled at you, and overcome it! This type of stimulation gives energy rather than draining it from you. It is wonderfully invigorating—*if* you are not under any significant personal stress.

The additional stressors in one's life are highly individualized, and each person must deal with them individually. Coping behaviors vary immensely, as one might expect. Whatever the method of coping, however, it is vital that it not become a secondary stressor, as is the case when drugs or alcohol are utilized.

We are all human beings with unique lives to live outside of the PACU environment. At any moment in time, many of us will be contending with such problems as marital separation or divorce, the death of a loved one, arrangements for adequate day care for children, financial debt, attendance at evening classes to earn a degree, an alcoholic spouse, an unruly teenager, or an aging parent. Yet, let us not forget the good stressors: marriage, pregnancy (hopefully), a promotion, vacations, and holidays. These joyous events are stressful because they challenge our adaptive capacities, even though they may bring other stressors with them.

Only you can decide how much stress is too much stress. If you have a considerable number of personal stressors to contend with, you may begin to feel you cannot juggle them anymore. You may become frustrated, angry, moody, tearful, or anxious. Coworkers may begin to notice your changing behavior and comment on it. At a certain point, you are likely to snap at them and use a few choice words in the process. In such a situation, it takes a truly sensitive and compassionate coworker or friend to break through the barrier. Depending on how stubborn you are, this may take quite some time, even with the most patient of friends and colleagues.

Provided your work does not suffer, you may continue in your overstressed state, but with a new reputation of being a grouch. Sooner or later, however, you will find yourself sitting in the office of your nurse manager, who will be understandably concerned. If you are not ready to share your burden, you will probably end up apologizing for your behavior ("I don't know what's gotten into me") and be on your way again. Now you have added another stressor to the load: the need to be careful not to discharge your anger on the PACU. It is almost inevitable, however, that if your personal situation remains unaltered, your work will suffer. In the PACU, this can be a potentially dangerous situation. When your mind is caught up with all your own problems and confusion and indecision sets in, caring for patients becomes very difficult, simply because you cannot concentrate effectively. Soon you may find that even the basic tasks become monumental. You may not be able to decide what to do first when a patient arrives: Take the blood pressure? Check the dressing? Check the airway? When this happens, some type of therapeutic intervention is a must.

COPING MEASURES

Dealing with Stressors

In coping with prolonged stress, there are three basic approaches:[7]

1. Completely eliminate the stressor.
2. Resist or minimize the stressor.
3. Accept the fact that some stress is inescapable but it can be managed or relieved.

Choice 1 is very tempting, indeed; however, it is not always possible. Also, ironically, the act of removing a stressor can in itself be stressful! A woman who files for a divorce is, in a sense, removing the stressor completely (provided she does not have children). What she is doing is removing herself from the source of her stress. The act of divorce is nevertheless stressful, even if she is better off without her husband. Similarly, you could quit your job, if that is the stressor; but you must find another, and that too is stressful. In short, stress is here to stay; hence, a combination of choices 2 and 3 seems to be the most logical approach.

One of the best ways of minimizing a stressor is to ask the question, What is the worst that can happen? Once you have dealt with this question, anything else that happens cannot be as bad. This is of course a simplistic approach, yet it deserves some consideration.

There are many other ways to resist and minimize stressors. First a clear and objective appraisal of the source of the stress is required. We can start by asking ourselves: To what extent are these stressors going to upset our plans, hopes, dreams, expectations, and, most important, our self-esteem?

Our ancestors, the cavemen, either fought or ran away from their predators. We too can adopt a "fight or flight" philosophy but we pay a high price if we choose flight. The problem is that no one can hide for very long; sooner or later action must be taken. This means confronting the situation and proposing solutions that will work for us. It requires serious and honest self-confrontation. We must decide what we can and cannot live with.

For example, if the stressor is an impossible work-study schedule, the solution may be to drop a few courses, work part-time and go to school full-time (if financially feasible), or postpone school until finances permit a full-time commitment. A job that causes more stress than it is worth may not be a desirable situation to be in, but it is always possible to go job hunting in the meantime; this will at least give you the satisfaction of knowing you are doing something to alleviate the stress. Once you have found a better job, you can terminate your present position.

The divorce or death of a loved one is a stressor that must be accepted. These are events that call upon your deepest emotions; however, the grieving process does eventually bring relief. Major stressors such as these also respond favorably to some type of psychological counseling. In fact, counseling and group encounters can serve as strong support systems for anyone dealing with marital problems, rebellious adolescents, chronic illness, alcoholic spouses, and other major problems.

Coping with stress is a matter of altering your response to it. Because stressors challenge your adaptive capacity, some form of readaptation is required. You alone can determine just how you will achieve this. It involves considerable self-confrontation—talking to yourself, if you will—and priority setting. Can you eliminate the stressor? If so, by all means, do it. Remember, however, that choosing this option will, in all likelihood, create additional stress. It thus is helpful to list on paper the advantages and disadvantages of such a move. Again, only you can decide whether or not the consequences are justified. If removing a stressor produces even greater anxiety and more stress, you may want to minimize it instead. Strategies for dealing with it in that way can then be employed. In the final analysis, the best solution is simply a matter of looking out for your own best interests.

Stress can rule your life, but only if you let it. A change of perspective (how you choose or want to react) must be followed up by a change in behavior, and this is often the most difficult part. It is so easy to say, "I am not going to let this get to me," or "I am not going to bring this on myself again," but these statements must then become the basis for action. When dealing with stress, actions do speak louder than words; let your actions speak.

There are countless annoyances that can drive all of us up the wall. There are also compulsions we all possess to a certain degree—compulsions that add unnecessary stress to our lives. Are you a compulsive cleaner? Do you fret if you are forced to leave unwashed dishes in the sink overnight? Does your bathroom have to sparkle like an ad in a magazine every day without fail? Can you tolerate a little bit of dust here and there without flying into a rage?

What about other high expectations you place upon yourself and others? Can you ease up a little? Can you be spontaneous and enjoy a bit of recreation, even though you are trying to meet a deadline? Can you appreciate your need to relax, to let up on yourself, and to let things slide for a while as being beneficial to your welfare and mental health? Or, do you feel guilty when you are not constantly tending to your work? Don't you feel you could use a break, if for no other reason than to preserve your own sanity? You may say, "This is fine in theory, but I do not have the time." Make the time, order your priorities, and start being kind to yourself.

Nurturing Yourself

Nurses are well-known for their ability to help and take care of others. When it comes to taking care of themselves, however, they often fall short. Frequently, those who take care of others very conveniently avoid taking care of themselves. Nurses who leave the PACU every day and go home, only to continue their nurturing function with spouses and/or children, are in a double bind. For these men or women, there is no reprieve; and the only ones who suffer are themselves.

Imagine, if you will, any person, place, or thing that brings you joy. What is your idea of a totally pleasurable experience? Think of the lyrics to the song "My Favorite Things." Besides identifying moments of happiness, the song also illustrates how thinking pleasant thoughts can replace stressful ones.

Despite busy schedules, most individuals do find the time for leisure activities. These activities can be as varied as the people who engage in them. The objective is to plan for them the same way you plan your work schedule. Often, when stressors are bearing down, aspects of personal growth are tossed aside: hobbies are dropped, meetings with friends are postponed, vacations are cancelled, and family members are ignored. It is precisely at such a time, however, that we desperately need support systems. We need to be distracted, if only for a brief time, from all the burdens we carry around with us. We need to relax and allow the child within us to take over for a while. To deny this very basic aspect of self-nurture is a very serious mistake. All work and no play will not necessarily make you dull, but it can make you sick!

Why is it that some people refuse to let up on themselves? Why do they continually overextend themselves, taking on one task after another without a thought of how they will manage it? Some people cannot say no, and one might wonder why. Such individuals may be out to prove that they are supercapable.

Deep down, however, they may be desperately seeking approval from others; the problem is that the seeking is at their own expense.

One of the biggest barriers to self-nurture seems to be low self-esteem. Very simply, if you do not like yourself, you are unlikely to reward yourself, because you really believe you do not deserve it. So you push yourself, making heavy demands upon yourself, setting unrealistic goals, neglecting yourself in the process. Once a better sense of self is achieved, however, taking care of yourself becomes second nature.

How does one raise self-esteem? By taking a long, hard, inward look and asserting, "I am a person of worth, and I am deserving of love and respect." This affirmation should be made daily while looking in the mirror; in about two weeks' time, you will feel the difference and actually begin to believe what you are saying. Too often, we beat up on ourselves and punish ourselves needlessly, and we end up hating ourselves. Why not praise, instead of degrade, for a change? The principle is quite simple: say anything to yourself frequently enough and you will incorporate it into your personal belief system. Affirm and believe in yourself. After all, you are the one who must live with you!

A Prescription for Self-Nurture

Whether or not you are under prolonged stress, the following guidelines are highly recommended; if you are currently experiencing a significant amount of stress in your life, they are mandatory:

- *Get plenty of rest.* Marathon work sessions are unhealthy. Allow yourself frequent breaks, get up and stretch, take a walk (fresh air is invigorating, while the exercise keeps you in shape), or call a friend. If you require eight hours of sleep each night, make sure you get it. Working into the wee hours will inevitably take its toll the next day. Plan your schedule accordingly; set a cut-off time and stick to it. Luxuriate in a hot tub or long shower at the end of the day. Do something nice for yourself, like getting a massage. In short, reward yourself for all your hard work.
- *Take time off.* Time off means time away from the task at hand. Go out to dinner with friends, or take a trip to an art exhibit you have been interested in seeing. You can also catch up on reading that book you have been postponing, seeing that movie, writing your memoirs. Engage in hobbies you enjoy—get out and ride your bicycle, try a new recipe, put together that scrapbook. Take a vacation, time permitting, and really get away from it all. The possibilities are endless.

- *Eat properly*. A diet of coffee and cigarettes does not provide good nutrition. Make sure you are getting a proper balance of protein, carbohydrates, fats, and vitamins. Vegetables are a great source of vitamins and minerals, and they are low in calories. Pay attention to protein. Limit your fat intake; but remember, a certain amount of fat is desirable. Avoid binges on junk food that is high in carbohydrates and fat content and has zillions of calories. However, an occasional cheeseburger and french fries will not kill you, as long as it is not a steady diet. Moderation is the key with any food. In fact, moderation is the universal key; too much or too little is never a good policy. Finally, regardless of how well-balanced your diet is, it is always beneficial to increase your intake of B vitamins during stressful periods.
- *Have an outlet*. If you are feeling particularly overwhelmed, get on the phone and call a friend who will listen. If your friend is not at home, sit down and write your feelings down on paper (this can be a very cathartic maneuver). Feel free to have a good cry, or to beat up a pillow and let your anger out. Any activity that discharges anger is fine provided you do not hurt yourself or anyone else in the process. Try to avoid displacing your anger onto an innocent party. Instead of engaging in a fight with your spouse, for instance, remove yourself from the premises and run around the block a few times.

Assertiveness

Unfortunately, we bring a lot of stress upon ourselves by our own actions. This happens, for example, when we do not say what we want at the time it is appropriate. By the time we muster up the courage to say what we want, it is often too late and anticlimactic. Stress has a nasty habit of lowering self-confidence; this makes it difficult to be assertive. Yet, when you are nonassertive, you merely set yourself up for further stress.

Being assertive, in contrast, leads to less stress and increased self-confidence. The aim, therefore, is to develop a more assertive approach, to stand up for our rights. We have the right to:[8]

- state needs and set priorities
- be treated with respect
- express feelings
- express opinions and values
- say yes or no
- make a mistake

- say, "I don't understand"
- ask for what we want
- decide what we are responsible for

It is up to us to put these rights into practice. We do not have to cope with every stressor that comes our way; we can learn to say no and set limits.

A valuable hint for avoiding unnecessary stress is to take notice of how it makes you feel. If, for instance, you find yourself agonizing over a certain situation that is making you uneasy, choose another strategy. There are always alternatives to explore. You are the judge of just how much you can safely cope with. Do not invite more stress; rather deal with the matter at hand, taking it one day at a time.

In sum, stress is neither good nor bad. But, it can motivate us to greater achievement, or throw us into the depths of despair. In any event, we play an active role in determining how we will react. We can use the power of our intellect to make the decisions that are most beneficial to us. When the balance shifts, however, and we feel overwhelmed, we can seek help:

> God, grant me the serenity to accept the things I cannot change . . . courage to change the things I can . . . and wisdom to know the difference.
>
> (St. Francis)

I wish you serenity, courage, and wisdom.

NOTES

1. H. Selye, *Stress Without Distress* (New York: Signet Books, 1974), 14.
2. J. Luckman and K. Creason Sorensen, *Medical-Surgical Nursing: A Psycho-Physiologic Approach,* 2d ed. (Philadelphia: W.B. Saunders, 1980), 50.
3. J. Wells, *Coping in the 80's: Eliminating Needless Stress and Guilt* (Chicago: Thomas Moore Press, 1986), 84.
4. Ibid., 85.
5. M. Bond, *Stress and Self-awareness: A Guide for Nurses* (Rockville, Md.: Aspen Publishers, 1986), 1.
6. Ibid., 2.
7. Wells, *Coping in the 80's,* 84.
8. Bond, *Stress and Self-awareness,* 99.

BIBLIOGRAPHY

Alberti, R., and Emmons, M. *Your Perfect Right.* London: Impact Books, 1974.
Bond, M. "Dare Your Say No?" *Nursing Mirror* (13 October 1982): 40–42.
Clark, C.C. *Assertive Skills for Nurses.* Rockville, Md.: Aspen Publishers, Inc., 1978.

Index

A

Abbott, Gilbert, 11
Abdominal abscess, 295
Abdominal surgery, 111-24
   case histories, 114-22
   diagnosis, 111-14
   postanesthesia care, 123-24
Abortion, elective, postanesthesia care for, 221
Abscesses, 292, 295
Accurbron, 281
Acetaminophen, 47
Acidosis, postoperative, 258-62
Acquired immune deficiency syndrome (AIDS) virus, 301, 302, 305 (table), 308
Active compression of blood vessels, 238-39
Acute intermittent porphyria, 207-8
Acute respiratory failure (ARF), 255
   intraoperative setting, 256-58
   oxygenation/ventilation to treat, 262-64
   postoperative setting, 258-62
Adenoidectomy, 55
Adrenalin, 281

Adult respiratory distress syndrome (ARDS), 92
   in pediatric patients, 201-2
Ageism in nursing care, 333-34
Aging process, 321-25
   normal physical changes in, 323-24 (table)
Agitation,
   in older patients, 329-30
   postoperative, 19, 208
AIDS. *See* Acquired immune deficiency syndrome (AIDS) virus
Air emboli, 16. *See also* Pulmonary embolism
   in head/neck surgery, 65-66
Airway maintenance, 18. *See also* Acute respiratory failure (ARF); Respiration
   in burn patients, 140-41, 147
   clearing of excessive secretions, 278 (table)
   in head/neck surgery, 52 (fig.), 63-64, 67-68
   improvement of airway size, 277 (table)
   neck anatomy, 52 (fig.)
   in oral/maxillofacial surgery, 43-44, 46-47
   in pediatric patients, 16-17, 199
   pressure patterns, 93, 94 (fig.)

Albumin, 86
Alcoholic cirrhosis, 246
Aldosterone, effect on kidneys, 173 (fig.)
Alignment in orthopedic patients, 158-64
Alkalosis, 89, 90
Alpha blockers, 208
Alupent, 199, 281
Aminoglycoside, 293
Aminophyllin, 199, 281, 283
Analgesics, 5, 83, 102
Ancef, 296
Anectine, 32, 40, 282
Anesthesia. *See also names of specific drugs*
  adverse respiratory effects, 256-57
  for burn patients, 146-49
  for cardiac patients, 76-77, 79, 80, 81, 315-17
  epidural (*see* Epidural anesthesia)
  general (*see* General anesthesia)
  head and neck surgery, 62
  local (*see* Local/regional anesthesia)
  in obstetrical patients, 218-20
  ophthalmalogic surgery, 38-40
  origins of, 11
  in orthopedic patients, 157-58
  preoperative, 5, 14-15, 38, 146, 282
  in renal/urological patients, 184-88
  residual effects in pediatric patients, 196-97
  for respiratory disease patients, 272-76, 282-83, 288-90
  technique, 15
  topical, 31
  for vascular surgery patients, 129-31
Anesthesiologist, 4
  reports by, to PACU/ICU staff, 82-83
  -surgeon team, 11-20
Aneurysm, 113, 127-28, 131
Angina, 312
Antibiotics, 121, 138, 197, 273, 292
  choice of, for infection, 293
  prophylactic, 296-97, 298-99 (table)
Anticholinergics, 5, 146, 282
Anticholinesterase, 108

Anticoagulation therapy, 78, 246
Antidiuretic hormone (ADH),
  excessive secretion of, in renal patients, 172
Aorta,
  acquired diseases of, 127-28
  insufficiency of, 78-79
  stenosis of, 77-78
Aortofemoral occlusive disease, 128
Apena monitor, 196
Aplasia of the bone marrow, 244
Appendicitis, 113, 114-16
  surgical technique, 116, 117 (fig.)
Apresoline, 28
Aramine, 86
Arfonad, 27, 84
Arterial blood gas, 19, 274
  in diagnosing respiratory failure, 255, 259, 284, 288
Arteries. *See also* Aorta
  bleeding, 26-28
  grafting of, 131-32
  splanchnic arteries, 128-29
Aspiration pneumonia, 264, 265
Aspirin, 245, 248
Assertiveness, to cope with stress, 350-51
Asthma, 276-85
  prophylactic treatment, 281, 286 (table)
Atelectasis, 259, 263
Atherosclerosis, 125, 126
Atracurium, 184, 283
Atrial fibrillation, 101, 214
Atropine, 5, 197, 211, 282
Avitene, 240

B

Bacteremia, 295
Baltimore Longitudinal Study of Aging, 322, 323-24 (table)
Barbiturates, 38, 208
Benadryl, 244
Benzocaine, 209
Benzodiazepine, 146
Beta blockers, 101, 209

Biopsy,
  lung, 107
  neck mass, 55
Bladder, 171
  cancer of, 180
  foreign bodies in, 180-81
  trauma to, 181
Bleeding. *See also* Anticoagulation therapy; Hemostasis in surgical patients
  abnormal, in surgery, 247-52
  in burn patients, 145, 147, 152
  control of, 237-40
  in cranial surgery, 26-28
  in oral/maxillofacial surgery, 45, 47-48
  in orthopedic surgery, 157, 160
  in pediatric patients, 203-4
Bleeding test time, 249, 250
Blepharoplasty, 34, 37
Blood,
  clotting, 234-37, 247
  gas (*see* Arterial blood gas)
  magnesium levels in plasma, 227, 228 (table)
  pressure (*see* Hypertension; Hypotension)
  transfusion, 86, 203
  transfusion-related infection, 295-96
  vessels, 231-32, 238-39
Blood smear test, 249
Body fluids,
  in burn patients, 137 (fig.), 152
  in older patients, 327 (fig.), 328
  in pediatric patients, 202-4
Bones,
  aplasia of marrow, 244
  categories of, 155
  composition of, 155-57
Bradycardia, 84, 86
Brain surgery. *See* Craniotomy
Brethine, 223, 281
Bretylium tosylate, 85
Bretyllium, 213
Bretylol, 85
Bronchitis, chronic, 269-70

Bronchoscopy, 54, 107
  for burn patients, 140
Bronchospasm, 199, 276
Bronkosol, 199, 281, 283
Buck's traction, 160, 161 (fig.)
Bupivacaine, 38, 255
Burn surgery, 135-53
  airway management, 140-41
  anesthetic considerations, 146-49
  monitoring criteria, 141-44
  postanesthesia care, 149-53
  "rule of nines," 138, 139 (fig.)
  surgical procedures, 144-46
  survival as a function of age and area burned, 326 (fig.)
  types of burn injuries, 136-38
  wound care/potential complications, 138-40
Bursa, 156
Butler, Robert, 334
Bypass surgery. *See* Coronary artery bypass grafting (CABG)

C

Caesarean section, 17, 224-25
Calan, 85
Calcium, and hyperthermia, 206-7
Calcium channel blockers, 101, 197
Calcium chloride, 86, 211-12
Cancer. *See also* Tumors
  bladder, 180
  leukemia, 244
  prostate gland, 179-80
Carbocaine, 38
Cardiac arrhythmias. *See also* Tachycardias
  in pediatric patients, 213-14
  postoperative, 19, 84-85, 86, 90, 101
Cardiac function,
  and acute respiratory failure, 264-65
  in pediatric patients, 193
Cardiac surgery, 16, 73-97. *See also* Coronary artery disease (CAD); Vascular surgery
  postoperative care, 81-96

Cardiac tamponade, 108-9
Cardiopulmonary life support, in
 pediatric patients, 210-14
 advanced cardiac support drugs, 212
 basic cardiac support, 210-12
 prognosis, 212
 treatment of tachyarrhythmias, 213-14
Carotid endarterectomy, 29, 131
Carotid sinus reflex, 65
Case histories,
 abdominal pain, 114-22
 nursing care for older adults, 335-37
Casts,
 for orthopedic patients, 159-60
Cataract surgery, 32, 35
Cautery of blood vessels, 239
Cefazolin, 296
Cefoxitin, 293
Central and peripheral nervous systems,
 in pediatric patients, 194
Central venous pressure monitoring, 17
Cephalosporin, 296
Cerebrovascular occlusive disease,
 126-27
Chemotherapeutic agents, for burns,
 138-39
Chest tubes, 103-6, 201
Childbirth, postanesthesia care after
 vaginal, 221
Chloroprocaine, 225
Chlorpromazine, 84
Chlorpropamide, 172
Cholecystitis, 114
Cholelithiasis, 112
Chronic illness in older adults, 331
Chronic obstructive pulmonary disease
 (COPD), 268-76
 anesthesia considerations with, 272-76
 chronic bronchitis, 269-70
 emphysema, 268-69
 types A and B, 270-72
Cigarette smoking, 125, 268-69
Circulatory problems, postoperative, 18
 assessing, in orthopedic patients, 158,
 159 (table)
Cleocin, 293, 296
Clindamycin, 293, 296

Closing volumes, respiratory, 256, 257
Clotting, blood, 234-37
 cascade, 236 (fig.)
 diffuse intravascular, 247
 factors, 235 (table)
Cocaine, 31, 240
Codeine, 206, 282
Collagen, 240
Compartment syndrome, 164-65
Compazine, 265
Confusion in older patients, 329-30
Congenital hemostasis defects, 241-43
Congenital heart disease, 208-9
Conley, John, 67
Continuous arteriovenous hemofiltration
 (CAVH), 186, 187 (fig.),
 187 (fig.), 188
Continuous passive motion (CPM), 163-64
Continuous positive airway pressure
 (CPAP), 93, 94 (fig.)
Continuous positive pressure ventilation
 (CPPV), 93, 94 (fig.)
Corneal disease and injury, surgery for,
 32-33, 35-36
Coronary artery bypass grafting (CABG),
 73-74
 indications/procedures for, 75-76
Coronary artery disease (CAD), 73-77,
 311-20
 anatomy/physiology, 74 (fig.), 313,
 314 (fig.)
 anesthetic considerations, 76-77,
 315-17
 pathophysiology, 74-75, 311-13
 postanesthesia care, 317-19
 preoperative evaluation, 313-15
 surgical procedures, 75-76
Coumadin, 78, 246
Craniotomy, 25-29
Cromolyn sodium, 281
Cryoprecipitate, 241, 243
Cytomegalovirus, 308

D

Dacryocystorhinostomy, 37
Dantrolene, 207

Decadron, 68
Demerol, 38, 220
Desmopressin, 243
Dexamethasone, 68, 199
Diabetes mellitus, 32
Diabinese, 172
Diazepam, 38, 220
Diffuse interstitial pulmonary fibrosis, 287-90
Diffuse intravascular clotting (DIC), 247
Digestive tract, 51, 52 (fig.)
Digitalis, 85, 264
Digoxin, 101, 214
Dilantin, 208
Diphenhydramine, 244
Disseminated intravascular coagulation, 223-24, 225 (table)
Diuretics, 92, 273
Diverticulitis, 113, 120-21, 122 (fig.)
Dobutamine, 86, 87, 212
Dobutrex, 86
Dopamine, 87, 96, 212, 293
Droperidol, 208
Drug(s). *See also names of individual drugs*
  antagonistic, 18
  to control bleeding, 239-40
  -induced agitation, 19
  interactions, 13
  older patients' response to, 328-29
  pediatric cardiac support, 212
  sensitivity to, 130
D-tubocurarine, 282
Duramorph, 225
Dyspnea, 287

E

Ear, nose and throat surgery, 18. *See also* Oral and maxillofacial surgery
Echothiophate iodide, 40
Eclampsia in pregnancy, 226-28
Ectopic pregnancy, 113, 223-24
Edema, *See also* Pulmonary edema and airway compromise, 44, 67-68, 199
  in orthopedic patients, 158, 160

Electrolytes, in pediatric patients, 197, 204-5
Emphysema, 268-69
Endarterectomy, 29, 131
Endocarditis, 78, 80
Endoscopy, 53-54
Endotracheal tube, obstruction of, 198
Enflurane, 26, 76, 273, 282
Ephedrine, 148, 222
Epidural anesthesia, 17, 224-25, 226 (fig.), 258
Epinephrine, 87, 199, 211, 239, 281
Epispadias, 178
Ergonovine maleate, 221, 225
Ergotrate, 221, 225
Erythromycin, 296
Esophagoscopy, 54
Esophagus, 53
Ethrane, 26, 148, 282
Expiratory positive airway pressure (EPAP), 93, 94
External fixators, for orthopedic patients, 162, 163 (fig.)
Extubation, of patients with respiratory disease, 289
Eye. *See* Ophthalmalogic surgery

F

Fascia, 156
Fat embolism syndrome (FES), 165-66
Fentanyl, 76, 80, 225, 317
  in pediatric patients, 196-97
Fever. *See also* Hyperthermia
  postoperative, 47, 296
  as a sign of infection, 292
Flagyl, 293
Fluid management. *See* Body fluids
Fluothane, 26, 256, 282
Forane, 24, 148, 282, 317
Functional residual lung capacity, 256
Furosemide, 200

G

Gallamine, 80
Garamycin, 293, 296

Gastroenteritis, 112
Gelfoam, 240
General anesthesia. *See also names of specific drugs*
  complications with, 32, 40, 65
  head and neck surgery, 62
  ophthalmalogic surgery, 39-40
Genitourinary tract surgery, 17
Gentamicin, 293, 296
Glaucoma, surgery for, 33, 36

H

Halothane, 26, 197, 206, 256, 273, 282
Hamman-Rich syndrome, 287
Head and neck surgery. *See also* Oral and maxillofacial surgery
  anatomy and physiology, 51-53
  intraoperative and anesthetic considerations, 59-66
  postanesthesia care, 66-70
  postoperative pain, 24
  surgical procedures, 53-59
Healon, 41
Heart. *See* Cardiac surgery; Cardiopulmonary life support, in pediatric patients; Congenital heart disease; Coronary artery disease (CAA); Vascular surgery
Hematoma, 69, 152
Hemilaryngectomy, 58-59, 60 (fig.), 61 (fig.)
Hemodialysis, 185
Hemophilia, 241-42
Hemostasis in surgical patients, 231-54
  abnormalities of, 240-47
  abnormal surgical bleeding, 247-52 (*see also* Bleeding)
  blood coagulation values in pregnant, normal and DIC patients, 225 (table)
  in cranial surgery, 26-28
  evaluating defects in, 251 (fig.)
  physiology of, 231-37
  surgical techniques to facilitate, 237-40
Heparin, 81, 201, 246
Hepatitis virus, 302, 303 (table)
Herpes virus, 300, 302, 303 (table)

Histamine, 276, 277, 279
Holmes, Oliver Wendell, 11
Hyaluronidase, 39
Hydralazine, 28
Hydrocele, urological, 176-77
Hydroxyzinc, 265
Hypercapnea, 257-58
  postoperative, 258-62
  signs of, 261-62
Hypercarbia, anesthesia-induced, 256, 257
Hyperkalemia, 205
Hypernatremia, 204
Hypertension,
  postoperative, 18, 28, 83-84, 152
  and vascular disease, 126
Hyperthermia, 263
  malignant, in pediatric patients, 206-7
Hypertonic solutions, 25
Hyperventilation, 89-90
  deliberate, 25
Hypocapnia, 89-90
Hypokalemia, 84, 205
Hyponatremia, 197
Hypotension,
  induced, to reduce blood loss, 26, 27, 47-48
  postoperative, 85-87, 96, 152
  during pregnancy, 222
Hypothermia,
  in burn patients, 138, 150
  in older patients, 327
  postoperative, 83
Hypoventilation, 151
Hypovolemia, 86, 95-96, 113, 114, 148, 172
Hypoxemia, 199
  causes of, 151-52
Hypoxia,
  anesthesia induced, 256-57
  in pediatric patients, 197
  postoperative, 258-62
  signs of, 261-62

I

Idiopathic thrombocytopenic purpura (ITP), 245

Immobilizers, for orthopedic patients, 163
Incentive spirometry, 91-92
Incisions, thoracotomy, 100-101
Inderal, 28, 85
Infectious diseases, surgical patients with, 291-309
  controlling infection spread, 297-301
  infections as a result of surgery, 293-97
  infectious hazards for PACU personnel, 301-8
  preexisting infection, 292-93
  pulmonary, 265, 273
Injuries. *See* Trauma
Inspiratory positive airway pressure (IPAP), 93
Intal, 281
Intermaxillary fixation, 45, 46 (fig.)
Intermittent mandatory ventilation technique (IMV), 91, 93, 94 (fig.), 96
Intermittent positive pressure ventilation (IPPV), 88-89, 93, 94 (fig.)
Intraaortic balloon pump (IABP), 87
Intraarterial cannulation, 101
Intraocular pressure, 18, 33, 36, 37, 41
Intropin, 96, 293
Intubation,
  of burn patients, 141, 142
  of infants, 210-11
Intuition in nursing care, 334-35
Invasive hemodynamic monitoring, 17, 18, 19
Isoetharine, 281, 283
Isoflurane, 24, 26, 76, 79, 80, 197, 273, 282, 317
Isolation from infection guidelines, 297, 300-301
Isoproterenol, 199, 212, 213

J

Jaudice, 113, 246
Joints, 156

Jugular vein, ligation of internal, 70

K

Ketalar, 282
Ketamine, 19, 199, 220, 256, 282
Kidneys. *See also* Urological and renal surgery
  anatomy/physiology, 170-73
  function of, in pediatric patients, 195
  renal hypertension, 128-29
  stones, 113, 182
  transplant, 182, 183 (fig.)
Koller, Carl, 31

L

Lactic acidosis, 205
Larnyx, 52-53
  cancer of, 57-58, 59 (fig.)
  edema of, 67-68
Laryngectomy, 57, 59 (fig.)
  reconstructive surgery for, 59, 62-64 (fig.)
Laryngoscopy, 54
Laryngospasm, 198
Lasix, 200
Left ventricular end-diastolic volume (LVEDV), 142
Leukemia, 244
Levophed, 212, 222
Lidocaine, 38, 39, 85, 197, 209, 213, 224-25, 282
Lids of the eye, surgery on, 34, 37
Ligaments, 156
Liver,
  diseases of, and hemostasis, 246
  function of, in pediatric patients, 194
Lobectomy, 107
Local/regional anesthesia, 31, 273. *See also names of specific drugs*
  complications of, 39
  in ophthalmalogic surgery, 38-39

M

Macrothrombocytic thrombopathia, 243

Magnesium sulfate, 227, 228 (table)
Mannitol, 25, 70
Marcaine, 38, 225
Mechanical ventilation, 93, 274, 283
  complications of, 89-90
  initial settings, 87-88
  weaning from, 90-91
Mediastinoscopy, 108
Mediastinotomy, 108
Mefoxin, 293
Meperidine, 38, 206, 220
Mepivacaine, 38
Metabolism,
  in burn patients, 138, 147
  in pediatric patients, 192-93
Metaproterenol, 281
Metaraminol, 86
Methemoglobinemia, 209-10
Methylene blue, 210
Methyl methacrylate, 16, 157
Metocurine, 283
Metronidazole, 293
Metubine, 283
Microembolization, 266
Mitral regurgitation, 80-81
Mitral stenosis (MS), 79-80
Monitoring of patients, 16-18
  burn injuries, 141-44, 148-49
  fetal, 222, 223 (fig.)
  of pediatric patients, 195-96
  postoperative, 66-67, 81-83, 101-2
  preoperative, 14
  during vascular surgery, 130-31
Morphine, 83, 92, 103, 151, 152, 197,
    206, 208, 220, 263, 282
  as epidural anesthesia, 225, 226 (fig.)
Morton, William, 11
Mouth. *See* Oral and maxillofacial
    surgery
Myocardial ischemia, 74-75
  prevention/treatment of, 315, 316 (table)
Myocutaneous flaps, 59, 62-64 (fig.), 69

N

Naloxone, 18, 103, 197, 208-9, 225
Narcan, 18, 103, 225, 263

Narcotics, 5, 28, 38, 102-3, 146, 273, 317
  overdose, 151
Narcuron, 283
Nasolacrimal system, 34, 37
Neck. *See* Head and neck surgery
Nembutol, 256
Neomycin, 296
Neoplasm. *See* Tumors
Neostigmine, 263
Neosynephrine, 86, 222
Nephron, renal, 170
Nesacaine, 225
Neurosurgery, 16, 23-29
  carotid endarterectomy, 29
  craniotomy, 25-29
  spine surgery, 23-24
Neurovascular integrity, 158, 159 (table)
Nifedipine, 28
Nipride, 27, 48, 83-84, 130, 264
Nitroglycerin, 28, 48, 84, 92, 209
Nitrol, 28
Nitroprusside, 48, 87, 130, 264
Nitrous oxide, 24, 32, 76, 273, 317
Norcan, 151
Norcuron, 148
Norepinephrine, 222, 293
Nurse practitioners in PACUs, stress
    management for, 341-51
  coping measures for stress, 346-51
  meaning of stress, 341-42
  pervasiveness of stress, 342-43
  nursing and stress, 343
  reactions to stress, 343-44
  stress in the PACU, 344-46
Nursing care,
  bias of ageism in, 333-34
  principles/attitudes in, 332-33
  use of intuition in, 334-35

O

Obstetrical surgery, 17, 217-29
  anesthetic considerations, 218-20
  general considerations in pregnancy,
    217, 218 (fig.), 219 (table)
  postanesthesia care, 220-28
  surgical procedures, 217

Older adults, nursing care for, 321-38
 aging process concepts, 321-25
 areas of nursing concern, 325-32
 case study, 335-37
 subtle influences on, 332-35
Oliguria, 19
Operating room experience. *See*
 Surgical experience
Ophthaine, 31
Ophthalmalogic surgery, 18, 31-42
 anesthetic considerations, 38-40
 general considerations, 31-32
 pathophysiological considerations, 32-35
 postanesthetic care, 40-41
 surgical procedures, 35-38
Oral and maxillofacial surgery, 43-49.
 See also Head and neck surgery
 airway assessment, 46-47
 postoperative care, 43-46, 47-48
Orbits of the eye, surgery on, 34, 37
Orthopedic surgery, 16, 155-67
 anesthetic considerations, 157-58
 complications, 164-66
 general considerations, 155-57
 specific problems/techniques, 158-64
 surgical considerations, 157
Osmotic diuresis, in pediatric patients, 205
Oxacillin sodium, 293
Oxycel sponge, 240
Oxygen,
 decreasing patient demands for, 280 (table)
 toxicity, 92-93
 transcutaneous monitoring, 102
Oxygenation and ventilation, for acute respiratory failure, 262-64
Oxytocin, 28, 172, 221

P

Pain, 19, 28, 83
 abdominal, 111, 112 (fig.), 207, 223
 in burn patients, 151
 neck, 24
 in ophthalmologic patients, 41
 in pediatric patients, 205-6
 during surgery, 24
 in thoracic patients, 102-3

Pancreatitis, 112, 113
Pancuronium, 80, 148, 283
Parotid gland, 56
Patients,
 monitoring (*see* Monitoring of patients)
 older adults (*see* Older adults, nursing care for)
 pediatric (*see* Pediatric patients)
 positioning (*see* Positioning of patients)
Pavulon, 148, 283
Pediatric patients, 191-215
 anatomic considerations, 191-92
 cardiopulmonary life support, 210-14
 fluid and electrolyte management, 202-5
 monitoring, 195-96
 pain control, 205-6
 physiology, 192-95
 postanesthesia assessment, 196-97
 respiratory management, 16-17, 198-202
 unusual problems in, 206-10
Pelvic inflammatory disease, 113
 vs. appendicitis, 116
Penicillin, 293
Penrose drain, 68-69
Pentobarbital, 256
Pentothal, 220, 256, 282
Percutaneous transluminal coronary angioplasty (PTCA), 76
Pericardial window, 108-9
Perioperative experience, 3-10
Peritoneal dialysis, 185
Peritonitis, 292, 295
Phenergan, 265, 318
Phentolamine, 84, 200
Phenylephrine, 86, 209, 222
Phenytoin, 214
Phospholine, 40
Pitocin, 28, 172, 221
Placenta previa, 17
Platelets, 232, 233 (fig.), 234 (table)
 acquired disorders of, 243-47
 congenital function disorder of, 242-43
Pneumomediastinum, 66

Pneumonectomy, 106-7
Pneumonia, 294-95
 aspiration, 264, 265
Pneumothorax, 66, 200-201
Pontocaine, 31
Positioning of patients, 7
 head, for ophthalmalogic patients, 40-41
 after ligation of internal jugular vein, 70
 for spine surgery, 24
 to treat air emboli, 66
Positive End-Expiratory Pressure (PEEP), 91, 92-96, 202
 application of, in cardiac patients, 92-93
 best conventional, 94, 95 (fig.)
 cardiovascular effects of, 95-96
 contraindicated, 274, 283
 ranges of, 93-95
Postanesthesia care,
 abdominal surgery, 123-24
 asthma patients, 283-85
 burn surgery, 149-53
 cardiac surgery, 81-96
 coronary artery disease patients, 317-19
 head/neck surgery, 66-70
 neurosurgery, 27-28, 29
 obstetric surgery, 220-28
 opthalmalogic surgery, 40-41
 oral/maxillofacial surgery, 43-46, 47-48
 for patients with respiratory disease, 274-76, 289-90
 in pediatric patients, 196-97
 thoracic surgery, 109
 vascular surgery, 132-33
Postanesthesia care unit (PACU), 18-19.
 See also Nurse practioners in PACUs, stress management for
 infection hazards in, 301-8
 postoperative transfer to, 8, 9-10
Posterior fossa surgery, 28-29
Postoperative period, 8-10, 18-19
 See also Postanesthesia care
Preeclampsia in pregnancy, 226-28

Pregnancy,
 ectopic, 113, 223-24
 preeclampsia/eclampsia in, 226-28
 respiratory changes in, 219 (table)
 surgery during, 221-23
 systemic changes in, 218 (fig.)
Premature ventricular contractions (PVCs), 84-85
Preoperative evaluation, 4-5, 12-14
 in asthma patients, 281
 in coronary artery disease, 313-15
Prilocaine, 209
Procainamide, 101, 207, 213
Procardia, 28
Prochlorperizine, 265
Promethazine, 265, 318
Pronestyl, 101
Proparacaine, 31
Propranolol, 28, 85, 209
Prostaglandins, 221, 225
Prostate gland, 171
 benign hypertrophy vs. cancer, 179-80
Prosthetic heart valves, 78
Protamine sulfate, 246
Pruritis, 225
Ptosis, eyelid, 34, 37
Pulmonary artery catheters, 102
 wave forms, 143 (fig.)
Pulmonary capillary wedge pressure (PCWP), 142, 143 (fig.)
Pulmonary diseases, 266-90
 classification, 266-67
 obstructive, 267-85
 restrictive, 285-90
Pulmonary edema, 92
 in pediatric patients, 200
 prevention/treatment of, 265, 266 (table)
Pulmonary embolism, 201
Pulmonary function, 99, 100 (fig.), 287-88
Pulmonary hypertension, 287
 treatment of, 279 (table)

Pulse oximetry, 101-2, 196

Q

Quinidine, 213

R

Radial keratotomy, 33
Regitine, 84
Renal stones, 113, 182
Renal system. *See also* Urological and renal surgery
  anatomy, 170-71
  disorder diagnosis, 173, 174 (table), 175-76
  failure, 19, 182-83
  function, 169 (fig.), 170
  normal blood flow, 171 (fig.)
  physiology of, 171-73
Reports and records,
  epidural anesthesia, 226 (fig.)
  operating room, 9
  postoperative, 12
Respiration. *See also* Airway maintenance
  changes in pregnant patients, 219 (table)
  complications, 92, 264-66 (*see also* Acute respiratory failure (ARF))
  function/management, in pediatric patients, 193-94, 197, 198-202
  in older patients, 328
  postoperative, in cardiac patients, 87-96
Respiratory disease, surgical patients with, 255-90
  pulmonary diseases, 266-90
  settings of acute respiratory failure, 256-66
Retalar, 220
Retina, surgery on, 33-34, 36-37
Rheumatic heart disease, 78, 79, 80
Ringer's lactate solution, 86, 137
Ritodrine, 223

Rubella, 303 (table), 208

S

Salivary gland, surgery on, 56
Scopolomine, 5
Secretions, management of, 278 (table)
  in oral/maxillofacial surgery, 45-46
Self-nurturing, to cope with stress, 348-50
Septic shock, 292-93
Serum values, normal, 176 (table)
Shunt, anesthesia-induced, 256, 257
Sialadenitis, 56
Sialolithiasis, 56
Sickle cell anemia, 207
Silvadene, 138, 139, 140 (table)
Silver nitrate, 138, 140 (table)
Silver sulfadiazine, 138, 139, 140 (table)
Skeletal traction, 160, 162 (fig.)
Skin,
  functions of, and injuries to, 136
  grafts, 144-45
Smoke inhalation, 138, 140
Sodium bicarbonate, 211
Sodium citrate, 220
Sodium hyaluronate, 41
Sodium mafenide, 138, 139, 140 (table)
Sodium nitroprusside, 27, 28, 83-84
Sodium thiopental, 76
Sodium warfarin, 78
Speech, 52-53, 57-58
Spermatocele, 177
Spinal fluid drainage, 25
Spine surgery, 23-24
SRS-A, 276, 277, 279
Steroids, 44, 244, 245, 283
Strabismus surgery, 34, 37-38
Stress,
  affecting PACU nurses, 343-46
  coping measures, 346-51
  general response of older patients to, 325, 326 (fig.)
  meaning of, 341-42
  pervasiveness of, 342-43
Stricture, urological, 178-79
Stridor, 67-68

Stroke, 126-27
Sublimaze, 225, 317
Succinylcholine, 32, 40, 148, 198, 200, 206, 282
Sulfamylon, 138, 140 (table)
Surgeon, 4
 -anesthesiologist team, 11-20
Surgical experience, 3-10
 anesthetic technique, 15
 intraoperative procedures, 7-8, 15-18
 OR holding area, 6
 patient admission to OR holding area, 6
 patient admission to OR suite, 6
 patient arousal and transfer to PACU, 8-10
 patient entry/positioning, 7
 postoperative period, 8-10, 18-19
 preoperative evaluation, 4-5, 12-14
 preoperative medication, 5, 14-15
 preoperative transfer routine, 5
Surgical team,
 cooperation of, 11-12
 members/roles of, 4
Surgicel sponge, 240
Suture control of blood vessels, 238
Swan-Ganz catheterization, 16, 17, 102, 130, 142

T

Tachycardias, 77, 85, 90, 151
 in pediatric patients, 213-14
 as a sign of infection, 292
Teaching health techniques to older adults, 331
Temperature, body. *See* Fever, postoperative; Hyperthermia; Hypothermia
 in burn patients, 138, 150
 in older patients, 327
 in pediatric patients, 194, 206-7
Tendons, 156
Terbutaline, 223, 281
Territoriality in older adults, 331
Testicle, torsion of, 178
Tetanus, 138

Tetracaine, 31
Tetralogy of Fallot, 209
Theophylline, 281
Thiopental, 147, 148, 220, 256, 282
Thoracic surgery, 99-109
 chest tube use, 103-6
 monitoring after, 101-2
 postanesthesia care, 109
 postoperative pain, 102-3
 procedures, 106-9
 pulmonary function, 99, 100 (fig.)
 thoracotomy incisions, 100-101
Thorazine, 84
Thrombasthenia, 242
Thrombin test time, 249
Thrombocytopenia, 243-44
Thrombophlebitis, 166
Thymectomy, 108
Thyroidectomy, 55-56
Tissue valves, 78
Tocolytics, 223
Tonsillectomy, 55
Toxemia, 17, 226, 227 (fig.)
Tracheostomy, 57
Tracheotomy, 53, 54 (fig.)
Tracrium, 184, 283
Traction, for orthopedic patients, 160, 161 (fig.), 162 (fig.)
Tranquilizers, 5, 38
Transphenoidal surgery, 28-29
Trauma,
 eye, 35
 patients in surgery, 17-18
 urological system, 181
Trimethaphan, 27, 28, 84
Tuberculosis, 306 (table), 308
Tumors,
 brain, 27
 colon, 122
 eyelid, 34, 37
 head and neck, 54, 55, 56-59

U

Ulcer, perforated, 114, 116-19, 120 (fig.)
Uremia, 245

Ureteral stones, 181
Ureterocele, 181
Urethral hypospadias, 178
Urinalysis, normal, 175 (table)
Urinary tract infection (UTI),
 113, 294
Urological and renal surgery, 169-88
 anesthetic management, 184-88
 patient history and physical findings,
  173-76
 renal system function, 169 (fig.), 170
 specific urological disorders, 176-83
 systems anatomy, 170-71
 systems physiology, 171-73

V

Valium, 38, 220
Valvular heart disease, 77-81
 aortic insufficiency, 78-79
 aortic stenosis, 77-78
 mitral regurgitation, 80-81
 mitral stenosis, 79-80
Vancocin, 296
Vancomycin, 296
Varicella-zoster virus, 302,
 305 (table)
Varicocele, 177
Vascular surgery, 125-34
 anesthetic considerations, 129-31
 general considerations, 125-29
 postanesthesia care, 132-33
 surgical procedures, 131-32
Vasodilators, 83-84, 87, 92

Vecuronium, 148, 196, 283
Venous bleeding, 26
Ventilation. *See* Respiration
Ventilation/perfusion abnormalities,
 256, 257
Ventricular fibrillation, 213
Verapamil, 85, 213, 214
Vistaril, 265
Vitamin K deficiency, 246
Vitrectomy, 33
Vitreoretinal surgery, 36-37
Von Willebrand's disease, 243

W

Warren, John C., 11
Williams, T. Franklin, 335
Wounds,
 care of burns, 138-40
 care of surgical head and neck, 68-69
 infection in surgical, 295
Wydase, 39

X

Xylocaine, 38, 85, 225

Y

Yutopar, 223

Z

Zero end-expiratory pressure (ZEEP), 93

About the Editor

Miss Luczun received her basic training at St. Vincent's Medical Center in Staten Island, New York. She subsequently earned a bachelor's degree in nursing at Cornell University and a master's degree in nursing at Hunter College of the City University of New York. She is the author of *Post Anesthesia Nursing: A Comprehensive Guide* (Aspen Publishers, Inc., 1984) and associate editor of research for the *Journal of Post Anesthesia Nursing*. Miss Luczun also contributed the chapter entitled "The Urological and Renal Surgery Patient" in the American Society of Post Anesthesia Nurses' Certification Review Text.

Miss Luczun is currently a clinical instructor at Hunter College-Bellevue School of Nursing in New York. She is an active member of The American Society of Post Anesthesia Nurses (ASPAN) and a member of Sigma Theta Tau National Honor Society of Nursing-Alpha Upsilon Chapter. Her name is listed in *Who's Who in U.S. Writers, Editors, and Poets*, 1986–1987 edition.